P9-CCX-861

Praise for Anthony William

"Within the first three minutes of speaking with me, Anthony precisely identified my medical issue! This healer really knows what he's talking about. Anthony's abilities as the Medical Medium are unique and fascinating."

— Alejandro Junger, M.D., *New York Times* best-selling author of *Clean*, *Clean Eats*, and *Clean Gut* and founder of the acclaimed Clean Program

"While there is most definitely an element of otherworldly mystery to the work he does, much of what Anthony William shines a spotlight on—particularly around autoimmune disease—feels inherently right and true. What's better is that the protocols he recommends are natural, accessible, and easy to do."

— Gwyneth Paltrow, Oscar-winning actress, #1 *New York Times* best-selling author of *It's All Easy*, founder and CCO of GOOP.com

"Anthony is a magician for all my label's recording artists, and if he were a record album, he would far surpass Thriller. *His ability is nothing short of profound, remarkable, extraordinary, and mind-blowing. He is a luminary whose books are filled with prophecies. This is the future of medicine."*

— Craig Kallman, Chairman and CEO, Atlantic Records

"Anthony's gift has made him a conduit for information that is light-years ahead of where science is today."

— from the foreword by Christiane Northrup, M.D., *New York Times* best-selling author of *Goddesses Never Age* and *Women's Bodies, Women's Wisdom*

"Anthony is not only a warm, compassionate healer, he is also authentic and accurate, with God-given skills. He has been a total blessing in my life."

— Naomi Campbell, model, actress, activist

"My family and friends have been the recipients of Anthony's inspired gift of healing, and we've benefited more than I can express with rejuvenated physical and mental health."

— Scott Bakula, star of *Basmati Blues*, *NCIS: New Orleans*, *Quantum Leap*, and *Star Trek: Enterprise*

"How very much we have been moved and benefited from the discovery of Anthony and the Compassion Spirit, who can reach us with healing wisdom through Anthony's sensitive genius and caring mediumship. His book is truly 'wisdom of the future,' so already now, miraculously, we have the clear, accurate explanation of the many mysterious illnesses that the ancient Buddhist medical texts predicted would afflict us in this era when over-clever people have tampered with the elements of life in the pursuit of profit."

— Robert Thurman, Jey Tsong Khapa Professor of Indo-Tibetan Buddhist Studies, Columbia University; President, Tibet House US; best-selling author of *Love Your Enemies* and *Inner Revolution*; host of *Bob Thurman Podcast*

"Anthony is a wonderful person. He identified some long-term health issues for me, he knew what supplements I needed, and I felt better immediately."

— Rashida Jones, actress, producer, and writer; star of *Angie Tribeca* and co-star of *Parks and Recreation*, *The Social Network*, and *I Love You, Man*

"Anthony William's God-given gift for healing is nothing short of miraculous."

— David James Elliott, *Camera Store*, *Scorpion*, *Trumbo*, *Mad Men*, *CSI: NY*; star for ten years of CBS's *JAG*

"Anthony William is the gifted Medical Medium who has very real and not-so-radical solutions to the mysterious conditions that affect us all in our modern world. I am beyond thrilled to know him personally and count him as a most valuable resource for my health protocols and those for my entire family."

— Annabeth Gish, *Scandal*, *The Bridge*, *Brotherhood*, *The West Wing*, *Mystic Pizza*

"I love Anthony William! My daughters Sophia and Laura gave me his book for my birthday, and I couldn't put it down. The Medical Medium has helped me connect all the dots on my quest to achieve optimal health. Through Anthony's work, I realized the residual Epstein-Barr left over from a childhood illness was sabotaging my health years later. Medical Medium has transformed my life."

— Catherine Bach, *The Young and the Restless*, *The Dukes of Hazzard*

"My recovery from a traumatic spinal crisis several years ago had been steady, but I was still experiencing muscle weakness, a tapped-out nervous system, as well as extra weight. A dear friend called me one evening and strongly recommended I read the book Medical Medium *by Anthony William. So much of the information in the book resonated with me that I began incorporating some of the ideas, then I sought and was lucky enough to get a consultation. The reading was so spot-on, it has taken my healing to an unimagined, deeper, and richer level of health. My weight has dropped healthily, I can enjoy bike-riding and yoga, I'm back in the gym, I have steady energy, and I sleep deeply. Every morning when following my protocols, I smile and say, 'Whoa, Anthony William! I thank you for your restorative gift . . . Yes!'"*

— Robert Wisdom, *Flaked*, *Chicago P.D.*, *Nashville*, *The Wire*, *Ray*

"Twelve hours after receiving a heaping dose of self-confidence masterfully administered by Anthony, the persistent ringing in my ears of the last year . . . began to falter. I am astounded, grateful, and happy for the insights offered on moving forward."

— Mike Dooley, *New York Times* best-selling author of *Infinite Possibilities* and scribe of *Notes from the Universe*

"Anthony is a seer and a wellness sage. His gift is remarkable. With his guidance I've been able to pinpoint and address a health issue that's been plaguing me for years."

— Kris Carr, *New York Times* best-selling author of *Crazy Sexy Juice*, *Crazy Sexy Kitchen*, and *Crazy Sexy Diet*

"Anthony William is the Edgar Cayce of our time, reading the body with outstanding precision and insight. Anthony identifies the underlying causes of diseases that often baffle the most astute conventional and alternative health-care practitioners. Anthony's practical and profound advice makes him one of the most powerfully effective healers of the 21st century."

— Ann Louise Gittleman, *New York Times* best-selling author of 30 books on health and healing and creator of the highly popular Fat Flush detox and diet plan

"I rely on Anthony William for my and my family's health. Even when doctors are stumped, Anthony always knows what the problem is and the pathway for healing."

— Chelsea Field, *The Last Boy Scout*, *Andre*

"As a Hollywood businesswoman, I know value. Some of Anthony's clients spent over $1 million seeking help for their 'mystery illness' until they finally discovered him."

— Nanci Chambers, co-star of *JAG*; Hollywood producer and entrepreneur

"Anthony William's invaluable advice on preventing and combating disease is years ahead of what's available anywhere else."

— Richard Sollazzo, M.D., New York board-certified oncologist, hematologist, nutritionist, and anti-aging expert and author of *Balance Your Health*

"Whenever Anthony William recommends a natural way of improving your health, it works. I've seen this with my daughter, and the improvement was impressive. His approach of using natural ingredients is a more effective way of healing."

— Martin D. Shafiroff, Managing Director of Barclays Capital; rated #1 Broker in America by WealthManagement.com and #1 Wealth Advisor by *Barron's*

"I had a health reading from Anthony, and he accurately told me things about my body only known to me. This kind, sweet, hilarious, self-effacing, and generous man—also so 'otherworldly' and so extraordinarily gifted, with an ability that defies how we see the world—has shocked even me, a medium! He is truly our modern-day Edgar Cayce, and we are immensely blessed that he is with us. Anthony William proves that we are more than we know."

— Colette Baron-Reid, best-selling author of *Uncharted* and TV host of *Messages from Spirit*

"Any quantum physicist will tell you there are things at play in the universe we can't yet understand. I truly believe Anthony has a handle on them. He has an amazing gift for intuitively tapping into the most effective methods for healing."

— Caroline Leavitt, *New York Times* best-selling author of *Cruel Beautiful World*, *Is This Tomorrow*, and *Pictures of You*

MEDICAL MEDIUM

LIFE-CHANGING FOODS

ALSO BY ANTHONY WILLIAM

Medical Medium: Secrets Behind Chronic and Mystery Illness and How to Finally Heal

The above is available at your local bookstore, or may be ordered by visiting:

Hay House USA: www.hayhouse.com®
Hay House Australia: www.hayhouse.com.au
Hay House UK: www.hayhouse.co.uk
Hay House India: www.hayhouse.co.in

MEDICAL MEDIUM

LIFE-CHANGING FOODS

SAVE YOURSELF AND THE ONES YOU LOVE WITH THE HIDDEN HEALING POWERS OF FRUITS & VEGETABLES

ANTHONY WILLIAM

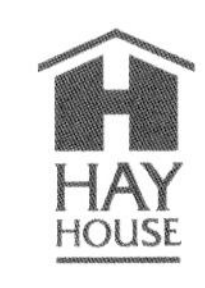

HAY HOUSE, INC.
Carlsbad, California • New York City
London • Sydney • New Delhi

Copyright © 2016 by Anthony William

Published in the United States by: Hay House, Inc.: www.hayhouse.com® • ***Published in Australia by:*** Hay House Australia Pty. Ltd.: www.hayhouse.com.au • ***Published in the United Kingdom by:*** Hay House UK, Ltd.: www.hayhouse.co.uk • ***Published in India by:*** Hay House Publishers India: www.hayhouse.co.in

Indexer: Jay Kreider
Cover design: Vibodha Clark
Interior design: Riann Bender
Recipe photos: Ashleigh & Britton Foster

Photos on pages 48, 52, 70, 74, 78, 82, 86, 86, 90, 94, 98, 102, 106, 110, 114, 124, 128, 132, 136, 142, 158, 164, 174, 186, 190, 194, 194, 198, 202, 206, 214, 218, 224, 232, 236, 240, 246, 254, 258, and 262 used under license from Shutterstock.com

All rights reserved. No part of this book may be reproduced by any mechanical, photographic, or electronic process, or in the form of a phonographic recording; nor may it be stored in a retrieval system, transmitted, or otherwise be copied for public or private use—other than for "fair use" as brief quotations embodied in articles and reviews—without prior written permission of the publisher.

The author of this book does not dispense medical advice or other professional advice or prescribe the use of any technique as a form of diagnosis or treatment for any physical, emotional, or medical condition. The intent of the author is only to offer information of an anecdotal and general nature that may be part of your quest for emotional and spiritual well-being. In the event you or others use any of the information or other content in this book, the author and the publisher assume no responsibility for the direct or indirect consequences. The reader should consult his or her medical, health, or other professional before adopting any of the suggestions in this book or drawing inferences from it.

Library of Congress Cataloging-in-Publication Data

Names: William, Anthony.
Title: Medical medium life-changing foods : save yourself and the ones you love with the hidden healing powers of fruits and vegetables / Anthony William.
Description: Carlsbad, California : Hay House, Inc., 2016. | Includes index.
Identifiers: LCCN 2016028077 | ISBN 9781401948320 (hardcover : alk. paper)
Subjects: LCSH: Functional foods. | Fruit--Health aspects. | Vegetables--Health aspects. | Fruit in human nutrition. | Vegetables in human nutrition.
Classification: LCC QP144.F85 W55 2016 | DDC 613.2--dc23 LC record available at https://lccn.loc.gov/2016028077

Hardcover ISBN: 978-1-4019-4832-0

17 16 15 14 13 12
1st edition, November 2016

Printed in the United States of America

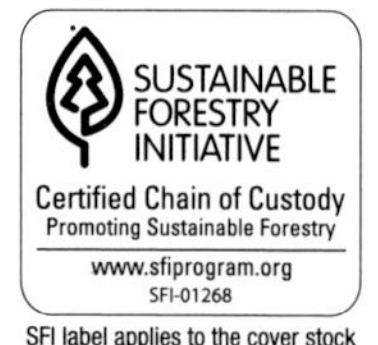

SFI label applies to the cover stock

For my wife

CONTENTS

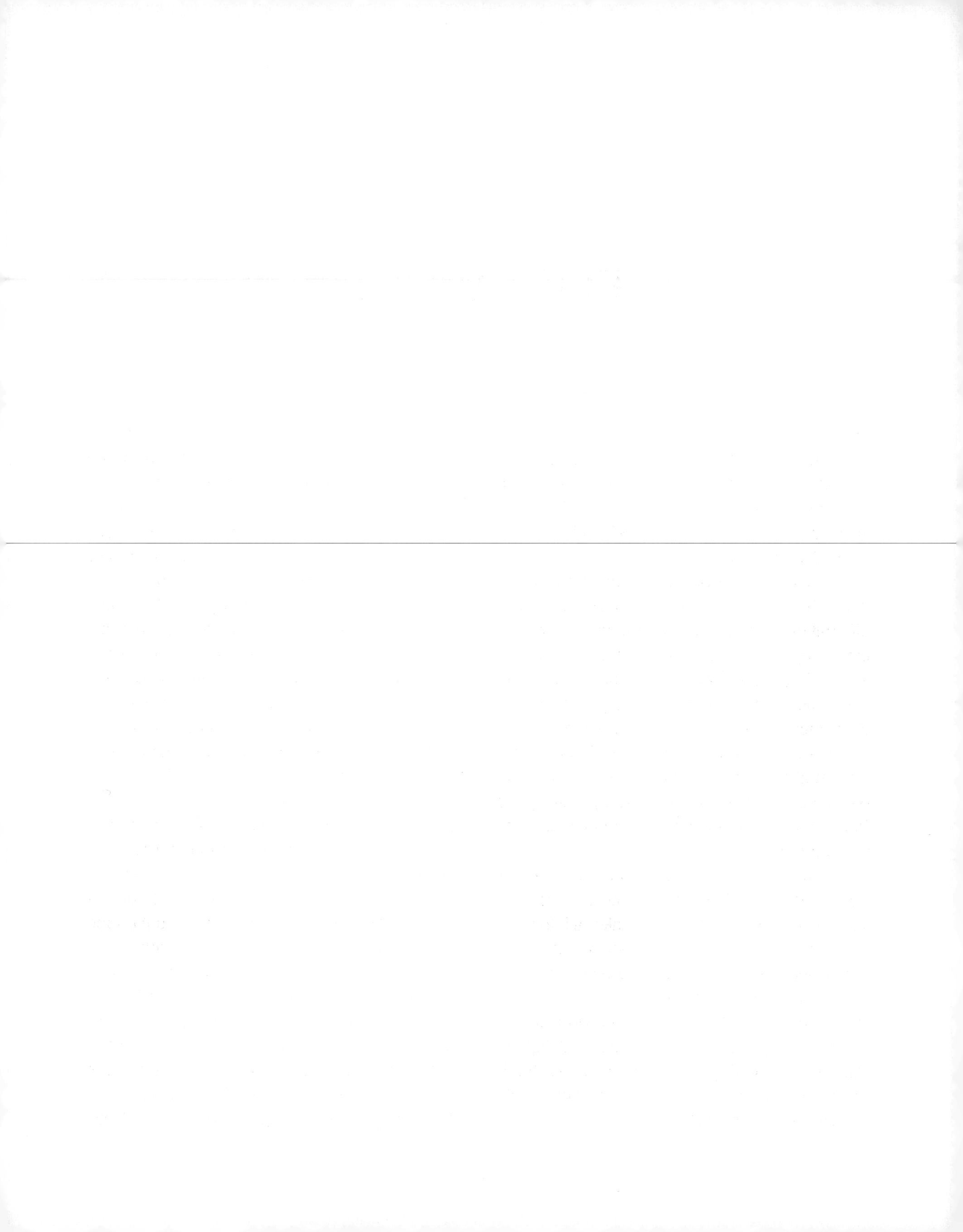

FOREWORD

I first met Anthony William a couple of years ago at a Hay House event. This unassuming, down-to-earth healer changed my life—including the way I eat and think about food, and about life on our Mother Earth herself.

As you may know, Anthony has been working with Spirit since he was a little boy. It's a gift that has made him a conduit for information that is light-years ahead of where science is today. A gift that has allowed him to see the vast amount of suffering on the planet and to do something about it. That something has to do with bringing the wisdom of Mother Earth and Mother Nature right into our bodies in delicious and healthy ways through eating the fruits and vegetables she has so lovingly provided for us.

Medical Medium Life-Changing Foods is about far more than eating "more fruits and vegetables," which tends to take all the joy and fun out of eating. That traditional advice is something you're "supposed" to do when you'd rather have a pizza. In this book, though, there is no judgment. No shaming. No food police. *Life-Changing Foods* is, instead, a delightful manual for bringing the vitality of these God-given gifts of the soil back into our lives. Deliciously, healthfully, joyfully.

Anthony, through Spirit, brings life-giving magic back into the subject of fruits and vegetables. It makes eating them a heightened experience of awareness that begins to transform you on all levels: body, mind, and spirit. Let me give you an example. When he tells us to eat wild blueberries, he's not just talking about the antioxidants in this delicious food, though they are certainly powerful (and there's a lot of science to back that up). Anthony is also referring to the amazing survival energies that are packed into these berries that grow and flourish in extreme conditions. Wild Maine blueberry bushes survive despite being burned periodically and having to cling to frozen rocks all winter, yet they are still capable of producing loads of sweet berries each year. When you eat wild blueberries, you are literally bringing into your body those same qualities—that same incredible tenacity of surviving against all odds. Spirit calls this the food of resurrection. Talk about a power food!

Now let's look at the lowly and much maligned potato. Spirit tells us that potatoes offer us a firm foundation of strength when we are feeling adrift or foggy in our lives. Part of this is their ability to draw high concentrations of macro- and micronutrients from the soil. They embody the qualities of grounding and stability.

And they remind us of our hidden gifts—those aspects of ourselves that, like the potato, are buried beneath the ground. Plus, we no longer need to fear them as a dreaded "white food" that will make us fat—as long as we know how to bring out the best in them. They can do the same for us. Until I met Anthony, I had avoided white potatoes for decades. Now they are a regular part of my diet. I have welcomed them back with open arms. And not a single unwanted pound!

As you read *Medical Medium Life-Changing Foods*, you begin to see fruits and vegetables in a new way. You find yourself excited and grateful for berries, onions, coconut, bananas, and all of the gifts that Mother Earth has provided for us. Hippocrates, the father of modern medicine—and the creator of the famous Hippocratic Oath that all of us doctors take when we graduate from medical school—said, "Let food be thy medicine and medicine be thy food."

But in today's fast-food world, how would you know what food to take for what? How can food be medicine? That's where this book truly stands out from every other food book I've ever read. For each food listed, from pears to celery, and many more, there is a list of the conditions and symptoms that that fruit or vegetable will help alleviate. But there's more. Each fruit or vegetable is also imbued with the specific emotional and spiritual support it provides when you eat it. Plus there are easy-to-follow, delicious recipes throughout.

More than that, *Life-Changing Foods* tackles the food fads and myths that have had so many of us confused for decades. This includes fruit fear (which I myself certainly had). Because of the sweetness of fruit, we mistakenly lumped its sugar in with all the other "bad" sugars out there that have contributed to so much obesity and ill health. Fruit is not the same. We need to be eating a lot more of it. Since adding more delicious fruit to my diet, my cravings for sweets (such as candy, cookies, and desserts) have pretty much disappeared. I have entered a whole new world of sweet delight through eating dates, berries, fresh oranges, and bananas. And frankly, that is a miracle.

When you follow the guidance in *Medical Medium Life-Changing Foods*, shopping and cooking take on new meaning, because the spirit of the fruit or vegetable starts to speak to you and to work in your body and in your life. You begin to feel truly supported by nature—and some deep primal part of you begins to wake up. You also become connected to unseen help by learning how to work directly with the life-changing angels who are responsible for our food supply. They fortify fruits and vegetables, help protect pollinators, encourage each apple and lettuce leaf and everything else to grow, help bring food to the hungry, work to disarm GMO food production, assist with and support the organic food movement, and even influence weather patterns. Talk about tapping into a power source. What a huge relief to know this.

Reading this book and tapping into the emotional and spiritual power of fruits and vegetables is potent medicine. As we take in this medicine, we begin to feel at one with the Mother who supports all of us—the earth. And as we align with the angelic realm, we begin to feel at one with the heavens, as well. Hope and vitality begin to flow back to us and through us.

And that, dear friends, feels like coming home to heaven on earth.

CHRISTIANE NORTHRUP, M.D.

INTRODUCTION

From an early age, you're taught to be careful. It starts when you're a baby and your caregiver pulls your hand away as you reach toward an electrical outlet or a can's sharp edge. It continues when a parent grabs on to your waist as you first try to stand on your own. On and on it goes—a mother who warns you to wash your hands before dinner, a teacher who scolds you for running in the hallway, an uncle who won't hear of you riding a bicycle without a helmet. As children, if all goes as it's meant to, we're surrounded by adults who monitor our comings and goings, who prioritize our safety—adults who care and who teach us to care.

As we grow up, we internalize these lessons. When we choose our first car, safety is a top consideration. Are there good airbags? Do the brakes work well? When we think about where to go to college, we ask ourselves if we feel safe on campus, if the professors truly care about the student body. And at a certain point, our concern branches out: We may meet a partner, and suddenly her or his safety is on the radar too. Together, we plan for the future, making each other's physical, financial, and emotional security a priority.

If children come along, we're right back where we started, only standing in a different position now. This time, we're the ones passing along the lessons. Some of them, like holding hands when crossing the street, are centuries old, while others, like cybersecurity, are unique to the time we live in. Eventually we may even become grandparents, with yet another generation to watch over. Meanwhile, as our parents age, we become their caregivers too. We are always looking out for one another.

Safety concerns never end. We lock our doors at night, purchase insurance, install alarm systems. We try different fad diets in hopes of preventing heart disease, cancer, diabetes. With the growing threats in the world, we practice shelter-in-place drills and walk through metal detectors. We are used to living within rules and regulations, because safety is the baseline. We understand that without it, we're lost.

This book is about another level of safety entirely, one we don't even realize we need, and yet one that we need more than ever. I'm talking about the safety of our health—in other words, survival. These are lessons that no one knew to teach us along the way about how to adapt to our changing times. Because even with everything we already know, *there is so much more to know.*

EAT OUTSIDE THE BOX

Today's information about nutrition—about what's behind those frightening illnesses like heart disease, cancer, diabetes, Alzheimer's, autoimmune disease, and the like, and what to do about them—is inside a box. Boxes make us feel safe. They make it seem like everything is contained, and containable.

They're deceiving that way. Threats to our safety are unpredictable; any IT specialist who's dealt with a zero-day computer virus or any emergency responder who's been called to the scene of an active shooter can confirm this. Safety threats aren't constrained by a box, so our thinking can't be, either. In order to protect our health, we need to think outside the limits of what we believe is known.

The way to truly protect yourself is by eating the foods in this book.

"Yeah, sure, Anthony," I can hear the doubters saying already, "fruits and vegetables—that's real original." Well, don't throw your rotten tomatoes at me just yet. This isn't the same old, same old. Fruits and vegetables aren't some cute hobby for people to occupy themselves with until scientists discover the big guns that will save the planet. These foods *are* the big guns. Their life-changing power is on a whole different level than has yet been discovered.

We take plant foods for granted. We think of eating them as a chore, one of those childhood lessons that we should have been allowed to outgrow by now. Or we've heard that we should fear cruciferous vegetables, nightshades, and fruit. Or, alternately, we're convinced of the virtues of fruits, vegetables, and herbs, yet have no idea how to harness their full power. It's a hodgepodge of food beliefs out there, all of them operating within a certain set of confines that limit your ability to protect yourself from health threats—and there are more health threats than ever in our current day and age. We need to be more preventative than ever before.

The information to come in these pages breaks out of the box of our modern-day understanding of nutrition. That's because these foods affect every single aspect of your well-being. It's not just about getting lutein for your eyes or calcium for your bones; although those are, of course, vital aspects of protecting your health, they're just the beginning. It's also about eating figs in groups of nine for maximum benefit, adding potatoes to your life to uncover your true nature, and wrapping up a date to take with you on a long journey as a talisman to help you find food along the way. It's about getting to the bottom of why conditions ranging from anxiety to colitis to dementia are taking hold of the population at record rates, and how to use these life-changing foods to protect yourself from vulnerability.

This information, which comes from a source called Spirit, is very often ahead of science, so when you read in the pages to come that, for example, onions help *alleviate* bad breath, not cause it, you aren't likely to find a scientific study or health-care expert who says the same thing, because no one knows this yet. Spirit understands that you don't have decades to wait for research to uncover these answers. Are you supposed to go another 20 years suffering with stomach pain, not knowing that celery juice is the most amazing digestive tonic? No—you need access to these insights now, so you can feel better and live your life.

When you do come across information in this book that is similar to what you've heard elsewhere—for example, that avocado is very similar to breast milk—keep in mind that over the course of more than 25 years, I've shared health information with tens of thousands of people, so as they have in turn shared that information with others, some concepts have made their way into the wider world. Spirit also likes to honor those discoveries that scientists have made about food and health, as well as health wisdom that's been around since ancient times, so here and there in these pages, you'll find information that echoes mainstream health knowledge. As I said, Spirit always takes it to another level. For example, yes, it's known that wild blueberries are antioxidant powerhouses. What isn't known is that wild blueberries are the resurrection food, capable of bringing us back to life when it seems like all is lost.

It all comes down to what you need to discover to tap into your greatest potential. So much earthly energy goes into searching high and low for answers about mental and physical health, safety, protection, and enlightenment. I am here to tell you that the answers have been hiding in the produce aisle the whole time.

ORIGINS

Those who know me know that I get my information from Spirit. When I was four years old, a voice that identified itself as Spirit of the Most High told me to announce at the family dinner table that my grandmother had lung cancer. I didn't even know what the term meant. However, I relayed the news, and medical testing soon confirmed it.

This was the beginning of what was to become a lifelong gift—although I can't say it's always felt like a gift. Spirit constantly speaks into my ear, filling me in on the symptoms of everyone around me. Plus, Spirit taught me from an early age to visualize physical scans of people, like supercharged MRI scans that reveal all blockages, infections, trouble areas, past problems, and even soul fractures.

This means that I am constantly zeroing in on suffering. Let me tell you, there's a lot of it in the world, more than we ever see on the news. There's a hidden epidemic of people dealing with extreme fatigue, brain fog, pain, dizziness, and more, and they don't know why. There are also people who get dire diagnoses and lose all hope in life. Far too often, those who are ill go on suffering for years without answers, and they end up feeling like they've somehow brought it upon themselves.

My job is to tell the truth about health. My job is to give people the answers medical science hasn't discovered yet, and to spread the message far and wide that you did not bring your ill health upon yourself, that you can get better. My job is to teach people how to protect themselves and the ones they love from the dangers of our modern world—dangers they may not even be aware are there. At first, I did this only one-on-one with people who were suffering and in need, as well as with doctors who needed help solving their most difficult cases. Eventually, Spirit told me it was time to take these healing insights to the wider world, which is how my radio show, books, and live events (where I'm able to offer light blasts to the entire audience to ignite healing) were born. The only way I can live my life is by knowing you're receiving this critical information that Spirit has offered.

You won't find citations or mentions of scientific studies in this book, because everything I've written in these pages comes from Spirit. You've no doubt read enough about scientific research everywhere else, and you've likely become confused in the process, wondering which of the competing claims to believe. The information I share here is not one more opinion in a world where everyone has opinions. It is truth. Spirit wants to elevate you above the sea of confusion, to offer you clear answers when you're not sure which theory to believe, and to share health information that's decades ahead of research.

That's because Spirit is the living word *compassion*. This Spirit of Compassion is the expression of God's compassion for humanity. I'm just an ordinary man who happens to hear Spirit's voice with clarity and precision, as if a friend were standing beside me and speaking. Every message I receive and relay comes from the voice of compassion, that place of deepest caring and empathy for humanity. It's not a gift I chose; it was chosen for me. And it's not about me. I don't have the answers—Spirit does. The only reason I've been able to help tens of thousands of people heal is that Spirit provides the information. And Spirit provides it so that *you* can get help. This is about you and your health. In the end, that's all that matters.

SPIRIT'S GOT YOUR BACK

If you type, "What is the highest mountain in the world?" into a search engine, you'll get a list of results pointing you to Mount Everest, along with some sites telling you that if you meant to ask for the *tallest* mountain, then they can direct you to the right place. If you type in, "How do you get from New York to California?" you'll get hits for cheap flights, driving directions, and exact mileage. What these searches have in common is that they're questions about explored terrain; they give you back the right answers.

Now what happens if you type, "What causes Alzheimer's disease?" into that same search box? You'll get a virtual smorgasbord of hits. Some sites will say it's unknown, others will list possible causes and risk factors, and a few will offer management tools. None will redirect you to the right results for alternate questions like, "Why are we losing our loved ones to this ruthless disease?"—because that's unexplored terrain. Instead of giving you a clear direction, the search results will lead you down culs-de-sac, roundabouts, and dead ends. I call these *non-results*, *non-truths*, and *non-wisdoms*. If you're persistent, you may find some beginnings of paths that are being forged in the wilderness—paths that will one day lead to the truth, though they're not there yet. What you won't find in a search about a chronic health issue are definitive answers.

"What gives you the right to say that?" you may be asking. I mean no disrespect to science or to the countless health-care professionals who fight every day for their patients. I have nothing but deep admiration for the practice of medicine and other healing arts. I am all for science. Spirit simply wants me to make you aware that something's missing in what science has discovered so far. In America alone, the more than 200 million people who are sick or have mystery symptoms are evidence of this. The mother who is ill in bed without any answers, too fatigued to look after her children, and at her wit's end wondering how to get better, will back me up. Ask her if medical science has come up with all the answers yet.

Illness is not something anyone likes to dwell on. We live in a time of positivity. That's because we all sense that something's amiss in our world today—so we try to keep our chins up, encourage each other to choose joy over despair, to seek wisdom and enlightenment so we don't get thrown off the ride. It's a powerful movement. At the same time, we have to be careful that our perpetual positivity doesn't give us an aversion to facing the truth.

I've found that when people question the epidemic of mystery illness, or say we don't have a widespread problem with misdiagnosis, or believe that the labels people get for their mystery symptoms are answers—that is, when people say that there's nothing wrong with the status quo—that's usually a sign that they haven't suffered from real health challenges. Maybe they've had the occasional headache, come down with the common cold, dealt with a urinary tract infection (UTI) that they didn't even think of as a real condition, or even broken a bone (where the cause and course of treatment were evident). Beyond that, they've been spared. I'm not saying that these people have somehow protected themselves from illness by not believing in it. Rather that, by luck of the draw, they've not been exposed to the factors that take other people down (factors that we'll explore in this book), and so illness seems like an experience that's "other" and distant to them, and something that can be warded off with the right attitude.

We can't pretend that non-truths are anything more than hypotheses, that sick people aren't really sick, or that the same fate doesn't await us if we don't take the right precautions—the precautions I cover in this book. I can't disrespect you as a reader, a human being, another soul on this planet, by delivering fluff. Before anyone can become enlightened, she or he has to see the world as it is. Wisdom is built upon a foundation of truth.

And the truth is that on top of the stress and nonstop pace of life today, we're up against a pernicious set of pollutants and pathogens that I call the Unforgiving Four (and describe in detail in the chapter to follow). If you're dealing with a health challenge, if you're beset by insomnia, stomach pain, vertigo, moodiness, brain fog, memory loss, bloating, fatigue, obsessive thoughts, or any of the other issues so common today, you are not to blame. It is Spirit's decree that you understand you did not bring it upon yourself. You did not attract or manifest your health problems with negative thinking. If you've been suffering, it is not in your imagination, and it is not your fault. In fewer than 0.25 percent of cases is an illness actually psychosomatic—and even then, what leads a person to induce her or his own symptoms is usually an underlying physical issue in the brain caused by Unforgiving Four factors or real emotional damage.

Along with acknowledging the reality that outside sources are behind the epidemic of chronic illness, it's vital that you learn your God-given health rights. These are rights that you were born with, and even if you didn't know they were there, they are yours: You have a right to be well. You have a right to mental peace. You have a right to get restorative sleep. You have a right to be free from pain. You have a right to heal from illness. You have a right to prevent illness. You have a right to adapt and thrive. These rights can never be taken from you. They are yours for life.

Spirit's mission is to make sure that you know how to protect these rights. This is not about rules, judgments, or punishment. Spirit is not some cosmic hall monitor, ready to give you a demerit for not following prescribed procedures. What good would that do, anyway? It would only serve to put you in a box, take away your sense of freedom, and make you feel worse than you already do.

Rather, Spirit is like a bodyguard. Spirit's number-one priority is that you make it through life in one piece. That doesn't mean slapping you on the wrist. It means instilling in you a sense of your own value. You are as important as anyone who walks around with a security detail. Part of protecting you is pointing out the threats to your peace and safety, and how you can be free from those threats. The rules we've learned up to this point are not enough.

As part of Spirit's security team, it is my responsibility to share the advanced information that will help you safeguard yourself, your children, and your children's children. These are lessons for a new era, secrets that should never have been secrets. It's time to tap into the wisdom that should have been yours all along.

HOW THIS BOOK WORKS

You know how when you make a major purchase, it often comes with a manual? Those manuals are never the whole story. Say you get a new all-terrain vehicle (ATV). No matter what safety precautions are written inside that manual, you're still liable to get hurt if an obstacle gets in your path. There's nothing to tell you, "Here's what to do if you hit a patch of ice at the same time that a fox darts out of the woods and distracts you, and you start skidding."

In the same way, the information that's out there about navigating life's health challenges isn't the whole story. It's not that anyone's holding it back—just that medical communities haven't yet gotten to the bottom of why fatigue and brain fog and chronic illness in all its many forms are plaguing so many people right now.

This book is meant to pack as much real, detailed, usable health information inside as possible. It's meant to warn you about the slippery patches and the dangerous distractions. It's geared for you to learn as much as you can, so that you don't get thrown off that ATV.

In Part I, "Rising Out of the Ashes," I give you a crash course on how we got to this moment in health history, and how to face it. The first chapter, "Save Yourself: The Truth about What's Holding You Back," introduces the Unforgiving Four and other major risk factors for our health, while the following chapter, "Adaptation: Move Forward with the World Around You," explains why the life-changing foods are the answer. Part I's final chapter, "Food for the Soul," gets at the emotional and spiritual side of food—including why we don't need to shun the idea of comfort food.

All of this is meant to be the primer for Part II, "The Holy Four." This is the heart of the book, and it's where you'll find Spirit's top information on 50 of the most transformational foods on the planet, in four categories: fruits, vegetables, herbs and spices, and wild foods. For each food, you'll find details about its health benefits, followed by lists of the conditions and symptoms it can specifically help, a section on its emotional benefits, a spiritual lesson it offers, and a few tips on how to use it. These features aren't meant to be comprehensive, telling you every possible detail about these foods—because that would require a book for each one. Rather, these are the highlights that Spirit has shared about each, so you can come away from this book with 50 new friends.

I've also included a recipe with each food, because I've found that many people think of fruits and vegetables within a box, and usually sharing space inside that box are unproductive ingredients that people are used to eating at the same time. How do you enjoy a potato, for example, without frying it in mystery oil or heaping it with sour cream and bacon bits? The answer is on page 162.

After you've filled your head with everything that the life-changing foods have to offer, turn to Part III, "Arming Yourself with the Truth." Here, I share more secrets about how to navigate our modern world. You can find out about fruit's connection to fertility, fads and foods to avoid, and one of my favorite topics, the life-changing angels who watch over us.

YOU CAN DO THIS

I'm sure you've been confused before in the realm of health. I'm sure you've puzzled over whether to believe the (false) claims that broccoli gives you goiters, or the recommendations to eat it to stave off macular degeneration. (Answer: Eat the broccoli.) And you've probably wondered whether you're supposed to push aside orange juice when you have a cold because its sugar supposedly feeds the virus, or to drink on up because the vitamin C will boost your immune system. (Answer: Drink the orange juice.) There's so much noise out there; there are so many contradictions, mixed messages, fads. It's impossible to know what to trust. If I didn't have Spirit's voice guiding me through life, I would have no idea what to believe.

What has always grounded me is that there *are* answers. *There is something you can hold on to in this world.* That something to hold on to is the information that comes from Spirit. It won't slip through your fingers like sand. If you follow Spirit's recommendations in this book, your life can change, and it can change tremendously for the better. I've seen it happen over and over again with the people who have come to me. And what Spirit always, always comes back to is the holy, healing power of food.

You can do this. You can connect to the person you are meant to be. It will take some letting go of what you've heard before, and it will take some getting used to new ideas. What it will take, more than anything, is trust.

I'm well aware that the worst way to convince someone to trust in the information you're sharing is to say, "Trust me." Trust is something that builds over time. You don't approach a horse for the first time, jump on its back, and gallop away—especially not if you've heard rumors that it's hard to handle. Instead, you take steps to develop a bond of trust between you and the horse.

In the same way, if you've had your doubts about the transformational nature of fruits and vegetables, you're unlikely to pick up a book about them and change your eating habits overnight. We've all learned to be careful with where we place our trust.

So what I invite you to do is read the pages to come, and turn over their messages in your mind. I invite you to pay attention to what it feels like in your heart to learn that the foods that grow from the earth are the gifts God has given us to save humanity. Just be with it, as if you're spending time with a horse, running a hand over its mane, sensing its true nature.

Before long, I hope you'll find that it all clicks into place. I hope you'll come to see that all along, a divine, benevolent force has been looking out for you, leading you to this time in your life—this time when you could finally climb onto the back of that white horse and let it take you farther than you imagined possible.

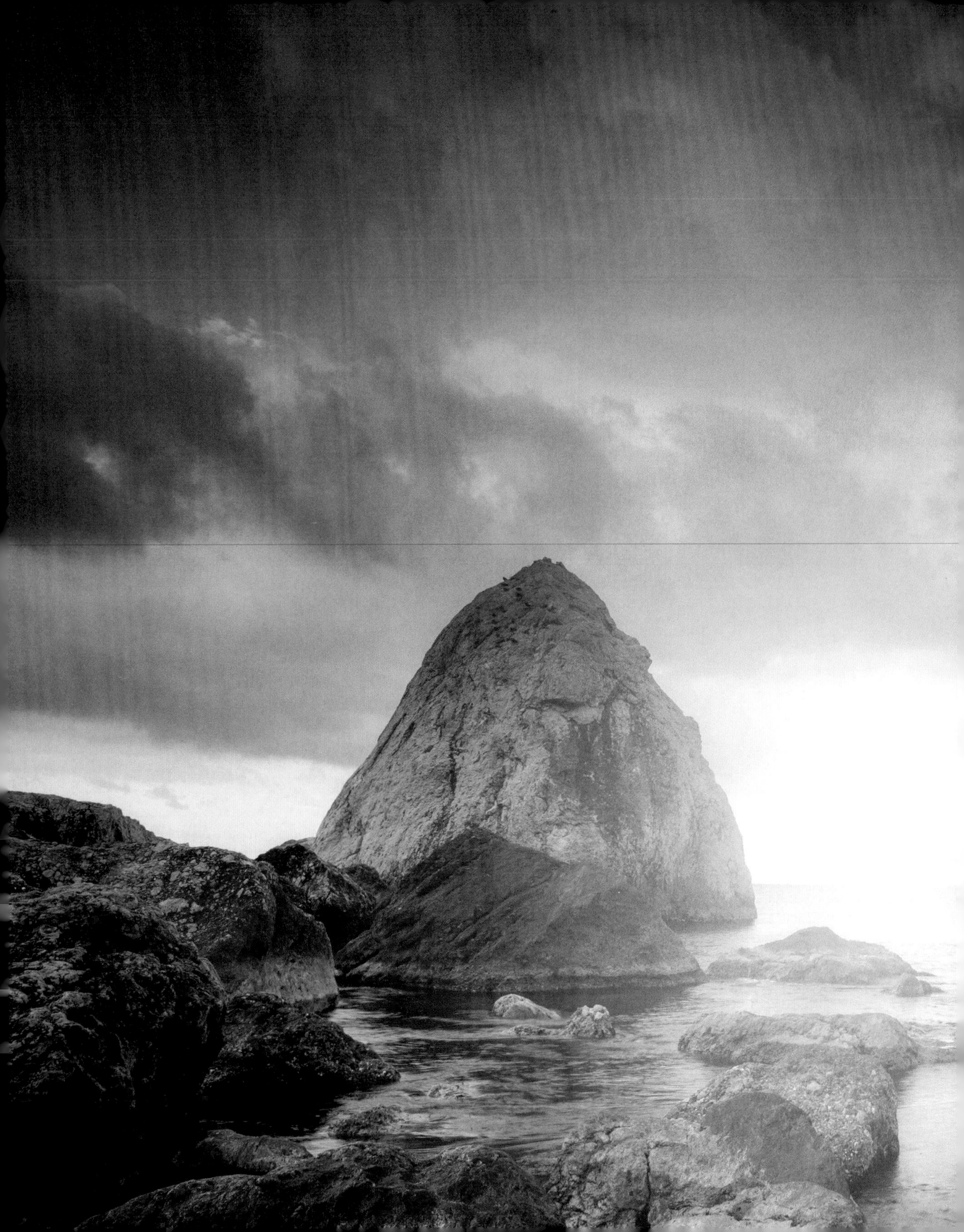

PART I

RISING OUT OF THE ASHES

SAVE YOURSELF:

The Truth about What's Holding You Back

There's a lot of fear out there in the world today, particularly when it comes to health. We fear cancer, Alzheimer's, Lyme disease, multiple sclerosis (MS), infertility, diabetes, amyotrophic lateral sclerosis (ALS). We fear losing our vitality, not performing at our best, being held back, suffering in pain, and missing out on life. We fear those unexplained symptoms that leave so many people feeling lost and hopeless. We lie awake at night worrying about losing our children, parents, friends, and partners to terrifying diseases. Or we live in denial.

I'm not going to tell you that it's just a matter of getting your mind right, that the real problem is fear, and that if you can get that under control, you'll be fine. Because in truth, we're right to fear. Our health is more susceptible than ever before in history. Chronic illness has become one of the most widespread issues of our time. In record numbers, people suffer from the conditions I listed above, plus rheumatoid arthritis (RA), chronic fatigue syndrome (CFS), thyroid disease, fibromyalgia, attention-deficit/hyperactivity disorder (ADHD), autism, autoimmune disease, Crohn's disease, colitis, irritable bowel syndrome (IBS), insomnia, depression, obsessive-compulsive disorder (OCD), migraines—and they don't know why. People experience fatigue, weight gain, achiness, brain fog, nerve pain, skin problems, numbness, digestive distress, body temperature fluctuations, heart palpitations, vertigo, tinnitus, muscle weakness, hair loss, memory loss, anxiety—and a visit to the doctor's office doesn't give them any clarity. The explanations they do get are usually about hormone levels or vitamin D deficiency, which don't give them much to hold on to. These individuals become sidelined from life, forced to put aside their dreams to deal instead with the singular task of survival. Sometimes they lose the fight.

We're dealing with an epidemic of *mystery illness*. That's not just a term that applies to six kids in Idaho who come down with an inexplicable respiratory disorder. As I wrote in my first book, mystery illness is any unexplained health issue—and there are a ton of those. More than 200 million people in the U.S. alone deal with mystery illness. The labels that medical communities have applied to conditions—think Hashimoto's thyroiditis, diabetic neuropathy, systemic exertion intolerance disease, and the like—may trick you into thinking that science has discovered explanations. Don't be fooled. Cancer and other chronic illnesses are still major medical mysteries.

None of which is a criticism of the medical establishment. Medical communities (by which I mean alternative, conventional, functional, and integrative practitioners) are heroes. I love doctors! Without them, we would be lost. They are behind some of the most important discoveries in modern times. They are doing the best they can with the information they have. It's just that research has left them in the dark about what's really going on with these mystery conditions and symptoms. And so with each passing decade, we don't make progress in this area. Some developments and insights get forgotten, buried, underfunded, or even hidden.

As we move forward in time, we've lost our sight. No one is getting a chance to learn the truth, because we're working off an old foundation of theories about chronic illness. Leading the pack is the medical industrial machine, which is really just made up of people who have no choice, because they're force-fed these outdated, misguided theories. Following them are people who don't have any better information to go on. Eventually they all fall into the pit of darkness and death together, and as a result, the masses suffer. This may sound harsh. I only say it so that you can be aware. The truth is that for decades upon decades, suffering has occurred because the causes and treatments for so many illnesses are unresolved or misunderstood. If we're not open-minded, equipped, and protected, then we, too, can be misled and hurt.

If you want to save yourself and your loved ones from this fate, you must learn what's really going on. It's the only way to end the cycle of affliction and fear. It is why I wrote this book.

TIME FOR THE TRUTH

It's not always easy to talk about the truth. Take your personal life: If you have some sort of behavior pattern or fixation that you know doesn't serve you, do you stop and face it, or is your instinct to keep repeating it over and over and just pretend it's okay? The same type of denial happens with medicine, on a much larger scale: We can all sense that something is amiss with the world health-wise, given that billions of people are unwell. And from time to time throughout history, we've stumbled upon reasons *why* people are suffering; for example, the once-revered insecticide dichlorodiphenyltrichloroethane (better known as DDT) was revealed over half a century ago to wreak havoc on public health. Mercury, which was once a coveted medical treatment, has long since been regarded as toxic. So wouldn't you think they're both in the rearview mirror?

We can't escape the past that easily. DDT is still in our environment and our bodies, and it's still behind illness today, even for those who were born long after its ban. Mercury that's thousands of years old continues to cycle through our current generations. These are just two examples of factors that medical research has yet to discover are still plaguing us today (I'll cover more soon). Until we turn a magnifying glass on what really happened in the past, history lives on, repeating itself. We make absolutely no progress by pretending the bad times are over and done with.

Just like we make no progress by pretending we're leading longer, healthier lives today. That's merely an illusion, because the overall population has grown exponentially across the globe. Meanwhile, the wave has crested. If you visit a nursing home today, you'll see that there are fewer residents in their 90s or 100s than there were 30 years ago, and that younger and younger residents are moving in. Twenty years from now, this transformation will be glaringly apparent. You'll be hearing and reading about this dramatic shift in longevity. On the whole, baby boomers are already facing many more life-threatening health challenges than their parents' generation did. Even with life-saving technologies being developed every day, life span is falling, not rising. And for those who do survive into advanced years, longer life often doesn't mean healthy life. While medications and procedures can prolong life in some circumstances, it can come with the price of prolonged suffering.

Do news reports have you worried about overpopulation? That won't be the real problem. Instead, we'll have trouble keeping population numbers up. It's a pretty stark reality to face: shorter life spans, mystery infertility preventing new life, more disease affecting a wider range of people.

One such disease, breast cancer, has everyone on high alert these days. Some women are undergoing genetic testing and choosing to have a double mastectomy if a BRCA1 or BRCA2 gene mutation is detected. It's a valid concern; in 30 years' time, every female born will practically be guaranteed to develop breast cancer. That is, unless she knows how to protect herself.

This is why the truth is so liberating. Sobering as it may be to learn about the risks of our time in the pages to come, the reward is your life. If you know that what I call the Unforgiving Four are threatening your health every day, you can mitigate the risks. If you understand how perilous our stress culture is, you can free yourself from the adrenaline trap. And if you discover just how central food is to saving yourself, it will change everything.

THE UNFORGIVING FOUR

If you're looking to point fingers about how things got so bad in the world, here's where to look: radiation, toxic heavy metals, the viral explosion, and DDT. I call them the Unforgiving Four, because they have shown no mercy in the decades, centuries, and millennia over which they have developed. They have, on their own and together, managed to ravage our bodies, make us question our own sanity, and push us to the breaking point as a society.

These four factors are responsible for the modern-day epidemic of mystery illness. Some of them, like mercury, have been wreaking havoc for thousands of years. Others, such as DDT, seem like open-and-shut cases from fairly recent but distant enough history. Throughout the centuries, events such as the industrial revolution and the invention of the X-ray have served as tipping points, moments in time when one or more of these factors could take particular advantage, gaining the momentum that brought us to this precipice.

The Unforgiving Four are the invisible intruders in our lives, the unknowns that keep us up at night, the reason that life has become so challenging and unpredictable. When I wrote in my first book about various chronic illnesses, I almost inevitably ended up mentioning at least one of these factors for each. They are that prevalent and threatening.

We have suffered from a what-you-don't-know-can't-hurt-you illusion in our current age. Even though everywhere we turn, people are suffering from persistent symptoms or grave illnesses, we try not to delve too deep into the why of it, hoping that if we keep some distance, the same fate won't befall us. Collectively, we quickly forget about those dangers we do hear about. The Unforgiving Four are prime examples: If we can't see radiation, toxic heavy metals, viruses, or DDT, and if they're not making the headlines every day, then we tell ourselves that it's okay not to think about them. We forget about society's old mistakes and instead forge ahead, not stopping to realize that without examining the past, we risk making brand-new errors.

In order to protect yourself, it's imperative to understand the Unforgiving Four. First, they tend to get passed down from generation to generation—an inheritance that's often confused with genetics. When we fall ill, and that illness is similar to something a family member went through, we automatically believe that we've been handed bad genes. It's an easy theory to subscribe to, because we look at the people we're related to and see similar traits. We figure that along with a certain nose shape or hair color or gait, we've inherited a susceptibility to a certain condition as part of the same gene package. Have you ever been told that your health struggle is genetic? Don't get wrapped up in the belief that there's something inherently wrong with you.

Rather, the reason that so many illnesses get passed down in families is because the Unforgiving Four are transmitted through the bloodline. Radiation, heavy metals, viruses, and DDT can all be passed along at conception and in the womb. That's the real story behind most illnesses that travel from generation to generation. We have to be cautious not to subscribe to ideas that hurt more than help us. Yes, we have genes, and yes, they play a pivotal role in our existence. The mistaken concept that you're dysfunctional on a genetic level, though, is just one more belief system that finds fault in your physical body's life-sustaining, sacred foundation. It's in the same league as believing that autoimmune disease is the body attacking itself. (It's not. For more on this, see the introduction to Part II, "The Holy Four.") Chronic illness is not about genes; it's about what your forebears were exposed to that got passed along to your parents, and later, to you. When you understand that the problem is a foreign presence such as a pathogen or toxin, it changes your perspective, because it means you can get rid of it and be free.

The second important point about the Unforgiving Four is that they amplify in combination, so the worst illnesses tend to be due to more than one of them. For example, a person could be exposed to radiation, either directly or through the family line, and because radiation weakens the immune system, she or he becomes more susceptible to coming down with a virus like Epstein-Barr, which can develop into multiple sclerosis. Or if a person inherits a high level of DDT, then gets exposed to heavy metals, particularly aluminum, it's a recipe for brain cancer. Also, toxic heavy metals are a favorite food of viruses, so a bug that would otherwise stay dormant or be flushed out of the system will instead proliferate if there's something tasty like mercury or aluminum nearby.

The third and most important point to keep in mind is that there is hope. With vigilance, it's possible to lower your exposure to these factors. With diligence, it's possible to detoxify them. And with the life-changing foods in the pages to come, you can protect yourself like never before.

Radiation

We've gotten to the point where we ignore radiation; we forget it's a problem. Even writing about radiation right now, I can anticipate what you may be thinking: *Who cares about radiation?*

Not too long ago, radiation concerns about cell phones were a big deal. Now we've brushed them aside. And while we worry about radiation exposure directly after a nuclear disaster, if we don't live near the site, before too long it leaves our consciousness again.

The truth is that every nuclear disaster has done irrevocable damage to our planet. To this day we're still under siege from the fallout of the atomic bombings of Hiroshima and Nagasaki in World War II, the 1986 explosion of the Chernobyl nuclear power plant, and the Fukushima nuclear power plant catastrophe of 2011. When radiation was released into the atmosphere in these events, it didn't all fall to earth immediately; most of it stayed there and still remains in the air we breathe, even if we live far away from Japan and Ukraine. The radiation that did fall entered our water supply and soil, so we're in nearly constant contact with it. Only a fraction of the radiation from Hiroshima has fallen so far. Much of it is still in the atmosphere; in 1,000 years, only half of it will have come to earth.

Then there's the radiation that people were exposed to before X-ray technology was fully regulated. In the mid-1900s, it was all the rage for a trip to the shoe store to include sticking your feet in an X-ray box called a fluoroscope. The idea was that the shoe clerk could help you find the best fit by looking at the internal structure of your foot. And because children's feet are always growing, kids, who are especially sensitive to radiation, would get subjected to the fluoroscope repeatedly, as would anyone who enjoyed shoe shopping often for pleasure.

Today, more radiation than ever before saturates our body systems. Whether from direct exposure, environmental fallout, food and water supply contamination, or inheritance of our parents' and grandparents' exposure, radiation is one of the major health risks we all face. It's a leading contributor to cancers, endocrine system dysfunction, bone diseases such as osteopenia and osteoporosis, bone spurs, immune system failure, and skin diseases. Radiation also acts as a *trigger* for every illness that can affect human beings—so if you have any underlying Unforgiving Four factors in your body, and then you get exposed to radiation, it can be the prompt that turns a dormant contaminant into a full-blown condition.

Toxic Heavy Metals

It's no secret that certain heavy metals are toxic. We all know to be careful of lead paint when renovating older homes, and we all learned at a certain point to switch over to mercury-free thermometers. What's less well-known—and in some cases, a complete secret—is that toxic heavy metals are behind some of the most widespread health issues today: ADHD, autism, Alzheimer's, infertility, Crohn's, ulcerative colitis, Parkinson's, depression, anxiety, cancers, seizures, and more. These metals are also fuel for the viral-related illnesses you're going to read about next.

Plus, we risk exposure in everyday contexts of which we might be unaware. Lead, mercury, copper, cadmium, nickel, arsenic, and aluminum can all build up in the body to create or contribute to illness. When was the last time you used aluminum foil, or ate out of an aluminum takeout container? Or perhaps you live in a house with copper pipes. Or you regularly walk through a park treated with pesticides (which often contain toxic heavy metals). Potential exposure is everywhere, and sometimes unavoidable. It's even falling out of the sky in vapors.

In some cases, the heavy metals in our cells have nothing to do with exposure in our lifetime.

Mercury, the most corrupting of the toxic heavy metals, can easily stick around in a bloodline for millennia, passed from generation to generation, amplifying as it goes. So the mercury in a child's cerebral midline canal that's causing his autistic symptoms could have been mined 3,000 years ago—and could be causing more trouble now than ever before. Or, if the inherited mercury has different placement in the brain, it can cause a person's depression instead. We're not just up against current exposure; we're dealing with ancient toxins.

On their own, these heavy metals are poisons. What's worse is that they tend to oxidize, causing even more problems, such as toxic runoff that damages any tissue in its path. And toxic heavy metals aren't just a problem in the brain. When they're present anywhere in the body, they lower overall immunity and act as fuel for viruses and bacteria.

The Viral Explosion

More than 100 strains and variants in the human herpesvirus (HHV) family are wreaking havoc on the population. Ninety-eight percent of the time, cancer is caused by a virus in combination with at least one other Unforgiving Four factor.

Plus, viruses such as Epstein-Barr (which, in an early stage, takes the form of mononucleosis), shingles, cytomegalovirus (CMV), HHV-6, HHV-7, and the undiscovered HHV-10, HHV-11, and HHV-12—including unknown mutations, offshoots, and varieties of each—are the true causes of some of the most debilitating and misunderstood chronic illnesses of our time. MS, Lyme disease, RA, thyroid disease, fibromyalgia, CFS, temporomandibular joint (TMJ) issues, migraines, diabetic neuropathy, Bell's palsy, Ménière's disease, frozen shoulder, and symptoms such as unexplained tinnitus, vertigo, twitching, tingling, tachycardia, atrial fibrillation, heart palpitations, erratic heartbeat, fatigue, hot flashes, and burning often have ties to viruses. And as with the other Unforgiving Four, we can't help but run into these infectious pathogens in our everyday lives—whether from sharing a soda with a friend or from eating a restaurant dish prepared by a chef with a cut finger.

These viruses often fly under the radar because they don't start truly causing problems until they've moved past the blood infection stage to take up residence in the organs, where doctors don't know to look for them. Over the more than 100 years since the Epstein-Barr virus (EBV) first took root in the population, it has mutated and spread like wildfire, accounting for the epidemics of people stuck in bed with unexplainable fatigue, muscle pain, and sometimes joint deformity.

All too often, though, patients are told that EBV can't be the problem, because their blood tests show antibodies that indicate a past infection, not a present one. If there were tools to measure for EBV in the organs, a huge lightbulb would go on for medical communities. They'd realize that for the person suffering from a condition such as fibromyalgia, CFS, or thyroid disease, that simple case of mono the patient had back in college never really left her or his system; it just took up a new residence within the body and started causing more serious problems.

Plus, there are many more strains of these viruses than medical science has discovered, so there's a lack of awareness about what to look for. In the human herpesvirus family, for example, the list doesn't stop at the documented HHV-8; it goes up to and past HHV-12. And countless patients suffer with the burning, immobilizing nerve pain of shingles—and have no idea that this virus is behind it, because studies have yet to reveal that there are non-rashing varieties of shingles, so doctors don't know to diagnose it.

When herpes viruses have their favored foods around (such as toxic heavy metals), they excrete poisonous waste products called neurotoxins, which disrupt nerve function and confuse a person's immune system as well as the doctor who's trying to diagnose the symptoms. Lupus, for example, is the body having an allergic reaction to EBV's neurotoxins. The condition ends up getting all the focus, while the underlying viral infection continues to grow.

If everyone knew what was going on with this viral explosion—knew that it was occurring and knew how to protect themselves—it wouldn't be the problem that it is today. Instead, people walk around in agony and don't know why, or how to stop it. While they may get labels for their illnesses such as lupus, Lyme disease, or MS, those labels don't give them answers about the true cause of their suffering.

DDT

People are rightly worried about pesticide exposure. It's important for your health to eat organic when possible, tend your lawn and garden without synthetic chemicals, and be wary of what the grass at your local park may be treated with to make it so green. All of this present-day awareness, though, shouldn't distract you from a dangerous chemical that was once so celebrated and widely used that it still exists in our surroundings, saturating our family lines and affecting our health decades after it was first discovered to be toxic. Of course, I'm talking about DDT.

It's easy to think of DDT as a thing of the past. Revealed over 50 years ago as contributing to cancers and other illnesses, wildlife endangerment, and environmental pollution, this toxic insecticide has been banned from widespread use in the U.S. for over 40 years. Trucks spraying DDT don't drive through every neighborhood anymore, and salesmen no longer show up at every door proclaiming its virtues for use in the garden.

Unfortunately, even decades after the pioneering efforts of those like scientist Rachel Carson, who in her 1962 book *Silent Spring* helped expose DDT's dangers and advocated to massively curtail its usage, we're still dealing with it every day. That's because DDT remains in the environment, which means it gets into our food supply, amplifying as it moves up the food chain. Further, as with the other Unforgiving Four, DDT gets passed down from generation to generation. So even if you weren't alive during DDT's heyday, chances are that your foremothers and forefathers who *were* around then came into contact with the chemical, which means you could have ended up with that old DDT in your system, wreaking havoc on your health. We're also being exposed to current-day DDT fallout, because not every country has outlawed its use. When DDT is sprayed, it gets into the air, and then winds carry it far and wide—even to other continents.

DDT, other pesticides, and herbicides are the major underlying cause of suppressed immune systems—they weaken people's bodies so that pathogens and contaminants can take advantage. Generation after generation, DDT can make family members susceptible to the same illnesses, so that what's really a condition that could be healed through detoxification is passed off instead as a genetic problem about which much can't be done. While DDT may be in history books now, it is still preying on us—for example, by making our livers hypersensitive (viruses are the other cause of major liver distress), instigating diabetes, enlarging spleens and hearts, causing poor digestion, triggering migraines and chronic depression, creating skin disorders, and disrupting hormones. This is tragic! It's exactly why I want you to have this information—so you can be proactive and take measures to cleanse your system with the foods in this book.

THE ADRENALINE ADDICTION

It would be one thing if today's health challenges stopped at the four threats above. Compounding it all, though, is the drug we're forced to use to keep up: adrenaline. The Unforgiving Four push our bodies to release more adrenaline than ever before as we fight off these invaders. Plus, the stress of the everyday has reached an all-time high; we're constantly drawing on our adrenaline reserves to put out fires in our working and home lives. And the toll it takes is not to be underestimated. When we live off adrenaline (also known as epinephrine), there's a serious price to pay.

It's like we're in a constant road race: To avoid being run over, we have to keep up, even if that's to our own detriment. In the racing world, when a souped-up engine isn't enough, street racers like to rig their cars with nitrous oxide. This colorless gas has its upside: All it takes is the flip of a switch, and the nitrous oxide releases to give the engine superpowers. The problem is that it's short-lived. You can only use it for so long before it will cause the engine to blow out, or send you into a spin, out of control. It puts your entire investment in the car in jeopardy.

Well, that souped-up engine is the equivalent of a high-energy, type A personality—the kind that's celebrated in today's culture. People use that sort of drive to get tasks done fast. However, they often find that it's not enough to keep up with demands, so they turn on the adrenaline switch—which, if we use it too often, can result in a health wreck. We have to be careful in this human race. If we want to protect our bodies, just like if those drivers want to protect those cars, it's important to understand the potential dangers of the decisions we make.

When Adrenaline Becomes a Drug

Our own adrenaline should be categorized as a Schedule I drug—that's how addictive it is. And like any drug, we become numb to adrenaline at a certain point. We lose our benchmark of what good, safe, happy, and normal feel like as we draw on ever more of it.

None of which is to say that adrenaline can't be good and safe at the proper levels. It is, after all, a completely natural part of how our bodies work, and vital to the survival of our species. In the past, we truly could function on low, healthy levels of adrenaline, with occasional surges when we were in danger. Think of it like taking a walk through a field of flowers on a beautiful day. With blue skies above, the sun shining, and birds singing, you could be in a state of calm—until you spotted a timber rattlesnake coiled in your path. Your adrenaline level would momentarily elevate as you figured out how to get past the snake without harm, and once you did, your adrenaline would come back down as you continued on your way. This is the equivalent of predigital life, and it's what our bodies were built for: homeostasis, punctuated by occasional adrenaline rushes to keep us safe.

Times have changed. We're still walking through that field of flowers; it's still a beautiful day with blue skies and sunshine and birdsong—except instead of one rattlesnake in our path, now there are hundreds. Every other step we take, we risk landing on one. It's the by-product of our technological age: With everything moving so fast, we encounter danger at a higher frequency, too. This means that our adrenaline levels have had to rise. Before, plowing a field or even a hard day at the office didn't jack up our adrenaline unless something life-threatening occurred. Being productive and maintaining physical balance didn't cancel each other out.

In our current age, we've lost the luxury of homeostasis. Constantly heightened adrenaline levels—not quite at crisis level, but on the edge—have become our new normal. Why? Because we're staving off potential emergencies all day long. We lie awake at night worrying about how to protect our families from the tragedies we see on the news. With the speed of modern communication, we feel we always have to be "on." Technology is changing in the blink of an eye, and we race to keep up. We have too much to do, too many directions to go in, and too little time. We see illness affecting our loved ones at higher and higher rates. And of course, pathogens and pollutants like the Unforgiving Four, passed down for generations, create baggage that pushes us past our limits emotionally, spiritually, and physically. All of this puts us into a state of perpetual stress. Then on top of it, true crises still occur. Our adrenaline spikes from the medium daily level to off-the-charts heights, and our lives become further defined by the hormone.

We also use adrenaline to self-medicate. Instead of medication, I call it *adrenication*. This is what I mean when I say adrenaline is a drug. We get so used to the sensation of this hormone coursing through our veins that we become addicted to it. We forget what a healthy level feels like. We associate an adrenaline rush with feeling "alive," so the moment we get a real chance to relax, we start to feel the letdown of coming off the ride, which prompts us to crave a hit of stimulation instead. This means we tend to keep ourselves over-busy and overstimulated in our "off" hours. It even almost feels like relaxation, because it keeps our minds from wandering to our overflowing inboxes, our never-ending to-do lists, and our fears about our own lives.

So this is where we are, and what we're up against: We live in an adrenaline-based culture, with adrenaline-inducing toxins in our environment, plus those passed down from generations before us. Adrenaline is our mainstay to cope with the changing times. The next question becomes: what is this doing to us?

This Is Your Brain on Adrenaline

Our adrenal glands produce 56 distinct blends of the hormone for all different activities and emotions. There's an adrenaline blend for bathing, another for dreaming, and dozens more for other neutral tasks that aren't associated with stress. Then there are the different adrenaline blends for crises. These types of overpowering adrenaline are only meant to be used for once-in-a-blue-moon, life-threatening emergencies—and when the adrenaline is released that infrequently, there isn't a health risk. When life always feels on the verge of crisis, though, as it tends to in our modern era, the balance starts to tip.

One way to look at adrenaline is like lighter fluid to our consciousness. Say you're starting up the grill at a cookout, and everyone's eager for their food. You might squirt the coals with some extra lighter fluid to get the fire started faster—to bring the coals to their most immediate potential. You'll probably get the result you want: The fire will ignite right away, and the heat from the glowing coals will be brilliant. There will also likely be a price to pay: The coals will burn out before their time. Without the lighter fluid, they would have lasted longer.

The same is true of adrenaline and the brain. Adrenaline lighting up our fires within means we're all getting a heck of a lot done. Collectively, we are accomplishing more tasks—and a wider range of tasks—in a shorter amount of time than ever before. Adrenaline is serving as the catalyst for accelerated intelligence and rapid-fire work levels, and it's expanding our capacity for developing technology. We're using all this adrenaline to push sports achievement to its highest, too—and we're using it to protect our children. There are more big, bad wolves to look out for now, and they come in all shapes and sizes. Drugs are one example. Whereas only 4 to 7 percent of a high school student body used to be on drugs, now in many parts of the country, up to 90 percent are using. Adrenaline helps parents keep on top of their kids, and keep them safe.

The flip side is that we're burning out faster, too. We're not yet balancing this unprecedented performance with advancements in self-care. The adrenaline that we're throwing onto our brains like lighter fluid is pushing our neurotransmitters, electrical nerve impulses, glial cells, and neurons past their full capacity before their time is due. It's part of the reason why we're heading into the land of Alzheimer's, brain fog, memory loss, disorientation, confusion, depression, lack of focus, depersonalization, forgetfulness, insomnia, and dementia. And it's putting us on the edge.

Our Most Precious Resource

We look for safeguards all the time. We get car insurance, health insurance, life insurance, disability insurance, property insurance. We seek out appliances with good warranties and refundable tickets for flights and events. We're always looking for a guarantee of protection—and we're willing to pay a premium for it. When it comes to adrenaline, though, there are no guarantees, paybacks, or insurance policies. If we're not aware of what our adrenaline is doing for us and what we're doing for it, if we don't realize what the risks are, we can get scammed into squandering our adrenaline. To avoid this, it's critical that we learn about just what price we pay for all this output.

It goes beyond brain burnout. Adrenaline is meant to protect us from acute, short-term damages. When we rely on it in the long term, though, it becomes a *source* of damage. Not unlike battery acid rushing through the body, too much adrenaline is corrosive and toxic. Consequences include adrenal fatigue, a compromised immune system, Addison's disease, elevated blood pressure, infertility, depression, vaginal dryness, weight gain, brain fog, motor ticks, twitching, spasms, blurred vision, migraines, loss of libido, moodiness, anxiety, fear, a sense of being lost, listlessness, malaise, paranoia, and a loss of the ability to trust. It's especially abrasive to the central nervous system and other nerve tissue. Further, it feeds the viruses I discussed above that are behind so many illnesses. More than any other toxin out there, excess adrenaline is taking us down.

I don't want you to think that our own bodies are to blame for the escalating levels of illness in the population. The *outside factors* are what's pushing our bodies past their limits. So we have to get wise about protecting ourselves; we have to reorient our thinking to value our reserves of adrenaline. Adrenaline is like liquid gold. With other valuable resources such as our finances, we know to balance expenditures with earnings to prevent being overdrawn. We know that we cannot spend, spend, spend and expect to remain solvent.

However, we forget this math with our adrenaline. We're bombarded with distractions, expectations, challenges. We become adrenaline spendthrifts without even realizing it. Then there are the adrenaline highs that so many people seek out. Bungee jumping, for example, may feel exciting in the moment, just like a shopping spree or a trip to the casino, yet it still registers as life-threatening to our bodies, which can then put us into deficit. For every adrenaline high, there's an adrenaline crash waiting. And the longer you stay on your adrenaline high, the longer the crash that's waiting for you.

More adrenaline spending means more work for our accountants (neurotransmitters) and money managers (neurons). It can, ultimately, overwhelm them, causing our adrenals to become underactive or overactive or to alternate between the two states. At that point, other parts of the body try to step in and bankroll us to prevent physical debt. The endocrine system and pituitary gland go into overdrive. The liver starts to release a large portion of its vital glucose reserves. The pancreas releases all the enzymes it can. It's as though every available body system tries to step in and print money to replace the liquid gold of adrenaline. It can deplete and burn out these precious body systems—unless we take steps to preserve our health, which I describe in the next chapter, "Adaptation."

THE FIGHT FOR FOOD

Along with the Unforgiving Four and excess adrenaline, we're dealing with a food crisis. I'm not just talking about overpopulation, monocropping, diminished and demineralized topsoil, GMO engineering, pollution that enters the food chain, and fewer, less bioavailable nutrients. While those factors are all too real, they're also getting all the blame, when far more is putting us in danger.

Here's what else we have to look out for: diminishing sunlight, a lack of living water, and—most important—the choices we make about what to eat. We live on a changing planet; the world is becoming more of a threat to our health every day. We need to be aware of the changes, and to look after ourselves and our families so that the major shifts don't take us down.

Diminishing Sunlight

We don't have the sunlight we once did. While news headlines focus on the dangers of sun exposure, warning us about ozone depletion and ultraviolet (UV) rays, the real danger is that we don't have *enough* sun. That's right; sunlight has diminished greatly over the past couple of centuries. What we think of as clear skies today are nowhere near as bright blue as they used to be. If you traveled back in time to a sunny day 200 years ago, you would be shocked—it would be like cleaning off smudged eyeglasses to reveal a crystal-clear world.

Pollution and chemicals now fill the skies. I'm not talking about clouds that block the sun; I'm talking about a white haze filled with barium that makes the sky dimmer and keeps the full strength of the sun from getting through. Given the widespread panic about the threat of

UV rays to our health, less sunlight may sound like a good thing. I assure you, it's not. Over the past decade in many parts of the country, critical growing periods during the summers have become colder, with lower yields on certain crops. While there are still hot periods in the summer, these temperature dips at key moments are disruptive to plant life. Less sunlight getting through is the culprit. Our skies are no longer as clear as they once were, and that's taking its toll on the economy, not to mention the health and livelihoods of so many in the U.S.

Similar negative effects of inadequate sunlight are threatening other parts of the world. It's rare in many places now to see a brilliant blue sky. Instead it's an almost smudgy haze caused by pollutants such as vaporized metals, radiation, and chemicals that are diminishing sunlight—even when technically, there may not be a cloud in the sky. This filmy haze that overtakes the sky is different from smog, which settles closer to the ground.

And it's not just a problem for plants. While we focus on vitamin D as the only benefit of the sun, scientific research has yet to discover that like plants, our bodies perform a type of photosynthesis. We rely on the sun to increase production of various enzymes, minerals, vitamins, and other nutrients to revitalize our body systems. Less sun means a shorter life span, and no proper sun exposure means we cease to exist. If we're going to stay safe in the face of this, we have to know it's happening.

Water Deficiency

The rain that once showered our earth was full of life. Alive with minerals and other nutrients, this water was brimming with vitality and operated on a frequency that, when it entered our bodies through our food, provided us with a foundational essence for our survival. Snow used to be called "poor man's fertilizer," because when it melted, it miraculously fortified gardens and fields with extremely high levels of living molecules and active trace minerals. There was enough life force in this water from the sky that there was no need to amend the soil—all the nourishment that crops needed was right there.

Today, our rain and snow are deficient. I'm not talking about a lack of precipitation, though of course drought is an increasingly problematic issue in certain places. I'm talking about the rain itself not having all the components it once did. Deficiency is a concept you're no doubt familiar with: Say you visit the doctor because you're experiencing fatigue and weakness. The doctor runs some blood tests and discovers that it's possible you're low in iron and vitamin D, explaining that this accounts for your symptoms.

Our rain is suffering in the same way, except this is not getting any attention. Other areas of planetary distress are getting attention—and rightfully so. This issue is equally important. A miraculous purification process naturally occurs as rainwater starts to fall, like a giant water filter in the sky. As the sky fills with ever more toxins, though, the purification process intensifies. For nature to disarm the harmful chemicals, radiation, and vaporized toxic heavy metals that are saturating the sky, it must also disarm the life-giving nutrients that are present in the water. The result is that the precipitation that makes its way to earth loses some of its life force and becomes deficient.

A True Food Crisis

You've just read about the risks of our modern world—the Unforgiving Four, the adrenaline pumping through our bodies as we rush to keep up with the unprecedented speed of daily life. You've also read about the hidden threats to our food supply—the changing nature of sunlight and water, two elements that are critical for life here on earth. This all puts us at a particularly precarious moment in history: our future as a species hinges on what we eat going forward.

Right now we are experiencing a food crisis. Not to be confused with food shortages that tragically put whole regions at risk, this food crisis is affecting places in the world where people have access to practically any type of food. This food crisis is about what people are choosing to eat when their choices are unlimited. While food has always been at the center of human survival, eating *healthily* used to be just a hobby for those few who cared and could afford it. And with so many mixed messages, contradictory studies, and fad diets out there, just *how* to eat healthily has always seemed like a giant question mark.

One factor that leads people astray with their eating is the search for emotional comfort. It's so easy to want to drown our sorrows in a hot fudge sundae or a double bacon cheeseburger, even when we know full well that we'll pay for it later with high cholesterol readings, a strained waistband, or worse. Temptation abounds in our world today, and the stress of overly full schedules means that the easiest, cheapest meal choice is often the most processed and detrimental. Even when we know better and have the means to purchase or grow better food, we reach for that inflammatory, ulcerative, blood-sugar-spiking, artery-blocking, liver-clogging, brain-fog-inducing, edema-causing, energy-robbing, pathogen-feeding, disease-promoting grub—because our souls have a real need to be nurtured, and these nostalgic foods have a way of shutting down our minds long enough to give us a moment of escape. (I'll talk much more about this in the next chapter, "Food for the Soul.")

At other times, we have the motivation to eat well, the support from family and friends, ready access—it seems like all the puzzle pieces are in place. However, even in this situation it's still very easy to choose unproductive foods, because fads and trends persuade us that secretly hazardous items are healthy. An example is canola oil: Tons of health food stores and restaurants celebrate canola for its so-called benefits, praising its low levels of saturated fat and saying that it can reduce the risk of heart disease. They don't know any better; it's just the common "wisdom" at the moment. In fact, canola oil causes inflammation, feeds pathogens, and is abrasive to the arteries. Cooking with canola, like other foods I covered in the "What Not to Eat Chapter" of my first book, leads people down a dangerous path. It's a completely hidden contributor to the food crisis we face.

There is mass misunderstanding about how to eat well, and how to feed our souls at the same time as our bodies. The truth is that it's not either-or, and it's not impossible. It's not even unpleasant. We can turn this crisis into an opportunity to learn what's truly best for us.

A WAY FORWARD

I don't want you to think this is all doom and gloom. Yes, we're up against some serious threats in our world today. Yes, it makes life scarier and more uncertain than ever before. The lack of information out there right now—camouflaged by the onslaught of misleading, attention-grabbing headlines—causes widespread suffering. That is simply the truth. When we try to ignore it, to bury our heads in the sand, or when we don't know the *why* of it, we're much worse off—individually and as a whole. We get stuck, and that makes us vulnerable. Only when we face reality can we truly move forward.

It's time for change, for you to learn what you were always meant to know about how to save yourself and your family from a beyond-challenging world. Your life is sacred and precious. You have an individual purpose here on earth, and I want you to be alive and well to see it through.

Now you know how we got to this place where our lives are threatened. You know what the specific hazards to your health are. After reading this chapter, you've become better equipped to protect yourself and your loved ones. And finally, armed with this knowledge, you can learn the secrets in the pages ahead of how to not only combat the danger but overcome it.

Keep a light heart. The time has come to rise up, to tap into the divine forces waiting to help us. The time has come to thrive.

ADAPTATION:

Move Forward with the World Around You

This time we live in has a name: the Quickening. It's an era when technological advancements fuel a faster-than-ever-paced life. In the blink of an eye, devices, platforms, and procedures race ahead. We walk around with tiny computers in our pockets, chat by live video with people halfway around the world, read articles about how robotic surgery has become commonplace . . . this is the future! And yet all this development still leaves us vulnerable if we don't adapt at the foundation.

Because here's the thing about progress: It doesn't always happen in perfect synchronicity. While some areas race ahead, others lag behind. Take cars, for instance. Today's cars are equipped with Wi-Fi, computerized dashboards, GPS, solar panels, remote starters, cameras that show you your blind spots, heated seats, televisions in the headrests, automatic transmissions, rain-sensing windshield wipers, and other features no one could have dreamed of a century ago, when Henry Ford unveiled the first Model T. Cars are basically spaceships at this point. We hear that soon, they will even be driving themselves.

Yet all of those advancements are carried around by massively outdated technology: rubber tires filled with air. That's the same as it was 100 years ago, when you had to crank the engine to get it started! And we all know just how common flat tires still are—and how debilitating. You can be driving along on the highway, grooving out to your satellite radio, enjoying the perfect individualized temperature from your dual climate control, with a voice telling you exactly which turns to take—and none of it will protect you from a pile of nails on the pavement. The tire will start to deflate, you'll feel the telltale bumpy ride, and you'll be forced to pull onto the shoulder, unable to continue until you get a whole new tire. Five minutes ago, you were on top of the world. Now, standing by the side of the road, it may feel like you're only a stone's throw away from the days of the wooden wagon wheel. Until there's a revolution (so to speak) in the conception of how cars get from point A to point B, automobiles are going to be stuck in the past no matter how decked-out they become up top.

This explains where we are health-wise as a society, too. Without our health, collectively and individually, the progress we make in other areas of our lives is less meaningful. Health is what carries us along the road of life. Health is the foundation. Health is *everything*. Without our health, we're stuck. And yet advancements in all kinds of other arenas are pulling the wool over our eyes, distracting us from how susceptible our bodies are. Potential dangers—nails in the road—lurk everywhere. You just read about several of them in the previous chapter.

So what do we do about this? How do we cope? We do something that's part of our human nature, written into our DNA, something we are all meant to do and that the universe wants to support us in: we adapt.

SEEKING ASSISTANCE

It's nobody's fault that the information isn't out there already about *how* to adapt. No one's to blame that advancements in preventative health care fall far behind the progress made in so many other arenas. It's just the way the world has developed over the years. One aspect of the Quickening is that the rapid-fire pace can get out of hand and start moving matters in a negative direction. So there *is* plenty of assistance out there—if you're in the business of destroying yourself. If you want to drink more, you won't have to look hard to find a bartender who will pour you the next cocktail. If you want to drive 100 miles per hour in a 50-miles-per-hour lane, just step on the gas; the car will assist you. If you want to bungee jump off a bridge, you'll easily find someone to secure the rubber cord for you. Help is boundless and readily available 24/7 if you want to put your life on the line.

The flip side is that finding help for improvement is a struggle. You've probably experienced what an uphill battle it is when you try to better yourself: how when you're on a diet, temptation lurks around every corner. Or how when you're trying to exercise more, 10 urgent issues suddenly pop up to get in your way. When real help *is* there, it's limited. You can only find one healthy restaurant near your office, say, so when you get tired of the food there, you cave to the burger joint. The advice you find on time management tells you that fitting in exercise is just a matter of "making time," so you beat yourself up for being lazy whenever you can't get in a workout. Then there are all the harmful health fads that deceive countless people—trends that advertise themselves as beneficial, when the truth is, they're anything but.

Of the seven billion people on the planet, six billion are lacking the help they need with their well-being. It's not because they don't deserve to thrive. It's not because they've manifested or attracted the wrong life circumstances. It's just chance. The world has gotten to the point where our natural ability to ebb and flow, and to maneuver around certain health obstacles, has been overridden by counterproductive forces. It's the car tire effect: innovation has left some gaps.

Let me be clear that this is not because God has left us on our own down here. It's human free will that's gotten us to this point. Groupthink and a series of uninspired decisions throughout history have led industries to toil with materials that are hazardous to our health, and led research to develop high-minded gadgets when it's our foundation that needs attention. Experts, teachers, authorities, and professionals in the health-care field can't show us the way in this area, because they haven't been given the data to teach the human race the most important answers about how to adapt. The Higher Spirit, the Holy Source, the Universe, the Light, angelic forces—whatever language for the great divine speaks to you—is there. God is looking out for you more than ever before. And connecting to that heavenly benevolence is what will elevate you above the sea of confusion so that you can gain control.

To begin with, we need to seek assistance—true assistance—from a most unlikely source.

DEALING WITH STRESS

Being alive during the Quickening is like being the proverbial frog in a pot of water. The temperature keeps going up and up, in increments we can't quite detect, until suddenly it's too much to bear. We didn't just jump right into this churning state of affairs; it's been building over time. If we don't wise up soon, though, we risk being boiled alive.

Stress as the Great Teacher

A critical step in adapting to our modern world is to stop seeing stress as an adversary. Yes, life these days can be distressing—big-time. We have so much to balance constantly, and women especially juggle more jobs and responsibilities than ever before. The pressure to be everything to everyone can be panic-inducing. If you feel overwhelmed by it all, under siege, you absolutely have every right to feel that way. It is 100 percent valid and real.

The only way to protect ourselves from the dangers of our changing world is to change along with it. We have to find a way to cope; it's the only way to stay alive and move forward. Some people de-stress with exercise, which is beyond a doubt beneficial. Others turn to meditation and prayer, which I think are so important that I devoted two chapters to the topic of soul and spiritual support in my first book. Still other people find success by cutting back in areas where they can afford to devote less attention. That's a great approach, if you can swing it; absolutely, give yourself permission to "work smarter, not harder," to back out of plans as needed, to delegate, to nap when your energy is flagging, and *not* to check off every item on your to-do list.

Many of us have tried all of the above, though. And much as we'd love to cut back on the obligations we have left, it's impossible. We're already not getting to everything we're supposed to, and we can't avoid many of the situations that come our way, nor can we wish them out of existence. It's the way of the world right now: there's a lot to be done.

This is where making friends with stress comes in. I don't mean this in a cutesy way, as though it's an easy thing to do. I mean it in all seriousness. This is the grave reality: If we spend each day burning through excess adrenaline, it will take us down. Too much of that corrosive substance running through our bodies will be the end of us.

You can learn to counter adrenaline reactions energetically by viewing stress as a messenger. What's the stress telling you? That you're needed on this planet, that you're useful, that you have a purpose. If you are stressed out to the max, if you feel up against it, like pressure is coming at you from every direction, then you are on the frontiers of purpose—you have a *purpose-plus*. Purpose-plus means you are engaged on the next level above ordinary living, that you truly touch others with your life. And that demands a lot from you.

Stress is not trying to kill you. It's a master teacher that is trying to communicate with you. It's trying to test you—though it's not about any sort of score. Just being chosen for this test makes you instantly successful. The world is becoming something new and different. You've been recognized as amazingly capable and a key player in seeing the world through this challenging age of the Quickening. We'll only come out on the other side of this era of rebirth if committed people like you learn to recognize stress as an honor and to use it to their advantage.

Did you ever have that teacher in school who really pushed you and often frustrated you, someone you now look back on as your best teacher? That's what stress is like. Rather than looking at stress as an invader, understand that stress is preparing you to be a master. Say hello to stress. Recognize it as a familiar face, someone you care about, and look it in the eye. Greet stress as your great mentor. Feel almost sorry for stress. After all, you will move past it, rise above it, succeed it—you'll leave it behind. When dealing with stress, it's key to remember this impermanence. No matter what, all things change. Nothing will stay the same. In the moment when stress is pushing you past your capacity, when you feel in dire need of relief, remind yourself that it will not last.

When stress *is* there, we can appreciate it. Without stress, where would we be? There would be no challenge to inspire us. With the weather always perfect, food always abundant, love always flowing, we wouldn't have anything to strive for, and life would grow boring. Without stress, we would lose our will, because will is built upon constantly succeeding, rising above, and breaking through to the other side of stress. Imagine all the birds suddenly gone from the planet. Not only would we miss out on everything birds do for the ecosystem, the experience of life on earth just wouldn't be the same if they vanished. That's how it would be if stress suddenly ceased to exist. If we didn't have all these stresses flitting through our lives, it simply wouldn't be right.

If you think about it, *stress* is just the name we give it in negative circumstances (or what we label as negative circumstances). There are plenty of moments in our lives that we think of as leisure or play that have elements of stress involved. When you're riding your bike on the weekend, giving it everything you've got to get to the top of a hill, that's stress—only you probably think of it as exhilaration or release. Or when you first learned to ride a bike, you probably thought of it in terms of the amazing end reward of riding a two-wheeler, so even though it was challenging and technically stressful, you registered the experience as exciting and fun, skinned knees and all. The point is, stress is natural. It's always been there, and it's always been a friend. No matter how intense or grave stress feels in a given moment, we have to remember not to fear it.

We hear the term *stress management* a lot. The issue with this concept is that managing stress can feel like one more job to do, and one more thing to feel bad about. So many people already walk around feeling inadequate for not being able to keep up with every single detail of their lives. On top of that, they're supposed to feel like they have one more task—to manage the way they're managing it all?

Staying sane is less about managing stress and more about interacting with it. Instead of trying to fight against stress, communicate with it. Even consider letting stress reside at your address. Welcome it to your table. Break bread with stress. Acknowledge it as you drink your warm bowl of soup with stress beside you, offering it honor and respect, as though it's a coach who has moved in to get you into prime shape. If you're used to getting physical symptoms such as tight muscles from stress, politely ask stress instead to zero in on those problem areas like a masseuse and send them the message that it's time to let go and work for you, because they're needed to help you fulfill your purpose-plus.

There is one boundary you need to set with stress: bedtime. When you retire for the night, that's when you tell stress, "You're locked out." No matter what's occurring in your life, you get to shut off your thoughts about it all when you shut off the light. This is when you call the angels in and create your sanctuary for the night, so you can navigate your dreams and be cleansed of difficult emotions that cropped up during the day. You need and deserve your rest.

The approach of seeing stress as a messenger, friend, teacher, mentor, body worker, and coach makes stress less stressful. It is a powerful technique to help us grow and adapt to the challenges of our time. When you feel sorry for stress, appreciate it, and recognize it as impermanent, it doesn't send the same jolt of excess adrenaline through your veins—it doesn't take the toll on your body that it would otherwise. So go ahead, watch what happens when you greet stress with this new perspective. I can't wait for you to feel the relief.

Stress Assistance and the Importance of Grazing

When we're feeling thrown off by difficult life events or too much to do, it's common to want to reach for something to eat. This isn't a bad instinct. It's the brain's way of saying that it could use some support in navigating a challenge. The key is to know which foods will actually help us. The foods you'll read about soon are masters of adaptation. Surviving out in the elements has granted them cell-deep knowledge of how to thrive in difficult circumstances, and this adaptability becomes a part of you when you eat them. You'll find that I give some foods in this book (such as sprouts) a special note about their adaptogenic nature, while others get extra praise for being potent stress-assist foods. These are the refreshments you want to stock in your kitchen and pack for work, because they offer true refreshment so you can deal with what's at hand. It gives a whole new meaning to the term *stress eating*. (For more on cravings and comfort food, see the next chapter.)

Another important way that we can protect ourselves from the mania of our overcharged world is by grazing. Eating something every one and a half to two hours is vital for dealing with the adrenal roller coaster that is life today. This goes against much of the macho messaging that's out there at the moment. Right now, it's all about energy drinks, skipping meals, and mainlining caffeine. We tend to congratulate ourselves for being able to go several hours without eating and feel weak-willed if we need a snack between meals. It almost starts to feel like we should become robots who require no food at all to meet the demands of the digital age.

It's time to rethink this conditioning. Even if you *can* last ages with no food, it doesn't mean you *should*. For one thing, what's the point of all our technological advances if we have to pay the price of acting inhuman? For another, it doesn't work for our bodies. If you eat a dense lunch at noon that keeps your stomach feeling full until dark, your blood sugar will drop regardless by about 1:30 or 2:00 P.M. Unless your liver has amazing glucose reserves (most people's don't) and your brain's neurotransmitters are strong, your adrenals will be forced to pump out adrenaline and cortisol to fill in for the lack of sugar in the bloodstream. As I've said, too much adrenaline is corrosive. And cortisol is no treat, either: an excess of it can dehydrate you, contribute to weight gain, and eat away at your body's reserves of building blocks like glucose, glycogen, iron, electrolytes, and amino acids.

As the adrenal glands themselves get strained (which I wrote about in the previous chapter), you have a recipe for fatigue and disease. The much preferable alternative is to graze. If you eat three meals a day, you definitely don't have to give up your routine. Just remember that if you want to maximize energy and prevent your body systems from becoming strained and susceptible to illness, then supplement your breakfast, lunch, and dinner with light, balanced snacks. You'll find dozens of suggestions for just what to snack on in the middle section of this book.

FOOD IS THE NEW FRONTIER

Remember that analogy from the previous chapter about the field of snakes? How even though we face potential dangers with every step, it's still a gorgeous day? It's the absolute truth. At the same time that we face so many challenges here on earth, there is great beauty. For one, there's the actual, physical beauty of nature. Even if we live in a city, we can look up at the wide, ever-shifting sky, or we can appreciate the subtleties of a tree's changing leaves at the park. For another, there's the art that people make to add to the splendor here. There's also animal companionship. There's love. There's kindness, compassion, and generosity—qualities sometimes brought out in our fellow human beings by the very adversity they face here.

There is also literal sweetness and light that we can take into our bodies to align ourselves with the divine beauty all around us. I'm talking about four holy food groups: These are the sacred assistance granted to us to make it through life here. These are the answers for humanity. These are what will save us. To counteract the Unforgiving Four and every other challenge we face, we must turn to the Holy Four:

- Fruits
- Vegetables
- Herbs and spices
- Wild foods

That's why the center of this book is devoted to them. You'll read many more details there about just how these foods counteract and detoxify the Unforgiving Four, help you handle stress, boost your immune system, and give you strength and agility to thrive. Don't worry, you don't have to stop eating everything else. No matter what type of diet works for you, adding more of the Holy Four to your daily rotation can change your life.

Rethinking What's Good for Us

What you will discover about food in these pages is unlike the traditional information you've heard before. It goes far beyond articles you might have read about the benefits of fresh produce. Paying attention to what you eat—which means bringing more fruits, vegetables, herbs and spices, and wild foods into your life—can have benefits beyond imagination. You've no doubt heard the expression "food as medicine." That's part of it. As the world advances, so does disease. If we want to stave off illness, we must be proactive and embrace the medicinal power of the 50 life-changing foods in this book.

The Holy Four food groups are more sacred and powerful than we can even comprehend. Because they grow from the earth and are showered by the sun and sky, enduring out in the elements day after day as they form, they are intimately connected to the holy forces of nature. They don't just contain the building-block nutrients that we need to function. They contain intelligence from the Earthly Mother and the heavens that we desperately need about how to adapt.

Long gone are the days when we didn't have to pay much mind to what we ate. The world has changed; we're more vulnerable than ever before. Now food is everything when it comes to survival. Also long gone are the days when that old, traditional food pyramid applied to us. In order to make it here, we have to turn our understanding of nutrition on its head. Even the updated food pyramid miscalculates the importance of the different food groups in relation to one another. It will be decades before that chart gets it right.

80,000 Meals

It matters what we eat. In a lifetime, the average person eats about 80,000 meals. That sounds like a lot—until you break it down. How many meals have you eaten that have been predominantly made up of fruits and vegetables? Usually, fresh plant foods are more like a garnish—a banana sliced over morning cereal, or a side salad with steak at dinner. We're so busy that we often lose track of how many days have passed without fresh fruits and vegetables. We think we're making healthy choices, because we remember something about some spinach leaves with dinner or a few slices of apple, and we forget that several days have passed since we ate them. When one of the Holy Four does have a primary role in a meal, it's often not in its freshest, most whole and unadulterated form. Instead, it's a twice-baked potato loaded with cheese and bacon, or strawberries in a dessert that's saturated with corn syrup and preservatives.

Interview a group of women and men in their 90s and ask them if fruits and vegetables were ever central in their diet, before fads and trends and ad campaigns took over to sway people's eating habits. Your interviewees are sure to answer yes—and tell you the story behind those foods. It was once part of our common wisdom to eat diets rich in fruits, vegetables, herbs and spices, and wild foods for longevity. It was once a thing of joy and community, rather than just another chore. Before long, a person of advanced age will be lucky if she or he has eaten enough of the Holy Four to equal 15,000 meals. That's less than 20 percent of a lifetime's meals. It's not enough—not if you want to protect yourself from feeling run down, maxed out, miserable, or sick. It is simply not enough to sustain you.

Which isn't to say that other food groups are bad—they certainly have their own unique value. It's just that foods in the Holy Four groups are adaptogenic in nature, filled with endless life-healing and life-repairing phytochemicals to protect you from the Unforgiving Four and other health threats that cause illnesses such as cancer and heart disease. It's all about making sure that you have a balance in your diet, and taking those opportunities to bring in the life-changing foods when you have the chance.

The Holy Four have a living past. Wild blueberries, for example, hold thousands of years of healing wisdom. They've survived environmental ups and downs for millennia. The very first wild blueberry plants to take hold in North America passed on their survival knowledge to the plants that followed them, so that the wild blueberries we blend into a smoothie today are rich with generations of information. The same is true of other whole plant foods: Adaptability is part of their DNA. Whether we eat their wild forms or the cultivated cousins, we are gaining access to ancient living wisdom that our bodies inherently know how to use to transform our health.

If you want to be healthy and live a long life, it is all about bringing more fruits, vegetables, herbs and spices, and wild foods into your life. Not just here and there—every day, multiple times a day. We can't get distracted by constant new claims about what we should eat. Right now everyone is worried about protein. While of course protein is important (and by the way, the best, most bioavailable and assimilable protein in the world comes from leafy greens), what we really need to focus on are nutrients such as minerals, trace minerals, enzymes, coenzymes, and omegas, as well as phytochemicals like anthocyanins, lycopene, chlorophyll, luteine, resveratrol, and flavonoids. These are the survival elements, and the Holy Four food groups are rich in them. Without these nutrients, we lose huge health opportunities. If you want your children to be well, it is all about making the Holy Four a cornerstone of what you feed them. Look no further for an answer, antidote, or silver bullet. *This* is the key.

If you've already eaten 40,000 of your 80,000 meals, and they were lacking in fresh plant foods, you have some making up to do. Make what's left of your 80,000 meals count.

Light-Filled Foods

The Holy Four aren't just filled with the nutritional components that have been discovered by science. They are rich with undiscovered elements that are fundamental to counteracting the challenges we face here on earth. As I mentioned in the previous chapter, we're in a bad place when it comes to sunlight. Far more of it used to get through to us; now a white haze of pollution in the sky blocks the sun's full force.

If you've ever lived through winter in a cold, dark climate, or had a job that kept you indoors and away from windows all day long, you know what light deprivation feels like. It's not pretty. Your mood drags, your skin pales, your immune system loses oomph—and those are just the easily detectable effects. Sunlight has countless other undiscovered benefits for your emotional and physical health; it does much more than boost vitamin D. With a little sunshine, we get more vitamin A, more B vitamins, more nutrients as yet undiscovered by science; our anxiety can lower, depression can ease. Getting sunlight on your skin even enhances the process of digesting food and methylating nutrients to convert them for your body's use.

So what can we do about less sunlight getting through? Given that dimming light is a reality of our changing world, how do we adapt?

We bring more light into our lives—in the form of the Holy Four food groups. As these vines and trees and other plants grow, they absorb sunlight, collect it, concentrate it, and—when we ingest these roots and shoots and leaves and fruits—pass it along to us. While ever murkier skies and other changing aspects of climate are making it harder for crops to produce at their full potential, the fruits, vegetables, herbs and spices, and wild foods that do make it are strong. They are fighters. They are built for endurance. They have used sunlight to its full advantage, and they contain its sacred magic. All of this is for you.

Historically, we understood this. An orange in a Christmas stocking was once a most valuable gift. We knew that underneath that peel, the sweetness and light we'd find was like nothing else on earth. Today, if a kid reaches into a stocking to find a navel orange, you'll probably see disappointment on her face; fruit just isn't the novelty it once was. It's no less powerful, though. It's time to connect to the knowledge of our predecessors, to reclaim whole plant foods as the miracles they are.

Better yet, we can take it a step further. Whereas our ancestors who lived far from citrus groves had to settle for one lonely orange at the holidays, most of us today aren't limited in the same way. We live near grocery stores that cart in truckloads of fruits and vegetables year-round. Snacking on spinach, no matter the season, can fuel you with renewed purpose. Tanking on a bowl of tangerine wedges, the juice running down your chin and making your fingers sticky, can alter your vibration. Eating a mango in your darkest hour (literally or figuratively) can turn your life around.

When we can't get the sunlight from outside of ourselves, it's time to adapt our approach. Taking in these foods is taking in sunlight. Our cells absorb the light, and it radiates throughout our bodies and brains, emitting its energy and life force. You can look high and low, and you will not find a truer answer for how to cope with our changing world.

Living Water

Water has everything to do with our food. If we don't have water, we don't have food. If we don't have food, we don't have life. And if we *do* have water, yet it's not as complete as it's meant to be, then we're in trouble, too. In the previous chapter, I spelled out a warning about the state of rainwater. It's the stark truth that our planet's water supply has lost much of its living force.

How do we cope? Again, by eating more of the Holy Four. These plant foods have the miraculous ability to bring water back to life. In the next chapter, I'll uncover secrets of how amazing the water in fresh plant foods is for us. For now, know that the Holy Four are on your side when it comes to the rainwater deficiency crisis. Unlike other food sources, the Holy Four food groups aren't stagnant; they are adapting right along with the world. The only thing these foods can't do is actually speak and tell us why we need them.

Our ecosystem knows that the rain is lacking, and plants in the Holy Four food groups know it, too. Science hasn't discovered yet that their roots and leaves and stems and buds and fruits pick up on every change in the environment, and that they adjust to compensate. When micronutrients from rain (that would otherwise be inaccessible to us) soak through the leaves and roots of plants, those plants activate and transform the nutrition so that when we eat them, we get the full healing power of the water, as it was meant to be. At the same time, the earth is working to revitalize the rainwater as it hits the soil.

If we eat enough fresh fruits, vegetables, herbs and spices, and wild foods, we'll adapt, too. It doesn't mean your diet has to consist solely of the Holy Four, just that more than ever before we need to get away from processed foods. In their place, we need to focus on eating a higher quantity of fresh, delicious, nourishing, water-rich plant foods. It's the only way to get the living water—and every other type of nourishment—that our bodies desperately need.

FIGHT THE UNFORGIVING FOUR WITH THE HOLY FOUR

I could go on and on about the nutrition that the Holy Four food groups have to offer. They are the ultimate when it comes to adaptation, giving us support in all areas that we can't get anywhere else. Plus, if you're worried in particular about fending off the Unforgiving Four of radiation, toxic heavy metals, the viral explosion, and DDT, then these foods are your answer. Each of these 50 foods fights the Unforgiving Four in its own way, whether by strengthening your body so you're less susceptible, or by dealing with these invaders directly so they can't do your body harm. Soon you'll read about the individual 50 life-changing foods and which nutrients and properties lend them their healing powers. First, though, let's take a quick look at just a few of the critical components that make these foods our particular allies when it comes to facing the Unforgiving Four.

Antioxidants for Anti-Aging

As you read about the phytochemicals in this book, know that most of them act as antioxidants. You've no doubt heard all about antioxidants. Their importance, though—and just how many different types exist and are abundant in fruits, vegetables, herbs and spices, and wild foods—goes beyond even what scientific research has discovered. Oxidation is a chemical reaction of the body's organ tissue with an invader—that is, a toxin. On top of the toxins themselves causing damage, the free radicals that the reaction produces wreak havoc on the body, deteriorating cells and causing aging. Oxidation of toxic heavy metals in the brain is especially damaging and frequently behind brain fog, memory loss, dementia, and Alzheimer's. And when radiation and DDT are present in the brain, they can kill brain tissue, causing it to oxidize at a rapid rate. Antioxidants fight all of this. When you think antioxidants, think anti-aging. They bond to both toxins and free radicals, sticking to these invaders like fly paper so they stop oxidizing—and bundling them up for express shipment out of the body.

Go-To Glucose

Your body relies on the brain and liver maintaining proper reserves of glucose. These glucose reserves provide vital functions such as stabilizing blood sugar levels when you go too long between meals and powering the brain through mental processing and emotional upheaval. With daily life moving so fast, our brains work harder than ever, which translates to a lot of electrical activity. In the same way that a computer can overheat from processing too much data, so can our brains. And since toxic heavy metals are heat conductors, when they're present in the brain, they even take that heat up a notch.

To counteract this, our brains need two to three times the amount of natural sugar they otherwise would. The bioavailable glucose and fructose in Holy Four foods—especially in fruit and raw honey—is the top fuel to help you meet the challenges of the day. Far from being something to fear, the natural sugar found in whole foods is like a cool breeze to counteract the electrical heat. It's also like a protective veil against the damage trauma can do to brain tissue. Without a steady flow of foods like melons, coconut water, fresh orange juice, and dates in the diet, it's far too likely that burnout will occur of multiple body functions that are working overtime to combat the Unforgiving Four.

The natural sugars that are present in the life-changing foods contain a traveling band of potent phytochemicals. So when your bloodstream delivers glucose to your organs, those organs not only get the benefits of the sugar itself, they also get a major dose of Unforgiving-Four-fighting power. Coupled with mineral salts, glucose is the reason we're even able to exist on Planet Earth.

Miracle Mineral Salts

For our bodies to function optimally, we need to have enough mineral salts in our diets. Lemons, coconut water, and vegetables such as celery and spinach provide bioavailable forms of potassium, sodium, and chloride that mean everything when it comes to keeping our systems strong so we can fight off the Unforgiving Four and other invaders. These foods are also rich in trace mineral salts that contain particularly bioavailable forms of the minerals that the body craves (and that science has not yet discovered).

Mineral salts allow information to travel throughout the body so it can keep itself in balance no matter what's occurring. They are instrumental in the electricity created by the heart and brain that governs all the other organs in the body. Mineral salts keep the heart pumping and create the neurotransmitters needed to take information from point A to point B in the brain—that is, from neuron to neuron. (Picture a thought as a boat and mineral salts as the ocean: if that ocean dries up, the boat can't go anywhere.) Mineral salts keep the kidneys and adrenals functioning and create hydrochloric acid in the gut so that your body can break down and assimilate what you eat.

Mineral salts are also temperature-regulating for the entire body; they stop us from overheating and prevent us from getting cold. Without mineral salts, we would be constantly susceptible to dehydration, severe edema, and unproductive diuretic conditions. They are that integral to keeping you alive and well so that you're in the best place to deal with whatever comes your way.

B_{12} Happy

What makes the Holy Four so valuable isn't just what's *in* them; it's also what's *on* them. A special probiotic film covers the leaves and skins of fruits and vegetables. I call these probiotics *elevated biotics*, or *elevated microorganisms*, because they cover the above-ground surfaces of raw, unwashed (or lightly rinsed) plant foods. Unlike factory-produced probiotics and soil-borne organisms, elevated biotics are able to survive your digestive process and make it to your ileum, the final section of your small intestinal tract that creates the vitamin B_{12} critical to your body's functioning.

Be selective about what produce you eat without washing; the best sources are your own organic garden, sprouts on your countertop, or a local organic farmer you trust. If you have a wax-covered, conventionally grown apple from the grocery store, you definitely want to scrub it before eating. It's not a good source of elevated biotics anyway, because the wax and pesticides used in the growing process have already interfered with the natural film of beneficial microorganisms. If, on the other hand, you have a piece of chemical-free, contaminant-free produce you'd like to eat but it has visible dirt on it, a light rinse with plain water is usually fine—the elevated biotic film should stay intact (after all, the microorganisms survive rainfall). Use your instincts about what is safe to eat unwashed.

Historically, it was the norm to eat fruits, vegetables, and herbs fresh-picked from the field, garden, or wild, so people were getting higher levels of elevated biotics. It's part of why brain issues, digestive disturbances, autoimmune disease, and so many other chronic illnesses were much less common in previous eras. Even though earlier generations had less access to fresh food in the winter months than we do now, the steady supply of elevated biotics in their diets from spring through fall carried them through when these vital microorganisms were scarce. Today, packaged foods and the fast pace of life have distracted us from getting elevated-biotic-rich foods.

Almost anyone reading this is likely to be deficient in B_{12}—even if your B_{12} levels are normal or high on your blood tests. (Learn more in the "Harmful Health Fads and Trends" chapter.) It's the way of the world right now. One reason to address that B_{12} deficiency (by getting more elevated biotics) is that B_{12} keeps homocysteine levels down, which translates to less inflammation in the body. Plus, the B_{12} specifically produced by elevated biotics is vital to brain health, because it fortifies our neurotransmitters, boosting mental function and keeping depression at bay.

Without B_{12}, we die. It's that critical. It's like B_{12} is a dam that holds back a massive reservoir of polluted water (the Unforgiving Four) that would flood the town (your body) and threaten life. When you have plenty of B_{12} in your diet, it makes that dam strong, so that the Unforgiving Four factors we can't help but encounter can't do us harm. Instead, they're held at bay, so that on the other side of B_{12}'s dam, critical processes can be accomplished, including the building of your immune system, the maintenance of your organs, and the recovery of your mental and emotional state from traumas big and small.

Which means that the elevated biotics responsible for producing B_{12} in our bodies make all the difference in adapting to our modern times. In so many ways, these friendly microorganisms lift us up and fill us with life. They're a major part of why the Holy Four are, in fact, holy.

ONWARD AND UPWARD

If you feel that you've been traveling along in life only to get stuck on the side of the road, then the foods in this book are for you. Holy Four foods are like that innovative tire technology I was talking about earlier that has yet to be invented for the world's cars. As I said, these foods are champions of adaptation and progress. When you bring them into your life, their adaptogenic nature becomes a part of you. Not only do they actively address the Unforgiving Four, stress, and other challenges that I mentioned in the previous chapter, they also help you become the best version of yourself, so you can handle the challenges you encounter on your path—and succeed.

While they may seem unassuming at first glance, you've just had a glimpse into how fruits, vegetables, herbs and spices, and wild foods are as advanced as it gets. You'll learn much more about those hidden powers in the pages to come—including how these foods are here to offer you emotional and spiritual support as well as physical transformation. So buckle your seat belts for the ride ahead. With these foods in your life, you're going places.

Food for the Soul

It is your divine right as a human being to derive a sense of solace from what you eat. You are allowed to take comfort from food and not have to pay for it later. Not just allowed to—*supposed* to. You are not meant to be above desire for food, somehow capable of operating beyond spiritual and emotional hunger.

It's also true that not every food can give you the support you're seeking. Those doughnuts that smell like bliss at the bakery on your morning walk to work? You already know that while devouring one may give you a momentary sense of enjoyment, shutting off worry and despair as the refined sugar and fried fat overpower your brain, there will be a price to pay when you come off the high: a poor cholesterol reading at the doctor's office, a strained waistband on your jeans, the feeling of being a little comatose for the rest of the day.

Certain foods, though—Holy Four foods, which come from the earth—have a whole host of benefits that go beyond physical nutrition. They can offer you a feeling of in-the-moment comfort and grounding, and they can also offer longer-term resolution you never knew possible. When you know how to unlock their secrets, these foods can even have an effect on the people around you—sometimes just by having them out on the kitchen counter during a difficult conversation!

That's why in Part II of this book, you'll find that each fruit, vegetable, herb, spice, and wild food has a segment on emotional benefits as well as a spiritual lesson. Feeding yourself isn't an escape from higher-minded pursuits; when you bring the Holy Four into your life, it is *part* of enlightenment. Just think about the mysterious forces that encourage a seed in the dirt to one day produce a glowing red grape. Nothing beats taking that miracle into your body. God created these foods to nourish you in ways you never thought possible, and angels watch over them to enhance these crops that they know are vital to the future of the human race.

Each life-changing food has a special set of healing characteristics. Just like we all know that the vitamin C in orange juice is handy when you're fighting a cold, there are foods for any manner of metaphysical ailments. There are fruits that prime us to find our true friends, vegetables that give us hope when we're grieving, herbs and spices that help us cultivate self-worth, and wild foods that make good memories stick. These are not just abstract lessons that the foods have to teach us when we spend time thinking of them; these are properties that become a part of us when we ingest them. Like tools in a tool kit, we can reach for these different healing foods in our different times of need.

There are also soul-boosting secrets of all the Holy Four foods, like the unknown fact that some of the water they contain is specifically geared toward our emotional and spiritual health. Further, there are techniques you can employ to amplify the healing effects of what you eat. I'll cover all that below. As you read the rest of this chapter and this book, then turn the last page and return to the world, remember: Food is meant to be a joyful part of your life. Healthful eating isn't meant to be an exercise in deprivation. We're so used to reading articles on nutrition that talk solely about fiber and blood pressure and sodium levels that it can be easy not to realize: when you know the right foods to eat, and how to tap into their benefits, food can feed you on every level—and you deserve that.

FOOD AND FEELINGS

When it comes to food and feelings, there are two ends of the spectrum. On the one hand, we've got the traditional concept of comfort foods: macaroni and cheese, fried chicken, pie à la mode. We have a stressful day or week or month, and that club sandwich or cheeseburger or pizza feels like exactly the choice that will take the edge off. For some of us, there's an element of addiction involved, a food-as-drug feeling, an out-of-control impulse to overeat. For others, it doesn't go into binge-eating territory, and yet we still don't feel so great afterward. In the moment, though, the smell of that cookie overpowers us, reminding us of that safe, warm feeling of sitting at Grandma's kitchen table as a child. And after the very grown-up phone call we just had to make about an aging parent's health, we feel the need to indulge.

Then there's the food-as-fuel approach to eating. On this end of the spectrum, we try to take all emotion out of mealtime and make decisions about what to feed ourselves based solely on nutritional content. We tell ourselves that it's a form of enlightenment not to need any comfort from what we eat, and that our emotions are there to be felt and not numbed out in any way. It's the mentality that drives people to shun snacks, spend hours without eating, and live off protein powders that taste like dirt. This viewpoint can veer into disordered eating when someone starts seeing her or his body in a negative light and restricting food to a point that causes stress. Food-as-fuel is also the approach that scares off a lot of curious onlookers. They want to eat healthier—they *know* they should eat healthier—and yet the idea of subsisting on carrot sticks alone takes all the enjoyment out of life.

I'm here to tell you that there's a balance to be found between these two poles. There's a secret element of the healing foods in this book that no one is currently tapping into, because no one knows about it yet. This is the key that can unlock healthy eating for you, the answer you've been waiting for about how to find a sense of both emotional comfort and spiritual fulfillment while simultaneously recovering and healing.

SOUL-CLEANSING COFACTOR WATER

You know how there's a huge difference between a plum and a prune? How you have to be careful not to leave lettuce out on the counter too long, or it will start to shrivel? And you know how droughts are one of the biggest threats to crops?

That's all because the water content of produce is a huge part of what defines it. And while dehydrated foods have their place, the water that's inside fresh fruits, vegetables, herbs, and wild foods possesses incredible healing qualities. Here's a distinction science has yet to discover, though: These plant foods actually contain two different types of water. Each type is structured differently, with different information stored within, and a separate system for delivering its healing benefits to you. The water doesn't all serve the same purpose, and it doesn't all go to the same place when it enters the body.

The first type of water that's inside all fresh Holy Four foods is *hydrobioactive water*. This is the water that holds life-giving nutrients to support your physical health. It's also the water that hydrates your cells better than any drink of plain water can. Hydrobioactive water—living water—is the reason people instinctively add a squeeze of lemon or cucumber slices to water, or reach for a coconut water or fresh juice or smoothie after a workout: because, like the name suggests, this water will replenish your body, feed your bloodstream, and keep you going.

Then there's undiscovered *cofactor water*. This other form of living water contains information to help restore your soul and spirit, and to support your emotions. Inside of a fresh piece of produce, hydrobioactive water and cofactor water are side by side, held apart on a delicate cellular level, almost the way a honeycomb has walls dividing each of its tiny compartments. If a bear comes along and claws down a beehive, the honeycomb will break, and the honey will all run together. The same is true on a micro level when we bite into, say, an apple: The cell walls dividing hydrobioactive water and cofactor water rupture, and the juice comes running together. Our bodies can still differentiate the two, though, and they put each to separate use.

However, this remains undiscovered by science, because when fruits and vegetables are under study in the lab, the tools used to take samples rupture the cell walls just like our teeth do. Even a minuscule syringe has this effect, so the water content of fruits and vegetables continues to be studied as one entity—and the spiritual side of food isn't exactly a hot topic in medicine, so all we keep hearing about is physical nutrition. What would truly advance research is if scientists approached the study of water in fresh, living plant foods the way they do blood and lymph in the human body—separate and yet aligned.

The takeaway is that cofactor water is just as important as hydrobioactive water, because it contains trace minerals, mineral salts, enzymes, and phytochemicals that specifically feed you spiritually and emotionally. Keeping your soul alive is just as important as keeping your heart pumping, so it's vital to understand that the living water in the Holy Four nourishes us on every level.

LIFE-ENHANCING FOOD RITUALS

The Holy Four foods are helping us out when we eat them, whether we know it or not. It is part of their purpose and mission to enhance all aspects of our lives, and they will go on doing that whether we wake up to it or not. However, there are specific steps you can take to enhance what they do for you, and to bring out their life-enhancing qualities.

Grow Your Own Healing Foods

Growing your own food can be the best thing you ever do for yourself—physically, spiritually, and emotionally. Gardening can be a transformative meditation. It's a soul-healing, soul-purifying method of getting in touch with the Earthly Mother. And you no doubt already know that it's great exercise, as well as a chance to access food at its freshest, keep chemicals off what you eat, and as you read about in the previous chapter, get critical elevated biotics into your system.

In addition to these amazing benefits, there's a secret you won't hear anywhere else: When you grow your own food, it grows for your specific needs. Each leaf of cilantro, each raspberry, each cucumber develops with your name written into it. When you plant a kale seed, the plant grows knowing exactly who you are and exactly what you need on every level. If you have an illness, the kale intuits what that illness is, even if you haven't been able to find a diagnosis for your symptoms, or aren't even aware that you're ill. As you tend to the plant—watering it, feeding it, and weeding around it—the kale picks up on who you are, and it develops with the right blend of nutrients for your individual requirements. When you eventually pick those curly leaves and turn them into a salad, it becomes the most healing salad you could possibly eat, because it delivers tailor-made nutrition to your body.

The same is true of your needs on a soul level. If your soul is fractured, if you're going through a difficult time, if you're questioning your purpose on earth—the plants you cultivate pick up on it. They want to help you come out on the other side of your distress, so they grow with the right elements and energy to mend your emotions. Food that you grow for yourself will protect you with fierce devotion. Sometimes we're trying our absolute best to enjoy the present moment, yet memories of the bad times won't let us relax. Often there isn't an obvious resolution: We can't always find the right listeners, the people who will truly hear our life stories and say exactly the right thing in response. We can't always make amends with people from the past. What we *can* do is tend to these tiny seeds in the soil that become symbols of vitality, plants that want to thank us for tending to them by tending to us.

Say you've always suffered from feelings of seeming invisible to those around you, and you read in this book that potatoes help when you're feeling trampled on. So in the spring, you plant some seed potatoes in your local community garden. During the months that you visit the plot, treating it to organic fertilizer, watering it when there hasn't been rain, and keeping your eye out for beetles that could ruin the crop, the potato plants pick up on your struggles. Plants like these are your true listeners, your true friends. They sense the childhood experiences that first kicked off your sense of being ignored, and the life events that followed in adulthood to cement your frustration. When the day finally comes that you can stick your shovel in the dirt to unearth your buried treasure, the meal you make at home with those steamed new potatoes will feed your soul like nothing else can—while going after the slight *E. coli* infection in your bowels that could turn into Crohn's disease if not eradicated early. As you continue to cook with those potatoes in the weeks that follow, they'll continue to protect your body from microscopic invaders and soothe those spiritual wounds. That is what I call the ultimate soul food.

Make Food Your Own

We can't always grow our own food, whether because of climate, time and space constraints, or other reasons of impracticality. And when we buy food from the market or grocery store, we still want to receive its maximum healing benefit. The trouble is, the very same principle that makes food from your garden so individually beneficial for you means that food you don't grow yourself has picked up other people's energy.

From the farm workers who planted the seeds and rootstock to those who tended the fields and orchards to the pickers to the shippers to the grocery store produce department employees to the shoppers who pawed through the food displays before you, a single peach or head of broccoli or sprig of rosemary has been in a lot of hands. It can pick up on all those people's needs and gear itself toward *their* healing. To counteract those effects and make your food purchases your own, here are a few techniques that go far beyond preparing food with love and gratitude. These practices truly make what you eat the most beneficial it can be for your specific struggles, on both a body and soul level. While it's best if you can do all three for your produce haul, just one of these techniques will have a powerful effect.

- A few times a day, run your hands over your precious produce. The fruit ripening on the counter, the items sitting in the fridge—take a moment when you're walking by to touch them, just as when walking by a beloved pet, you would connect and make contact.
- Talk to your produce like the dear ones they are: "You were grown for me. We were meant to be together. There was just a delay in that process, and now we're finally united."
- Before cutting into (or otherwise prepping and eating) a fruit, vegetable, herb, spice, or wild food, hold it in your hands for 30 seconds to give it the chance to attune to who you are and what you need.

INTERPRETING CRAVINGS

I wish I could tell you that cravings are always a message from your body about what food you need most in the moment. Unfortunately, that's not always the case. Our minds and bodies have been conditioned by years of advertisements, misinformation, social eating situations, and less-than-healthy snacks and meals, so that we lose touch with how to truly feed ourselves. Usually, cravings have much more to do with what's going on emotionally at a given point in time than what would be beneficial for us to eat. Sometimes, they're not so much telling you what you *need* as what you *want.*

As I said earlier, eating for your emotions is actually okay. It's just that you have to break free from the cravings trap and first learn with your head (in Part II of this book) what will really help your heart. Cravings aren't as straightforward as they seem. They have their own language, and we have to learn how to interpret them.

Say you're feeling underappreciated at work. All morning, you've been waiting to hear whether you were picked for a project you think you'd be perfect for. At 11 A.M., the e-mail arrives with the list of those assigned to the task, and your name isn't on it. By the time lunch rolls around, you're craving a bacon cheeseburger. You tell yourself you'd better go out and get just that, because your body must be telling you that you need the iron for strength.

In that situation, a bacon cheeseburger is not going to make anything better. Rather, the high fat content is likely to make you sluggish all afternoon, slowing down your brain so that work seems even more depressing in the wake of the morning's letdown. It's important to look at the craving beneath the craving. What were you really looking for from that meal? The feeling of comfort and pride you used to get from going out for bacon cheeseburgers with your parents when you'd gotten a good report card?

The food that would truly help in this situation is going to sound surprising, maybe even laughable: grapes. Believe me, I know that in the face of rejection, the idea of popping a few grapes into your mouth to soothe your wounds may seem a little dinky. That's only because we haven't been conditioned to see fruit's true value. Again and again in the middle of this book, you'll read about foods that have been taken for granted, and grapes are just one example. Grapes actually contain micronutrients that are critical to emotional support when we're dealing with disappointment. They also hold divine information to help us forge a new path and create better opportunities for ourselves.

What's more, the bioavailable fructose and glucose in grapes is amazing for the brain. Our brains thrive on natural sugar, so grapes serve as a pick-me-up rather than as a depressant, which most standard comfort foods do. If, instead of a bacon cheeseburger, you were to opt for grapes with a fig and "goat cheese" salad (see the recipe in "Figs" in Part II) for lunch on that tough day, you would be giving your mind and body amazing resources to cope. Rather than feeling traumatized by not being selected for the project, you would have a much better shot at finding the silver lining.

Think about it: When you've experienced a tough turn of events, is comfort all you really want? Maybe it's more like validation and solace, as well as the wherewithal to handle the situation with grace, and to transform it into something new and better. The Holy Four help us do that. I've seen it time and again when someone adds more of these life-changing foods to her or his diet and starts to use them as tools for emotional needs.

What Sugar Cravings Really Mean

Which brings me back to sugar. A yearning for sweets is one of the most common cravings. First thing in the morning, during an afternoon slump, or after upsetting news, we often reach for a pastry filled with cream and sugar, a candy bar, or pizza. In this case, the craving *is* communicating something specific biologically: your brain wants sugar. This may sound like a bad thing, because we're trained to think of sugar as bad. Not so. Like I said, natural, unadulterated sugar from whole plant foods is key for brain function, because the glucose cools the engine of the brain and prevents brain tissue from scarring when you experience stress or trauma. A sugar craving is your brain telling you that it's taxed and needs some support.

We just have to make sure that it's natural, unadulterated sugar from whole plant foods that we reach for when we have our sugar cravings—rather than pastries, candy, or pizza. Which reminds me: I know that pizza may not seem like a high-sugar food. However, with all that dairy and tomato sauce that's often sweetened with cane sugar or high-fructose cane syrup, plus the highly refined flour used for the crust, pizza's sugar content is through the roof. That's right: A dairy craving is usually a sugar craving, because the lactose (sugar) in dairy is quite high. The problem is, dairy is often high in hidden fat, and the fat-sugar combo can be a one-two punch for your insulin-regulating body mechanisms. True brain foods like dates, figs, melons, grapes, citrus, raw honey, and smoothies with coconut water will give your body what it's really asking for when you feel the need for a sugar fix.

A Need for Caffeine

Those brain foods are also fantastic alternatives to caffeine. When people are trying to cut back on caffeine addictions, they often sub in caffeine-free soft drinks for energy drinks and caffeinated soda. While of course that's a great step, it only helps by replacing the experience of drinking a sweet, icy-cold can or bottle of your old favorite—it doesn't help in the energy department. If you relied on these beverages for the energy boost, then fresh, juicy fruits will give you what you crave. Again, it's all about the bioavailable glucose (plus all the other amazing nutrients) to wake up your brain. If you're sensitive to changes in your blood sugar levels, then eating celery sticks, cucumber slices, or leafy greens along with your fruit—or just making a green smoothie—will help you avoid those highs and lows.

Cravings During Detox

When you add more produce to your diet, it's common to undergo some detoxification. This is exactly what you want. Ridding your body of toxic heavy metals, pathogens, viral by-product, radiation, chemical buildup, and damage done by unhealthy foods is precisely the path to wellness.

Eating more fruits and vegetables will also probably mean you're eating less of other types of foods that didn't serve you as well. It could trigger very valid feelings of loss as you distance yourself from unhealthy food choices that glimmer with nostalgia.

When you're on the detox path, a craving for baked ziti, a BLT, or some other food you associate with comfort can hit from seemingly out of nowhere. It can feel random, intense, and like maybe not the biggest deal if you just make this one exception and eat the deep-fried cookie that's calling your name at the street fair. This is the exact moment when you want to hold your ground. Instead, take a breath and reach for the packet of gooey dates you stashed in your pocket for just this scenario. You'll be rewarded in the long term.

It's not because you need to prove yourself morally. It's because when you're detoxing, a very specific craving for a food you know doesn't serve you means your cells are releasing old toxins from that very food. As the toxins release, it can feel like a bubble bursts in your consciousness, along with any emotions that you were using the food to stuff down when you used to eat it. (For example, maybe deep-fried cookies were your solace back in high school, when friends teased you.) On top of which, there are whatever environmental or pathogenic toxins your body was trying to process and expel at the time and couldn't because processing the unproductive food took priority—and so those toxins stayed buried deep inside your organs.

An intense craving during detox means your body is finally getting a chance to rid itself of all that old gunk. The last thing you want to do is interrupt that process. If you can find a way to ride the waves of detox cravings, you will find yourself a renewed person afterward. On the other hand, if you cut yourself off in the middle of that process by eating the food because you figure the craving means your body really needs it, you will cut yourself off from healing and enlightenment. And I really do mean enlightenment. The emotional, spiritual, and physical aspects of your being are infinitely interconnected. You cannot maintain a healthy state of mind without the Holy Four.

Coexisting with Cravings

To deal with cravings, plan meals ahead and keep healthy snacks on hand as much as possible. Each time an urge arises, act as its interpreter. What's it really saying? If there's an emotional or spiritual need that you can identify, page through the middle section on the Holy Four to find the food that can help your situation. If it's your brain crying out for fuel, sink your teeth into a creamy avocado or a ripe, sweet fruit. And if it's an overpowering longing for a food from your past, try to ride it out and tend to yourself in the meantime with a delicious, healthy substitute such as any recipe in this book.

And take heart. When you switch to a healthier diet, cravings do change over time. At a certain point, when your body has processed out enough toxins, your brain's glucose reserve has been replenished, and you've experienced the emotional and spiritual teachings of the Holy Four, you'll find yourself in touch with your deepest needs. Some cravings will vanish altogether, while others will feel more distant and manageable, and yet others will be true messages of what's right for your body, soul, and spirit.

RISE UP

If you were to take a walk past a field of ash, with the only thing in sight the blackened stubs of stems, what would you think? If it were me, I would assume I'd stumbled upon the scene of a devastation, that I was looking at some unlucky farmer's ruined year of crops. And yet if it happened to be a wild blueberry field, the truth would be the complete opposite. In areas where wild lowbush blueberries grow natively, it's common practice to set a controlled fire across the field to manage the plants. Native Americans were the first to discover that wild blueberries not only survive under fire but thrive. The year following a burn, the plants come back healthier than ever. They rise from the ashes.

This is why we need Holy Four foods like wild blueberries in our lives. Who hasn't felt soul-challenged by this world, and at one point or another, like all was lost? Who hasn't needed inspiration to come back from adversity, whether health-related or otherwise? As we navigate the Quickening, we must hold close the story of the wild blueberries' rebirth. This is a critical time in the history of our species, and of the planet. The choices that we make today to nurture our bodies and souls with the Holy Four will influence every era to come. If you're unwell, overwhelmed, or on the edge, you're not alone. It's not too late to turn it all around.

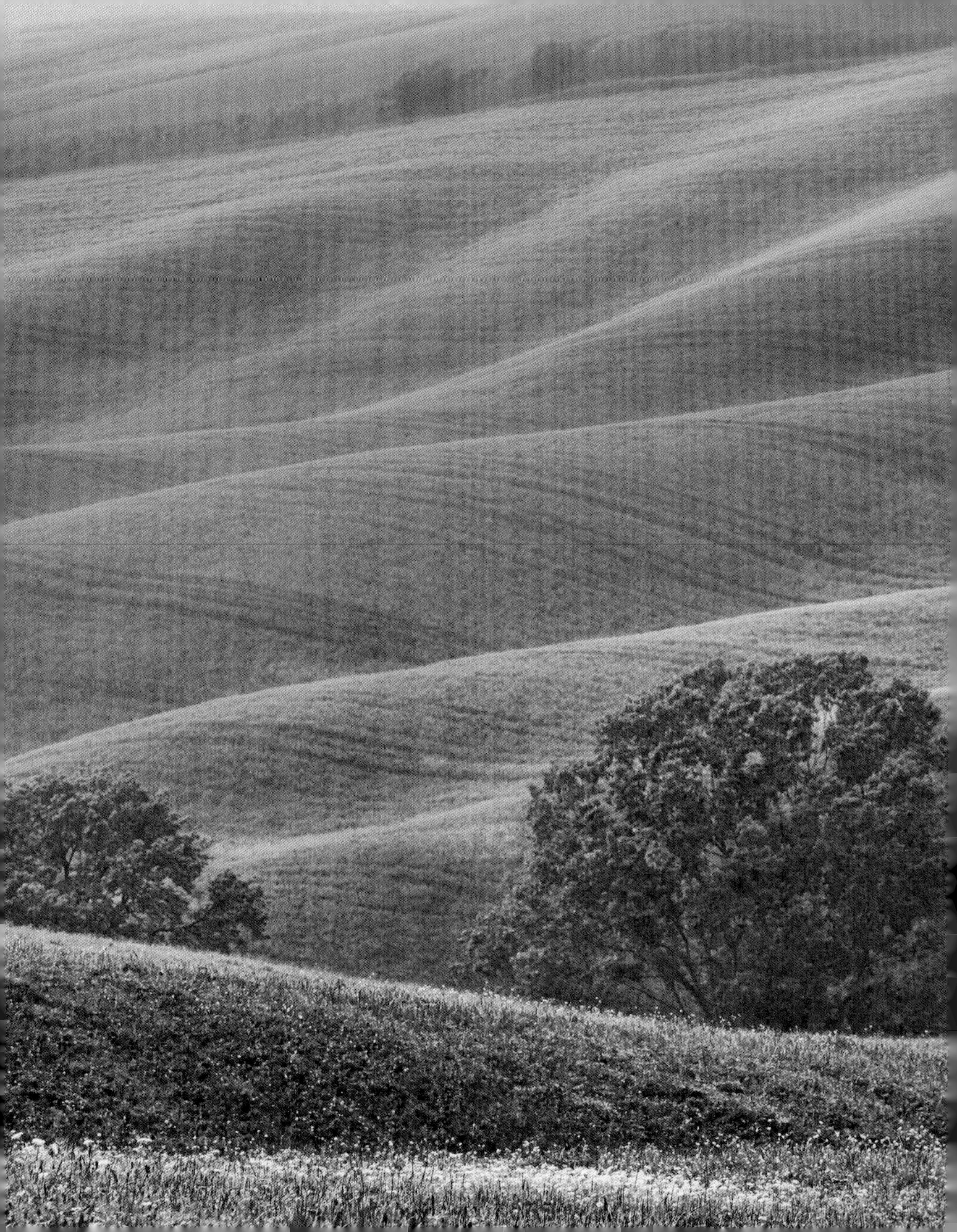

PART II

THE HOLY FOUR

FRUITS
VEGETABLES
HERBS & SPICES
WILD FOODS

An Introduction to the Life-Changing Foods

To benefit from the foods to follow, it doesn't matter what diet you subscribe to, or whether you subscribe to any diet at all. We're all different, so the particular combination of foods that works for each of us is going to be different. What it really comes down to are your individual needs. Are you struggling with cold sores? Then you could really benefit from potatoes. Are you looking for thyroid support? You'll probably be interested to read about cauliflower and its cruciferous cousins.

Now what happens if you subscribe to a particular diet that leaves out fruit, and yet you have a calcium deficiency and read here about how oranges are chock-full of the mineral in its most bioavailable form? Again, it's about your individual needs—you're going to be much better off eating oranges than avoiding them. And if you want to find relief from insomnia, then you're going to be missing out on an opportunity for that relief if you skip eating mangoes and bananas (top sleep aids) just because a particular diet tells you to avoid them. It's all about you. What particular health challenges do you deal with, or want to prevent? Symptoms and conditions are communications from your body, telling you what it needs. That's what determines the best foods for you. A particular food belief system never trumps that—you can't impose a food belief system over your body's needs.

One of the keys to reaping the benefits of these foods is to eat plenty of them on a regular basis. Any little bit helps, so you can certainly choose to use them supplementally. If you want more rapid results, try to go one day eating meals entirely made from the life-changing foods, while also avoiding the items in the chapter "Foods That Make Life Challenging" in Part III. Or try a whole week of life-changing foods, or a whole month. For support with this, I offer information on a 28-day cleanse in my first book. People who have tried it report amazing results.

Just knowing what these foods do for you can make all the difference. When you understand that fruits are cancer fighters, vegetables flush out acidity, herbs and spices build the immune system, and wild foods help us adapt to stress, reaching for these foods transforms from a chore into an opportunity.

There are also many more life-changing foods than I had room to fit here. I know there will be readers disappointed to find squash, mint, tomatoes, nuts, seeds, and countless other favorites missing from these pages. Rest assured that the 50 life-changing foods (really, 50-plus, since some are grouped) are just the beginning.

And keep in mind that the benefits of each life-changing food you're about to learn are just the highlights. Inevitably, I couldn't cover every detail, because it would take a full book on each food to give you the whole picture. So instead I focused in on what's unknown or not understood well enough about their health benefits.

Color, for example, has recently become a popular topic in diet. It's true that color matters. The deep purple-blue skin of the wild blueberry has the highest ratio of antioxidants in existence; the phytochemical pigments that give it that antioxidant power mean everything for brain health. It's just that color is not the sole defining characteristic across the board that makes fruits, vegetables, herbs and spices, and wild foods beneficial. Colors are important for some conditions and symptoms, while other nutrients are vital for other conditions and symptoms. We're used to thinking of "white" foods as bad, because we've learned by now that bleached and processed flours aren't health-promoting. When it comes to the life-changing foods, though, we have to be careful not to think that "white" translates to "devoid of nutrition." Apples, bananas, burdock root, some onions, many potatoes, certain radishes, and cauliflower are all white when you cut into them. And yet every single one of these foods, while partially lacking in the pigmentation department, is bursting with hidden healing powers. So while you'll read some details here about color as it applies, this is not a book all about color—that would leave out too much.

LABELS FOR CONDITIONS AND SYMPTOMS

You can use this section in the book in any way you'd like, whether reading from front to back or flipping through to find foods that list a particular condition or symptom you'd particularly like to prevent or alleviate. Note that the lists of conditions and symptoms for each food are not comprehensive; like the health benefits of each, these are the highlights that deserve particular attention.

A note on the names of conditions: If you've read my first book, or if you come to my live events or listen to my radio show regularly, then you know that I find certain labels for what I call *mystery illnesses* misleading. These are illnesses not yet understood by medical science, though the labels will make you think they're better understood than they are. However, I know that many readers will be coming to this book fresh. If you're one of them, it won't make sense to you if you see a reference to "the collection of symptoms mistakenly labeled Lyme disease" or "a high level of *Candida* that doesn't mean anything in and of itself, so you have to figure out the underlying cause first." In those cases, you'll just see "Lyme" and "*Candida*" listed. There are many other examples of this. As you look at these lists, especially if you already know my work, understand that I haven't changed my position on mistaken labels. I simply respect that people know illnesses by their mainstream names, so I've opted to use those better-known terms.

Another note: There are some illnesses that go by several different names. For example, for the sake of brevity I refer to chronic fatigue syndrome, or CFS, throughout the book—although of course I respect that the term you most identify with may be *myalgic encephalomyelitis/chronic fatigue syndrome* (ME/CFS), *chronic fatigue immune dysfunction syndrome* (CFIDS), or *systemic exertion intolerance disease* (SEID). The same goes for any condition that's known by multiple names.

The Inflammation and Autoimmune Confusion

There's a widespread misconception that autoimmune disease means the body is attacking itself. The term *autoimmune* itself is a mistake. *Auto-* comes from the Greek for "self," so the word is saying that your immune system goes after you—your own self! That makes "autoimmune" merely a tag that puts the blame on you and your body. It's a misnomer that means we can't even talk about the truth of autoimmune disease without perpetuating the misunderstanding. The body never attacks itself. It attacks pathogens. A more fitting term would be *virus-immune*, or *pathogen-immune*, because the immune system is going after an invader such as EBV, shingles, CMV, HHV-6, other herpetic viruses, or even certain bacteria.

Keep this in mind as you read the pages to come. As with other misbegotten labels for illnesses, I sometimes refer in this book to autoimmune diseases and disorders by the term *autoimmune* and by the common names of various illnesses considered by medical communities to be autoimmune, including RA, Hashimoto's thyroiditis, and lupus. Know that there's a much deeper story behind these illness names.

Inflammation is another term thrown around without true understanding. Deemed by medical communities to be the cause of everything from cancer to obesity to heart disease, it's become a catch-all word that we no longer question. We need to question it. Not because inflammation isn't real—as anyone who's dealt with its pain and swelling can attest, inflammation is all too real. What needs our examination is why that inflammation occurs. In itself it doesn't *cause* anything. When inflammation isn't the result of an injury, it's the result of a pathogenic invader. In the case of autoimmune disease, where inflammation is a defining characteristic, as I said earlier, that invader is viral. In colitis, for example, the shingles virus burrows deep into the lining of the colon, which prompts the immune system to try to fend off the invasive microorganisms. And in Hashimoto's thyroiditis, as I revealed in my first book, EBV invades the thyroid tissue, resulting in inflammation that's a sign of the body working to protect the thyroid gland from the virus. You'll hear from some sources that autoimmune responses happen when your body is defending itself against a trigger (such as a virus or gluten) and becomes confused in the process, unable to tell the difference between a foreign presence and your own body tissue. This is *not* how triggers work. Let me be clear: Triggers for autoimmune disease are direct fuel to viruses already present in a person's system. The body does not go haywire and start destroying itself. Any antibody activity is your immune system actively attacking a pathogen, not your own body. It's an important distinction.

Note that so-called inflammatory foods such as grains often get all the blame. Especially in the alternative-health community, grains are pegged as directly causing inflammation and even creating autoimmune disease itself. The buzzword is *mycotoxins* (toxic substances produced by fungi that can infect grain crops), and it's the explanation many sources use for why grains are problematic. The issue with this logic is that plenty of people eat grains and feel fine. How else to explain the 90-year-olds who have spent their lives eating grains and processed foods and have never had a health complaint?

What's really going on is that people with autoimmune disease have viruses and/or other pathogens in their bodies, and those bugs feed on the grains and mycotoxins, in the process creating more powerful neurotoxins that cause inflammation. So someone who's perfectly pathogen-free won't react to grains, because the grains don't set off a pathogen feeding frenzy. Someone with Hashimoto's, Sjögren's, scleroderma, MS, fibromyalgia, lupus, or RA, though, will likely feel foggy-headed and fatigued from eating something like bread or bagels. The food itself is not inflammatory—it just triggers inflammation. Which is not to say that grains such as wheat are an ideal food for anybody's health. (I explain more about why wheat is problematic in the chapter "Foods That Make Life Challenging.") Still, it's important to understand what's really happening in the body when someone has a reaction to wheat.

There are other types of triggers that can either give fuel to viruses and other pathogens in the body or weaken a person's immune system so that a dormant virus can take advantage. These triggers include exposure to radiation, DDT and other pesticides, herbicides, paint fumes, or mold; nutritional deficiencies; drug abuse; bad bug bites or stings; physical injury; toxic heavy metal exposure; and emotional trauma.

In order to make progress with your health, it's not just about keeping out foods that fuel the pathogens or avoiding exposure to other triggers. It's also about bringing in the foods that specifically target and cleanse you of viruses, bacteria, and the toxins that fuel them. So if you struggle with an autoimmune condition, or any form of inflammation, don't stop at just those food features that mention your specific condition or talk about calming down inflammatory responses. Any food that's listed as antiviral and/or antibacterial can help you heal. Dealing with these underlying issues is what alleviates inflammation and reverses autoimmune disease.

FRUIT FEAR

A fear of fruit stops far too many people from protecting their health. It mostly stems from the major misconception that the sugar in fruit is the same as refined table sugar and high-fructose corn syrup. This is absolutely not the case. The natural fructose and glucose in fruit and raw honey is very different from processed sugar. The natural sugars found in the Holy Four are bound onto antioxidants, including resveratrol and other polyphenols that are vital to keeping you healthy. Contrary to popular belief, fruit does not feed *Candida* and other fungi, cancer, viruses, bacteria, or anything else unproductive to the body. Fruit *fights* all of this. Because fruit digests so easily, fruit sugar leaves your stomach and enters your bloodstream within minutes after being eaten—so it doesn't even reach the intestinal tract.

What does feed disease is too much fat in the diet. Despite fads that may try to convince you otherwise, an overload of fat strains the liver and pancreas, makes detoxification sluggish, contributes to diabetes and fatty liver, promotes edema and weight gain, speeds up oxidation of toxic heavy metals, slows down digestion, and feeds pathogens. This is not to say that you don't need fat in your diet. You do—and two of the life-changing foods in this book (coconut and avocado) contain especially valuable forms of fat. It's just that too much fat, especially when it's from poor-quality sources like fried food, is not your friend.

If you're truly worried about disease and you want to feel your fittest, lower the fat in your diet a bit and eat lots of life-changing foods—especially an ample amount of fruit and leafy greens. And if you have any lingering doubts about any aspect of eating fruit, check out the "Fruit Fear" chapter in my first book.

WILD BENEFITS

Every single food in this book will feed you on every level: physically, emotionally, and spiritually. The foods in the first three groups—fruits, vegetables, and herbs and spices—are mainstay foods. They support us, fuel us, heal us, teach us, fight disease, and keep us going.

Wild foods take all of this to the next level. The wild foods in this book—we're talking aloe vera, Atlantic sea vegetables, wild blueberries, and more—have survived extremes. By the time they get to us, they are experts at thriving under pressure, and that's an expertise they pass along to us. Wild foods are amazing for reversing the damage caused by excess adrenaline, unproductive foods, and especially the Unforgiving Four. As a group, wild foods are the missing piece, the Holy Grail, and the secret to getting a fresh start. These powerful anti-agers are packed with adaptogens—that is, they're crucial to helping our bodies adapt to what life throws at us. Wild foods not only retain the vitamin and mineral levels that nature intended, they also carry critical survival information in their cells. When we ingest them, the wisdom that's allowed them to thrive out in the elements becomes a part of us.

While the idea of wild foods may seem foreign, don't be a stranger to them; you need these to make the other life-changing foods click into gear. Don't worry, you don't have to spend all of your time foraging in pristine locations to eat wild. Many wild foods (or foods so close to their wild form that they provide the same benefits) are actually waiting for you at your local market. You'll learn more details soon.

ONE FINAL NOTE

As you read about these 50-plus foods, you're going to see me use the word *miracle* a lot. It's not because I use the term lightly. I could use the term for every single food here, and it would not be an exaggeration. Right now, scientific understanding of the benefits these foods have to offer amounts to a handful of information, compared to the silo of knowledge yet to be gained. And even if science someday discovers the thousands of phytochemicals and other nutrients that these foods really contain, and the hidden powers they have to address health conditions, it will not touch the greater mystery of how these foods bring us healing on every level. That's because each of these foods possesses a miracle aspect that comes only from God and the universe. Over the decades of sharing Spirit's healing wisdom about the Holy Four food groups, I've watched these miraculous qualities transform so many people's lives—that's why I call these the life-changing foods. If you make a commitment to bring them into your life consistently and in abundance, they can do the same for you.

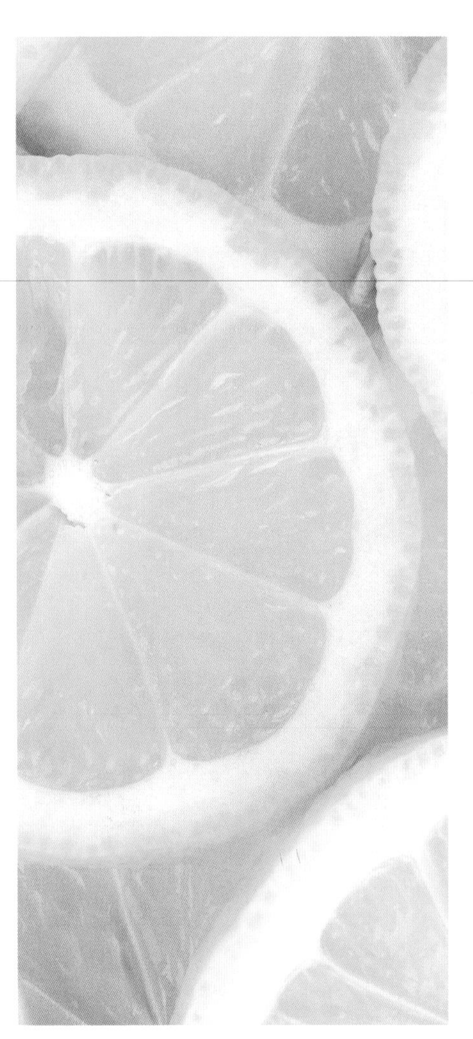
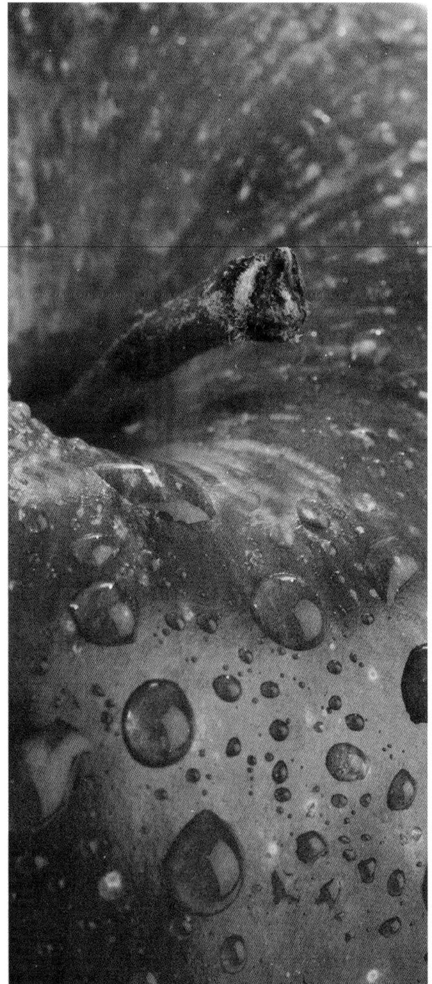
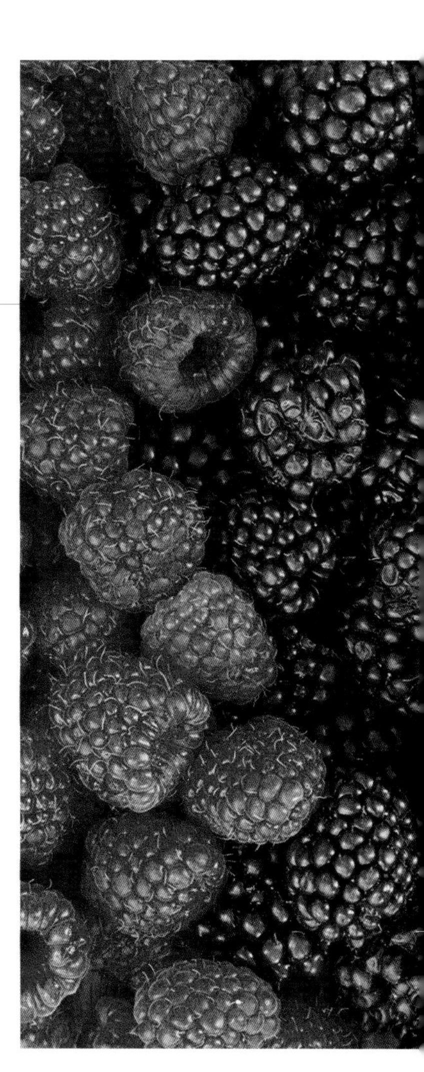

FRUITS

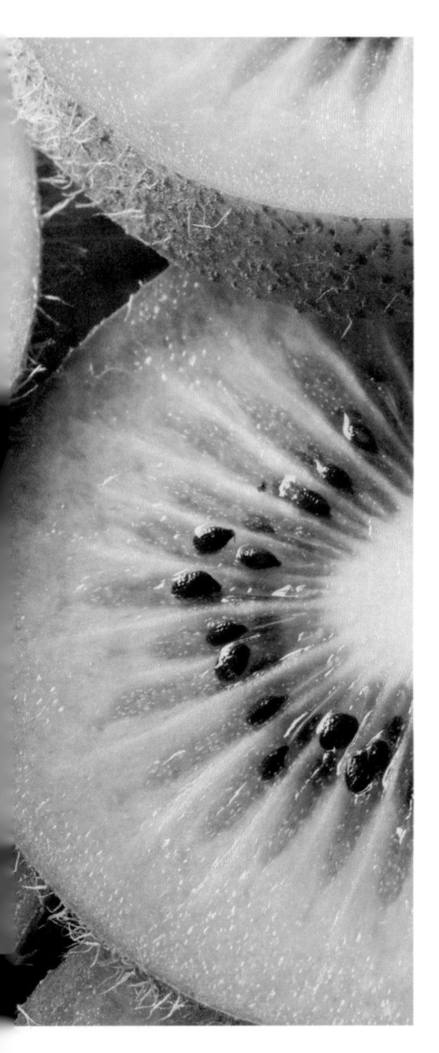

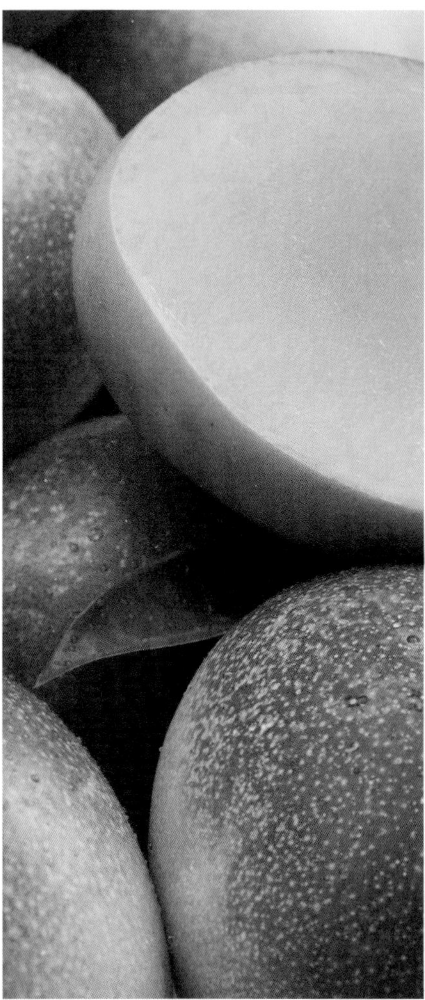

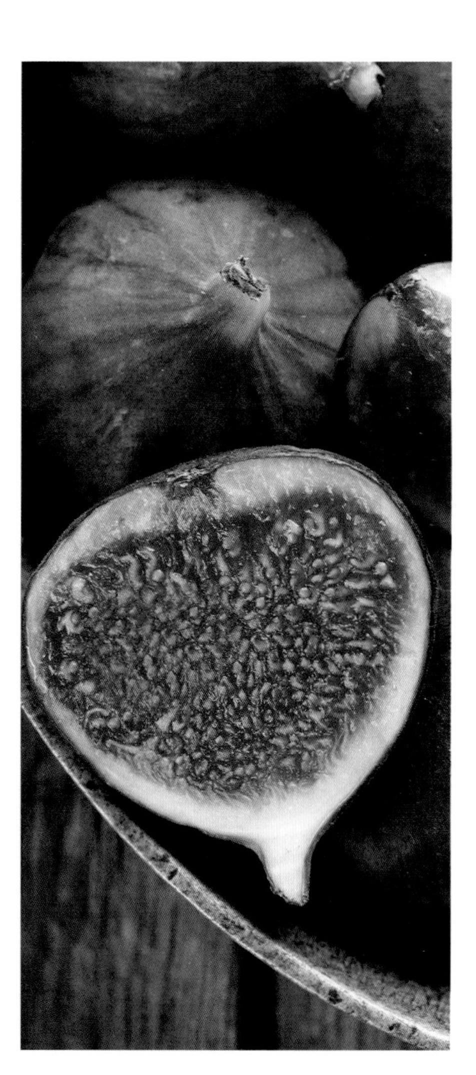

Apples

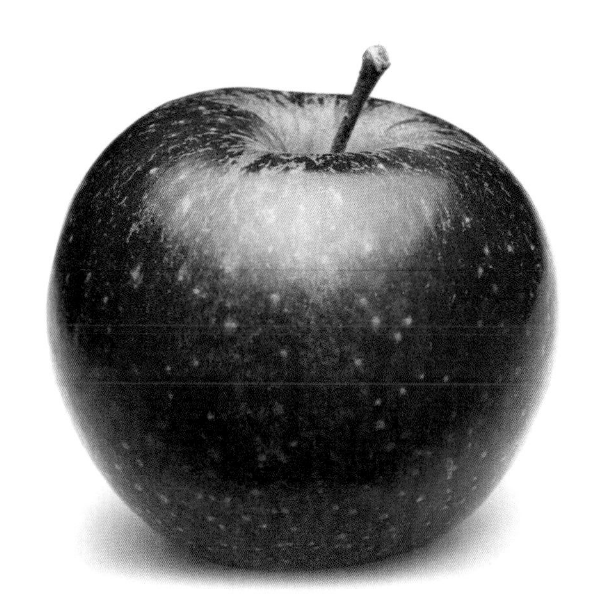

Never underestimate the power of an apple. This fruit's anti-inflammatory properties make it a top pick when you're faced with practically any illness. Encephalitis (brain inflammation), IBS (intestinal inflammation), and viral infection (which can result in nerve inflammation) are just a few conditions in which apples can play the critical nutritional role of calming your system by reducing viral and bacterial loads that create inflammation.

The phytochemicals in apples make them a true brain food, feeding neurons and increasing electrical activity. Apples with red skin contain anthocyanins and even traces of malvidin (a type of anthocyanidin), which are partially responsible for the red color. These pigments have anti-obesity properties and compounds that increase digestive strength, encouraging weight loss. Apples also have traces of flavonoids, rutin, and quercidin—phytochemicals that are responsible for heavy metal and radiation detoxification—as well as the amino acids glutamine and serine, which help detoxify the brain of MSG. This fruit helps cleanse and purify the organs, improve circulation in your lymphatic system, repair damaged skin, and regulate blood sugar.

Apples are the ultimate colon cleanser. As the pectin from an apple moves through your gut, it collects and rids your body of microbes such as bacteria, viruses, yeast, and mold. It also gathers and expels putrefied, impacted protein and debris that's been hiding in intestinal pockets and feeding colonies of harmful bacteria such as *E. coli* and *C. difficile*. This makes apples an excellent antiproliferative for healing SIBO (small intestinal bacterial overgrowth) and other digestive disorders.

Apples are also hydrating on a deep, cellular level. They provide precious trace minerals such as manganese and molybdenum, as well as electrolytes and critical mineral salts that help the body rehydrate after exercise or stress of any kind.

CONDITIONS

If you have any of the following conditions, try bringing apples into your life:

Kidney disease, liver disease, Alzheimer's disease, arthritis, seizure disorders, multiple sclerosis (MS), thyroid disease, hypoglycemia, diabetes, transient ischemic attack (TIA), urinary tract infections (UTIs), adrenal fatigue, migraines, shingles, mold exposure, obsessive-compulsive disorder (OCD), osteomyelitis, attention-deficit/hyperactivity disorder (ADHD), autism, post-traumatic stress disorder (PTSD), acne, amyotrophic lateral sclerosis (ALS), Lyme disease, obesity, small intestinal bacterial overgrowth (SIBO), anxiety, tinnitus, viral infection, vertigo

SYMPTOMS

If you have any of the following symptoms, try bringing apples into your life:

Ringing or buzzing in the ears, diabetic neuropathy, dizzy spells, room spins, balance and equilibrium issues, heart palpitations, acid reflux, hypoglycemia and other blood sugar imbalances, mineral deficiencies, body odor, premenstrual syndrome (PMS) symptoms, rib pain, fatigue, bloating, gas, constipation, nervousness, anxiousness, frozen shoulder, weight gain, back pain, blurry eyes, brain fog, body pain, confusion, ear pain, body stiffness, brain inflammation, dandruff, menopause symptoms

EMOTIONAL SUPPORT

The apple is an ancient food that brings us back to the source. It is one of the very first foods to have comforted us, and so apples connect us to a sense of sanctuary. This makes them ideal for when you're feeling depressed, alienated, invalid, powerless, useless, worthless—you get the idea. If the time ever comes when you feel you aren't being validated, eating apples can help change your course.

Apples open up a part of you and change the energy within and around you to attract happier and brighter things. They can bring back your vibrancy, elevate you, lighten your spirit, and make you more energetic. This is because for thousands of years, we've stored apples to get us through the winter months. The fruit is a ray of hope that puts us in touch with the good life. It's instilled in our bodies that when the outside world seems bleak, an apple can reconnect us to life, rebirth, sunlight, and summertime.

SPIRITUAL LESSON

Apples teach us not to get burned by the frost of insensitivity from others. Unlike crops that risk damage from autumn temperatures, many apple varieties continue to grow and ripen through the cooler months, protected by their frost-resistant skin. When a cold front from a friend, lover, or colleague comes upon you, take heed from the apple and draw a protective shield around yourself until conditions improve.

TIPS

- Red-skinned apples with the most color are best.
- Try eating three apples a day. If you commit to this routine, you could see your health improve in unexpected ways.
- At least once a year, go to an organic orchard that allows you to pick apples yourself. As I discussed in further detail in my first book, the skin of fresh, unwashed, pesticide- and wax-free produce contains elevated microorganisms that are critical to the health of your gut and immune system. The act of picking fruit is also one of the most powerful, grounding meditations that exists.

APPLES WITH "CARAMEL" DIP

Makes 1 to 2 servings

This is the perfect snack to have waiting when your kids get home from school: crispy apple slices laid out alongside a gooey caramel dipping sauce. You may want to double the recipe, because this dish will disappear before you know it.

1 large apple, sliced
6 dates, pitted
¼ teaspoon cinnamon

Arrange the apple slices on a plate. Blend the dates and the cinnamon with a splash of water until combined. (If working with dry, firm dates, soak them in water for 2 hours beforehand until they are softened.) Spoon the mixture into a serving cup alongside the apple slices.

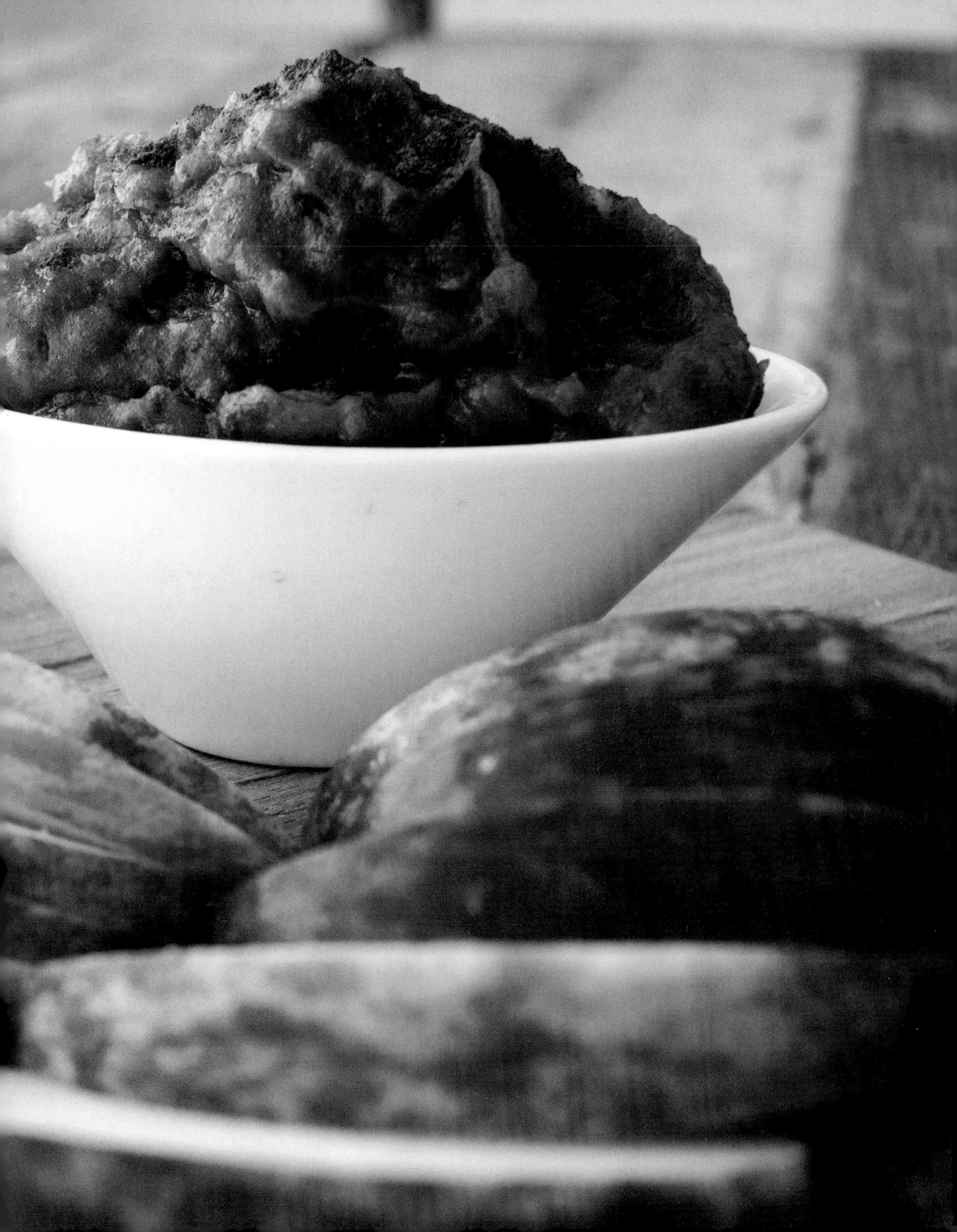

Apricots

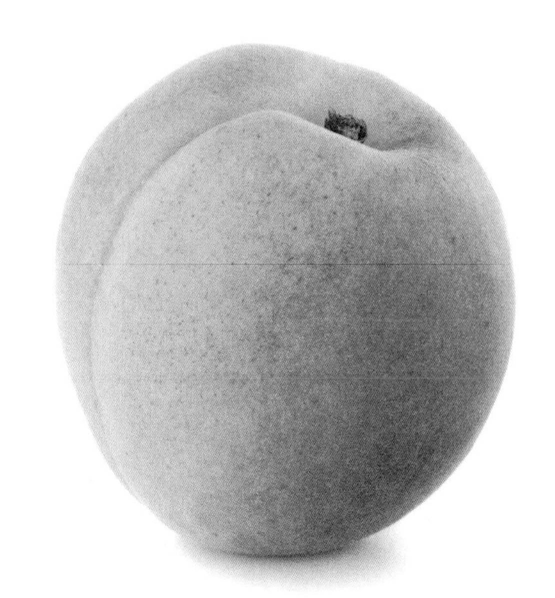

The apricot is an amazing food for rejuvenation. It's high in amino acids such as cysteine and glutamine, as well as minerals such as selenium and magnesium in their most bioactive forms. The fruit is also loaded with more than 40 trace minerals, some of which are bonded to each other as cofactor trace minerals, creating bioactive natural alloys that science has yet to uncover. Apricots have phytochemical compounds that attach and bind themselves to chemical molecules such as DDT deep within the body, lowering the risk of many cancers.

Apricots are a B_{12}-enhancing food, meaning they eliminate unhelpful elements in the digestive tract that get in the way of the body's healthy B_{12} production. When you eat an apricot, the skin collects and destroys mold, yeast, unneeded *Candida*, and other detrimental fungus in the body, plus the skin is high in enzymes and coenzymes that are DNA-protecting. An apricot's flesh thwarts the gut's production of ammonia, a destructive gas that can leach through the walls of the intestinal tract and cause problems throughout the body, from brain fog to dental issues. (This condition is called ammonia permeability, and it is as yet unknown to science. I cover it in detail in *Medical Medium.*)

Apricot is a warming food and an energy stabilizer that boosts the growth of red blood cells, strengthens your heart, and nourishes your brain. When your reserves are low from pushing yourself to the limit, turn to apricots—they're a sensational life bring-back food.

CONDITIONS

If you have any of the following conditions, try bringing apricots into your life:

Cancer, gallstones, gallbladder disease, bursitis, celiac disease, diverticulitis, Lyme disease, acne, anemia, hypertension, asthma, arthritis, depression, chronic fatigue syndrome (CFS), fibromyalgia, mold exposure, yeast infections, postural tachycardia syndrome (POTS), Raynaud's syndrome, hypoglycemia, hyperglycemia, diabetes, parasites, ammonia permeability

SYMPTOMS

If you have any of the following symptoms, try bringing apricots into your life:

Temperature sensitivities, fatigue, lightheadedness, body aches, chronic nausea, unquenchable thirst, gum pain, shortness of breath, food allergies, *Candida* overgrowth, sweating disorders (whether not capable of sweating at all or sweating too much), itchy skin, brain fog, bloating, body pain, colon spasms, congestion, cravings, flatulence, headaches, loss of energy, weight gain

EMOTIONAL SUPPORT

Apricots help us bring heart to life. They open us up, making us more kindhearted and helping those of us who have trouble with trust to tone down any nervousness or skittishness. Apricots calm us when we feel threatened and regulate a defensive nature, putting us in touch with our intuition so that we know when to keep our guards up and when to drop our defenses. When we become frustrated in any type of situation, apricots are excellent soothers.

SPIRITUAL LESSON

Apricots have been taken for granted in this century, overshadowed by shinier, flashier, and tastier food items. As you learn to appreciate this fruit for its health offerings—which top so many other foods—open your eyes and heart to the work opportunities, friends, and family that you've also taken for granted.

TIPS

- Apricots are so energy-shifting, so transformative, that you only need to eat one to enjoy its benefits. When dealing with a health condition, though, try to consume four apricots daily for support and healing.
- An apricot offers its greatest benefits from 3 P.M. onward. This is when the fruit's nutrients are at their highest levels—and most bioactive and assimilable.
- Have patience with apricot ripening. Wait until an apricot is well ripe before eating; do not eat the fruit underripe. Don't worry about juiciness, though. An apricot doesn't need to be dripping with juice to be beneficial.
- When fresh apricots aren't in season, sulfur-free dried apricots are an incredible alternative. While not every dried fruit is valuable, apricots tend to hold all their medicinal qualities when dehydrated. The potassium actually increases—unlike many other fruits—when apricots are dried.

APRICOT BARS

Makes to 2 to 4 servings

If you're always looking for a quick, easy snack to grab as you go about your day, these apricot bars will be perfect. They're sweet and chewy, with a subtle crunch of almonds. They only have four ingredients and take just a few seconds to make, and they'll keep in the freezer for up to a month.

1 cup dried apricots
½ cup dates, pitted
½ cup almonds
¼ cup coconut

Place all the ingredients in a food processor and process until well combined. Line a baking tray with parchment paper and press the mixture into a large, flat rectangle about half an inch thick. Chill in the freezer for at least 30 minutes before cutting into bars. Store the bars in the refrigerator for up to 1 week or in an airtight container in the freezer for up to 1 month.

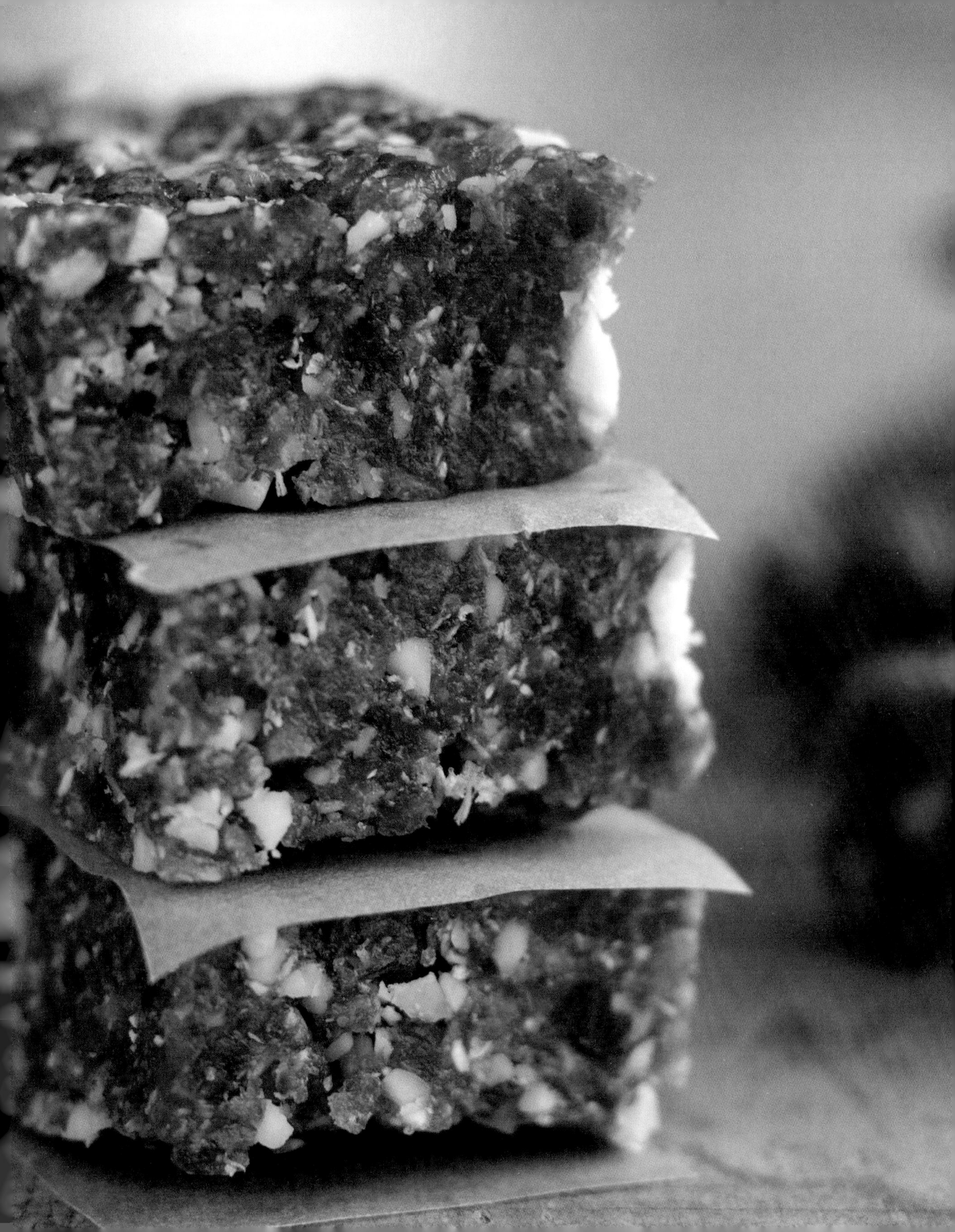

Avocados

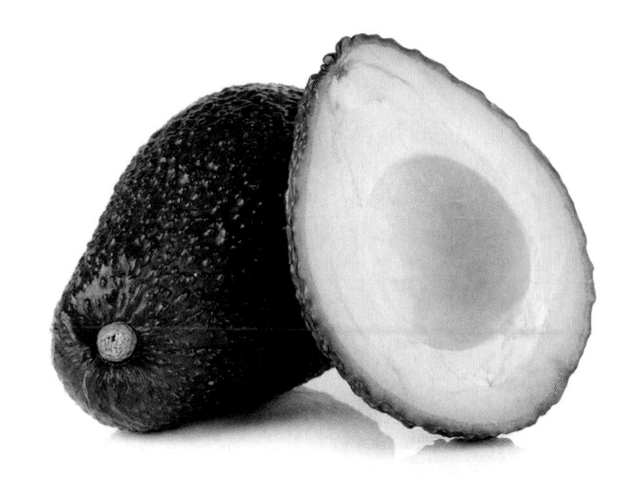

The avocado is the mother fruit. Whether you have a taste for it or not, it's vital to appreciate avocado as the foundation of the pantry, the conductor of the symphony, the strongest link in the chain, the landmark, the soul of all other foods. It's wonderful that avocados have gotten attention in recent years for their health benefits. They go far beyond what's reported, though. You don't know food until you understand the avocado.

Even though the skin of most avocados is inedible, it is loaded with hundreds of undiscovered phytochemical compounds, many of which are infused into an avocado's flesh as it grows. Some of these phytochemicals are isothiocyanates, which are involved with the color of the yellow-green flesh and help restore stomach and intestinal linings. When you are suffering from digestive disorders of any kind, avocados can come to the rescue. Easy to digest, their creamy flesh is the ultimate gut soother for those with food sensitivities, Crohn's disease, colitis, or IBS. Avocados possess anti-inflammatory compounds that have an aspirin-like quality without thinning the blood; this reduces narrowing and swelling of the digestive tract. This fruit also has polyp-reducing properties, helping you to prevent or rid yourself of these small growths of the intestinal lining.

Avocados are amazing for the brain, too. A healthy source of omega-6 fatty acids, they can help restore the central nervous system and alleviate Alzheimer's and dementia. Eating avocados also has an anti-aging effect on the skin, reducing dryness, giving you a healthy glow, and contributing to the disappearance of dark undereye circles. They also contain anti-radiation agents that are phytoestrogenic, meaning that they can stop estrogen-related reproductive and colon cancers. Avocados' benefits go far beyond what I have room to include here. Suffice it to say, you want avocados in your life!

CONDITIONS

If you have any of the following conditions, try bringing avocados into your life:

Heart disease, mystery infertility, human immunodeficiency virus (HIV), kidney disease, stroke, epilepsy, chronic fatigue syndrome (CFS), alopecia, brain cancer, Crohn's disease, colitis, irritable bowel syndrome (IBS), low reproductive system battery (see the chapter "Fertility and Our Future"), endometriosis, fibromyalgia, anxiety, sciatica, Alzheimer's disease, dementia, herpes, thyroid disease, adrenal fatigue, anxiety, attention deficit/hyperactivity disorder (ADHD), autism, depression, shingles, sleep disorders, polyps, urinary tract infections (UTIs), insomnia, hemorrhoids, ovarian cancer, uterine cancer, colon cancer, postural tachycardia syndrome (POTS), scleroderma, lichen sclerosus, radiation sickness, vertigo

SYMPTOMS

If you have any of the following symptoms, try bringing avocados into your life:

Memory loss, menopause symptoms, headaches, *Candida* overgrowth, muscle cramps, muscle pain, panic attacks, anxiousness, back pain, dizziness, balance issues, tingles and numbness on the extremities, gas, bloating, rashes, abdominal cramping, premenstrual syndrome (PMS) symptoms, gastroparesis, fatigue, food allergies, food sensitivities, trigeminal neuralgia, eye floaters, weakness

EMOTIONAL SUPPORT

Have you ever felt that you're not living life as your true self? That this is keeping you from standing up to challenges as you wish you could? That it's putting distance between you and those you love? Avocados help us find our way back to ourselves. When we need emotional strength and connection to who we really are, when we need to heal a broken heart, avocados fortify us to become strong links in the chain of human interaction. When we're dealing with those who are needy, aggressive, or destructive—weaker links in the chain—avocados help us pass along caring and mettle so we can uphold the integrity of our connections and teach others how to survive life's tests.

Avocados are also a pivotal tool when you're struggling with guilt. If you need to rewire and redirect feelings of shame and remorse, avocados will be your allies, nurturing you like a mother's love and helping to extract painful emotions from your heart and soul.

SPIRITUAL LESSON

Avocados are all about nurturing. As I said above, avocado is the mother fruit. Why? It's the closest food on the planet to breast milk. This means that in addition to the ways avocados help our bodies, they fill us spiritually with nurturing, motherly love. When we need to offer care to others—for example, when helping a friend or loved one through tough times—eating avocados helps us pass along this maternal energy. And when we're the ones who need love, either to keep us going as we tend to those around us or because of upheavals in our own lives, avocado is the ultimate comfort food. Bring avocado into your life as a teacher of unconditional love, both toward yourself and toward others, and watch your capacity for compassion grow and flourish.

TIPS

- For noticeable benefits, eat one avocado a day. For extreme benefits, eat two per day.
- Along the way, from harvest to display, people handle the avocados that you eventually buy in the store, and with each person who handles it, an avocado takes on some of her or his energy. Before you cut into an avocado that you've purchased, hold it in your hands for 30 seconds. This will identify the avocado as yours and connect its cells with your individual energy, being, soul, and DNA, making it the most nutritious it can be for your personal needs.
- When we think of travel foods, we often think of packaged snacks: trail mix, energy bars, potato chips, crackers. Yet the avocado is an amazing travel food. Try packing a few on your next trip as a fresh alternative to the norm of stale, greasy, or dehydrating road food. All you'll need to do when you get hungry is slice and twist open an avocado, then spoon out the flesh.

SALSA AVOCADO BOATS

Makes 2 to 4 servings

Beautiful and simple, these avocado boats are the perfect appetizer or snack to share. All the bright, bold flavors of your favorite salsa are nestled inside of a cool, creamy avocado. Make a double batch of the salsa ahead of time and have it on hand for any time the urge strikes.

2 avocados
1½ cup diced tomato
1 cup diced cucumber
¼ cup diced onion
¼ cup minced cilantro
1 garlic clove, minced
1 lime, juiced
⅛ cup minced jalapeño
⅛ teaspoon sea salt
⅛ teaspoon cayenne (optional)

Halve the avocados and remove the pits. Combine all the remaining ingredients in a small bowl. Scoop the salsa into the center of each avocado half and serve!

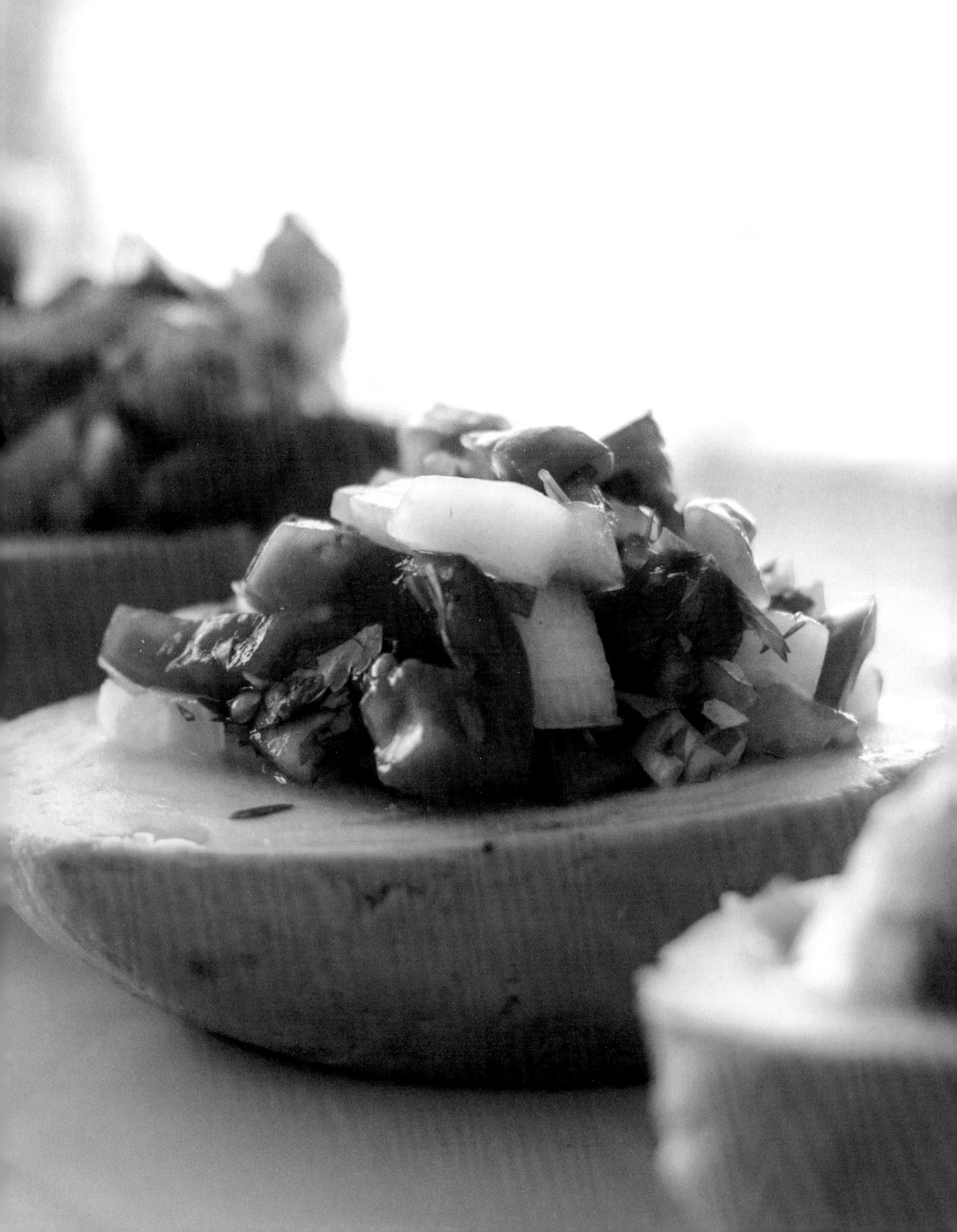

Bananas

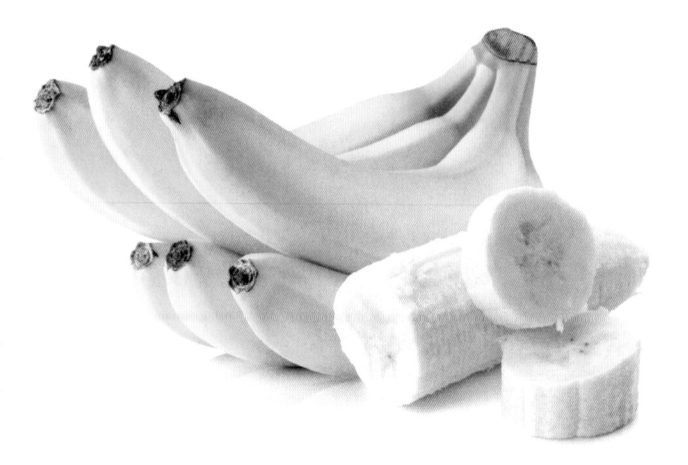

Bananas have gotten a bad rap lately, blamed for being too high in sugar. The reality is that the sugar in a properly ripened banana is completely different from the cane sugar and other processed sweeteners in cookies, cakes, and doughnuts. Unlike processed sugar, the fruit sugar in bananas is bonded to critical life-supporting trace minerals such as manganese, selenium, copper, boron, and molybdenum, and large amounts of minerals such as potassium, which is one of the most critical nutrients for neurotransmitter function. Bananas are also high in amino acids that work side by side with the highly bioavailable potassium as a catalyst for abundant electrolyte production. Rather than thinking of bananas as all sugar, we have to remind ourselves that bananas are made up of fiber, pulp, and water, too—and that their fruit sugar content is the very reason bananas have rich supplies of antioxidants, vitamins, and other phytonutrients to help us fight disease.

Bananas are a powerful antiviral food—so powerful that they have the capacity to repel growth of the retrovirus HIV. High in tryptophan, bananas can help soothe sleep disorders, create calm, reduce anxiety, and alleviate depression. And those who worry about *Candida* have no need to fear bananas. They are the ultimate fungus destroyers, removing unproductive bacteria while feeding beneficial microorganisms in the intestinal tract. This also makes them B_{12}-enhancing, because microbes in the gut can interrupt the ileum's rightful process of producing vitamin B_{12}.

When it comes to digestive aids, nothing beats bananas. They are truly an antispasmodic for hyperactive colons and small intestinal tracts. Bananas can alleviate gastric cramps and stress-related gastrointestinal disorders; they are a secret weapon in reversing colitis, IBS, and Crohn's disease. Bananas are also wonderful blood sugar stabilizers, have stress-assist phytochemicals to get you through your day, and help you balance your weight no matter where you are on the spectrum.

CONDITIONS

If you have any of the following conditions, try bringing bananas into your life:

Colitis, irritable bowel syndrome (IBS), Crohn's disease, celiac disease, autoimmune disease, heart disease, gastroesophageal reflux disease (GERD), adrenal fatigue, Alzheimer's disease, bipolar disorder, diabetes, carpal tunnel syndrome, depression, diverticulitis, gallbladder disease, hemorrhoids, human immunodeficiency virus (HIV), infertility, Parkinson's disease, arthritis, attention-deficit/hyperactivity disorder (ADHD), low reproductive system battery, sleep disorders, posttraumatic stress disorder (PTSD), fungal infections, shingles, tendonitis, anxiety, hypoglycemia, hyperglycemia, edema

SYMPTOMS

If you have any of the following symptoms, try bringing bananas into your life:

Loss of taste and/or smell, weight gain, weight loss, temporomandibular joint (TMJ) issues, enlarged spleen, blurred vision, fatigue, *Candida* overgrowth, diabetic neuropathy, bruising, tachycardia, constipation, bloating, diarrhea, headache, apnea, blurry eyes, blood sugar imbalances, food sensitivities, ear pain, jaw pain, muscle weakness, anxiousness, sensations of humming or vibration in the body, abdominal cramping, abdominal pain, Bell's palsy, back pain, tingles and numbness

EMOTIONAL SUPPORT

Bananas strengthen the core of who we are, encouraging us to peel back our false shields and expose our true selves. They can help reverse a state of mind that's saturated with fear (eating three or more a day can help reduce PTSD), and they help us express our true desire to be productive, overcoming procrastination and other unproductive behaviors in the process. If you think a friend is holding on to resentment, offer her or him a banana, and it will help dissolve the feelings of ill will.

SPIRITUAL LESSON

At times of spiritual growth, we may find ourselves feeling indestructible and completely absorbed in the moment. If we're not careful, though—if we haven't planned ahead and fortified ourselves for the future—the strong wind of challenge may take us down.

Learn, then, from the banana plant. Not technically trees, banana plants form thick and wide root mats, with underground corbs (stems) continually surfacing as suckers ready to grow. Because banana "trunks" are not actually wood—rather, they're formed from layer upon layer of leaves—they grow fast, with new offshoots able to rush to the rescue whenever weather has taken down another stalk.

As you reach for the sky, blossom, and bear fruit, remember to cast your own root system wide and deep. Let every lesson learned become a spiritual offshoot that may someday rescue you.

TIPS

- While you may like your bananas hard and green or mushy and brown, the optimal stage at which to eat bananas for peak nutrition is peak ripeness. When a banana's skin is still green, enzymes prevent absorption of any of the fruit's nutrients. And an overripe banana with entirely brown or black skin contains fermented fruit. The safest point at which to eat a banana is when its skin is yellow, with brown speckles. (The definitive test is that the banana won't give you a fuzzy feeling on your tongue.)
- Bananas are the best food for travel—whether on long car rides, flights, or errands around town. When you know you have a trip coming up, buy bananas ahead of time so they'll be at just the right stage of ripeness when you need them.
- Bananas are also the most powerful exercise food. Eating a banana before and after exercise can replenish the body more than any other food out there.

BANANA "MILKSHAKE"

Makes 1 to 2 servings

This "milkshake" is the classic childhood favorite without the dairy—and you won't miss it, because the drink is cold, creamy, and perfect. The hint of fresh vanilla bean and the dusting of cinnamon make it even more incredible.

1½-inch piece of vanilla bean pod, split lengthwise

2 frozen bananas

4 fresh bananas

2 dates, pitted

1 cup coconut water

⅛ teaspoon cinnamon (optional)

Scrape the seeds from the vanilla bean pod and place them in a blender.* Place the remaining ingredients in the blender; blend until smooth and drink up!

*Save the exterior of the vanilla bean pod for use blended into a smoothie or dessert. (Note that a high-speed blender will be necessary to break it down thoroughly.)

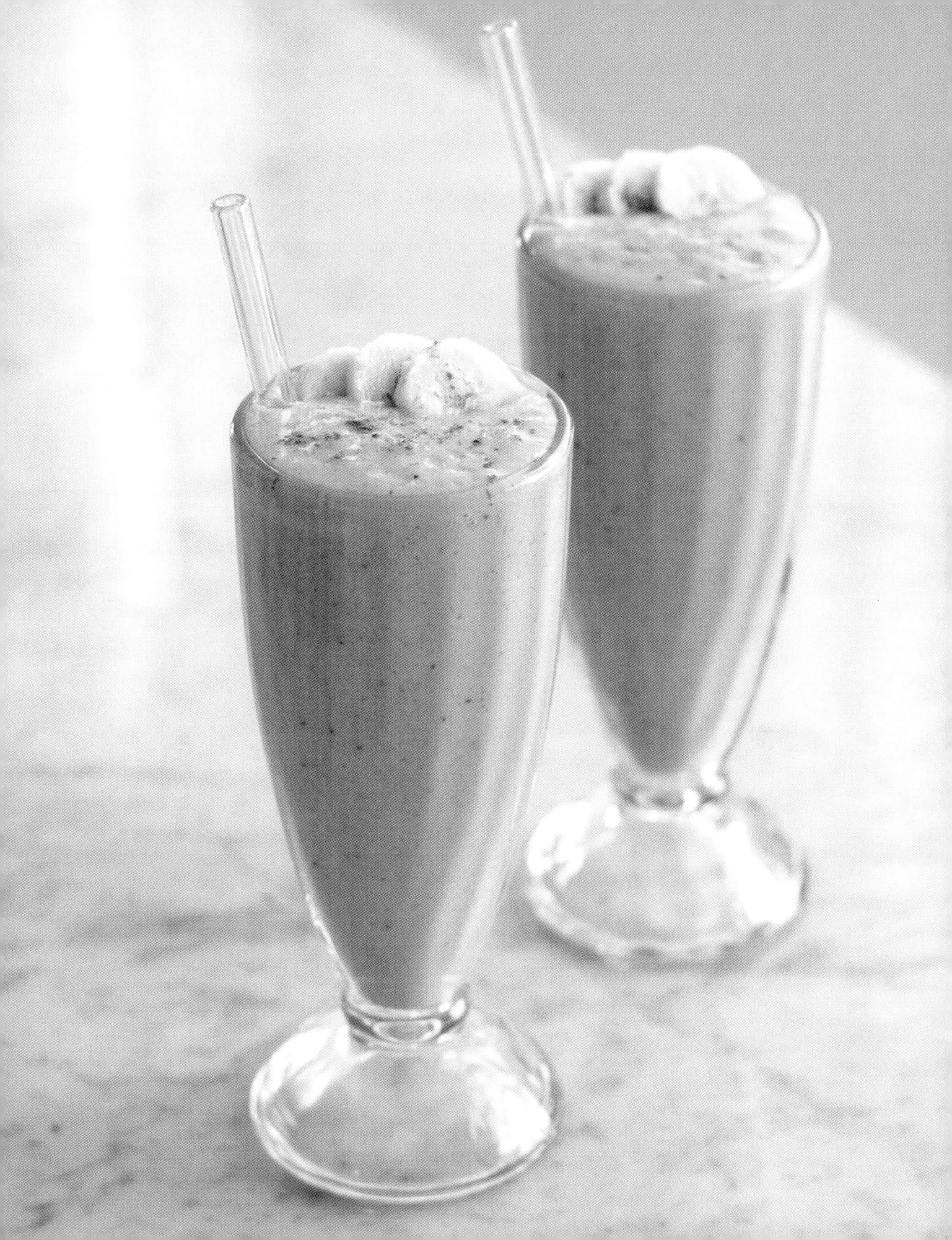

Berries

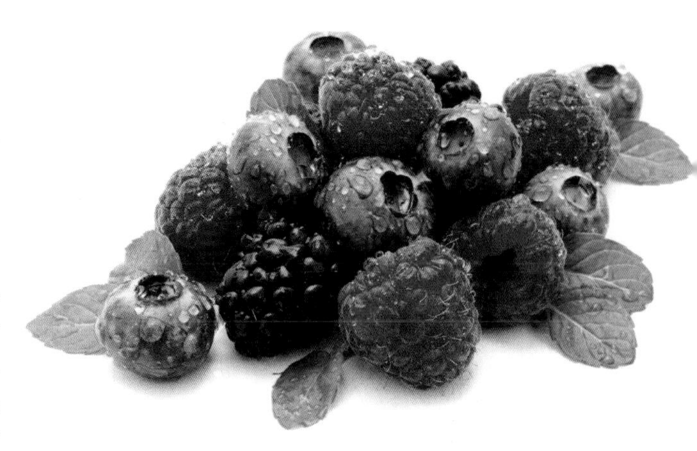

Berries are a saving grace. Their main power comes from antioxidants, the miracle fighters of free radicals. Antioxidants mean life, while oxidation means death. We need these antioxidants to fight the aging (oxidation) process, and to stay alive in the face of constant threats to our health. Berries broadcast their health value with their deep purples, blues, and blacks, which come from the polyphenols known as anthocyanins (including malvidin) and anthocyanidins. They're also rich in dimethyl resveratrol and dozens of other phytochemicals, amino acids, coenzymes, and co-compounds that have yet to be discovered by science and are more plentiful and bioavailable in berries than in any other food.

An excellent source of iron, magnesium, selenium, zinc, molybdenum, potassium, chromium, and calcium, berries also have traces of omega-3, omega-6, and omega-9 fatty acids. Plus, they have hidden compounds that stop excess adrenaline from causing damage to organs. This makes blackberries, raspberries, strawberries, elderberries, schisandra berries, and the like critical for life on earth. (For cranberries, see the separate feature on them.) Wild berries, especially, pack an anti-aging, disease-fighting, life-giving punch.

And wild blueberries are in a league of their own—you'll find information on them specifically in the "Wild Foods" section. Whenever possible, choose frozen wild blueberries instead of clamshells of fresh, cultivated blueberries. Make it part of your habit, after shopping in the produce section of the market, to swing by the frozen food aisle, where bags of wild blueberries are readily available. You'll be providing your body with the greatest chance of recovery and healing.

Berries are true brain food. Not only are they B_{12}-enhancing; they have the power to reverse stains on the brain—lesions, gray areas, calcifications, heavy metal deposits, white spots, scar tissue, crystallizations, and adhesions created by damaged, expanded blood vessels. For protection against all brain disorders and diseases, including brain cancer, ALS, Alzheimer's, dementia, Parkinson's, stroke, aneurysm, and migraines, turn to berries. For *any* illness with neurological symptoms, berries are the answer.

When you think of heart health, too, think berries. Nothing compares to the way berries protect heart valves and ventricles and remove plaque by dissolving hardened fat deposits within veins and arteries. The humble berry reigns supreme for keeping people out of the cardiologist's office.

And we can't ignore what berries mean for fertility. In the near future, scientific research will discover a group of compounds that specifically promote fertility. These pro-fertility compounds, which derive from a single variety of polyphenol, are responsible for a woman's reproductive system's ability to maintain a constant balance, so that the "low battery" behind so many cases of mystery infertility does not occur. (For more on this phenomenon, see the chapter "Fertility and Our Future.") Berries truly are an answer for the future of humankind.

CONDITIONS

If you have any of the following conditions, try bringing berries into your life:

Brain cancer, benign brain tumors, amyotrophic lateral sclerosis (ALS), stroke, aneurysm, migraines, Parkinson's disease, Alzheimer's disease, dementia, attention-deficit/hyperactivity disorder (ADHD), autism, encephalitis, epilepsy, Huntington's disease, narcolepsy, osteomyelitis, Tourette's syndrome, cerebral palsy, multiple sclerosis (MS), atherosclerosis, heart disease, tachycardia, ovarian cancer, atrial fibrillation, prostate cancer, uterine cancer, polycystic ovarian syndrome (PCOS), mystery infertility, endometriosis, pelvic inflammatory disease (PID), tinnitus, insomnia, depression, anxiety, posttraumatic stress disorder (PTSD), low reproductive system battery, obsessive-compulsive disorder (OCD), acne, adrenal fatigue, thyroid diseases and disorders, fibromyalgia, chronic fatigue syndrome (CFS), weight gain, bladder infections, fibroids, hypoglycemia, diabetes, Lyme disease, viral infection, eczema, psoriasis, adenomas, edema, thyroid nodules

SYMPTOMS

If you have any of the following symptoms, try bringing berries into your life:

High cholesterol; ovarian cysts; thickening uterus; inflamed uterus, ovaries, and/or fallopian tubes; irregular menstruation; hormonal imbalances; hot flashes; heart palpitations; fatigue; tingles; sensations of humming or vibration in the body; numbness; blurry eyes; swallowing issues; headaches; nerve pain; mineral deficiencies; cramping and spasming; chest pain; chest tightness; frozen shoulder; dizziness; panic attacks; phobias; malaise; listlessness; ringing or buzzing in the ears; brain lesions; spinal lesions; eye floaters; ear pain; jaw pain; neck pain; blood sugar imbalances; fatigue; brain fog; sluggish liver; anxiousness; myelin nerve damage; calcifications; scar tissue; *Candida* overgrowth; brain adhesions; back pain; knee pain; poor circulation; swelling; brain inflammation

EMOTIONAL SUPPORT

For those who feel distracted, unsure, unfocused, mixed up, foggy, disordered, blurred, adrift, dizzy, confused, or too often puzzled, berries hold unique powers to offer relief. These states of being are both conscious and subconscious, physical and metaphysical—conditions of the mind and soul. When you apply berries with the intention of self-treating all aspects behind your muddled feelings and perceptions, your issues can reverse, and miracles can come your way.

SPIRITUAL LESSON

If you seek abundance, become a student of the berry. From late spring to late fall, there's never a gap in berry offerings—as one field of strawberries wanes, blackberries in a nearby bramble begin to plump. It's all about replenishment, about not panicking when one source dries up, because more jewels are to be found just around the corner.

Berries are selfless. You won't find them high up, out of reach. Rather, they grow low to the ground, where they're accessible to all varieties of animals, from bears, deer, humans, squirrels, and birds, to mice, voles, rabbits, and even snails. Berries are all about sharing, about providing enough to go around for everyone. When we bring berries into our lives, their kindness and generosity becomes a part of us, so that we become providers in the cycle of abundance, not just takers.

TIPS

- Eating your favorite berries shortly after sunrise will boost your energy and vitality throughout the day.
- Grazing between meals with some handfuls of berries can raise your body's frequency to bring you to a more positive, peaceful state.
- Picking berries from an organic farm, your own backyard, or a wild source in nature, and then eating them unwashed, will allow their elevated biotics to restore much-needed beneficial bacteria to the gut, re-enabling the body's ability to self-produce all the coenzyme varieties of vitamin B_{12}.
- Berry picking is also an unmatchable grounding technique. Plucking blueberries from a bush or raspberries from a thorny cane, concentrating on selecting only the ripe ones and not getting pricked, forces you to be present. It's a sacred state of being that both connects us to our ancestors and brings us into unity with the singing birds and rustling leaves of the here and now.
- For the most powerful prebiotic possible to nurture all beneficial bacteria and other microorganisms in the gut, add raw honey to a bowlful of berries.
- Eating berries on a sunny day increases adrenal strength and helps balance blood sugar. Eating berries on a cloudy day increases cleansing of the liver and helps break it out of sluggishness.
- Invite a friend over to share a big bowl of berries. You'll be surprised at how emotional wounds start to lift and clear for both of you as your conversation becomes pleasingly sacred, deep, healing, and, in the end, happy.

BERRIES AND CREAM

Makes 2 servings

Beautiful and enticing, these berries-and-cream bowls are perfect for brunch, entertaining, or dessert. The coconut milk whips into a cloud of light, fluffy whipped cream, and the hint of ginger and lemon zest completes the dish. Enjoy impressing those you love with these beautiful berry bowls.

1 cup blueberries

1 cup blackberries

1 cup raspberries

1 cup strawberries

2 13.5-ounce cans full-fat coconut milk, refrigerated

¼ teaspoon grated ginger

1 teaspoon maple syrup

Lemon juice (from about ¼ lemon)

1 2-inch piece vanilla bean pod, split lengthwise

1 teaspoon lemon zest

4 leaves fresh mint, minced

Rinse the berries, mix them together, and divide them evenly into 2 bowls. Open the cans of coconut milk, being careful not to shake them. Coconut milk naturally separates in the can, leaving a thick, heavy layer on top. Scoop out the solid cream from each can and place it in a small mixing bowl. (You will need ½ cup of cream.) Discard the thin liquid that remains. Using a fork, whisk together the coconut cream, ginger, maple syrup, lemon juice, and the scraped seeds from the vanilla bean pod.* Whisk until the mixture is well combined and smooth. Scoop a generous dollop of cream over the berries in each bowl. Top with the lemon zest and mint.

*Save the exterior of the vanilla bean pod for use blended into a smoothie or dessert. (Note that a high-speed blender will be necessary to break it down thoroughly.)

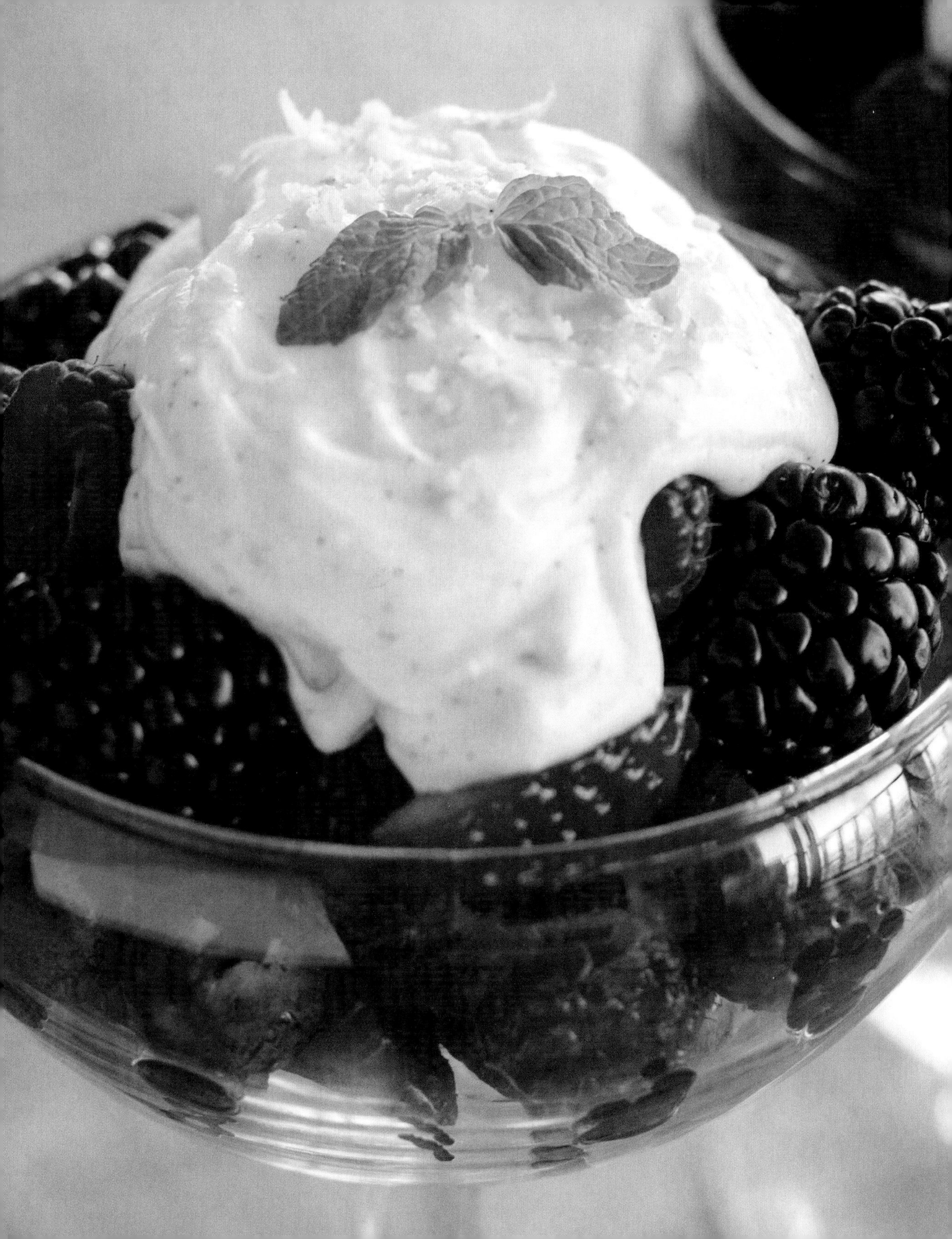

Cherries

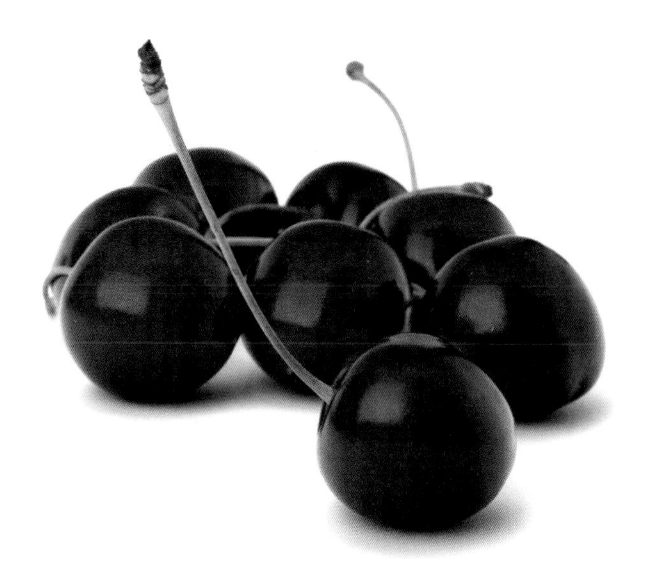

In this day and age, our livers are more burdened than ever before in history. With toxins in our environment and foods that stress our bodies, sluggish and fatty livers are becoming rampant. While certain liver-cleansing techniques have become trendy, a handful of cherries can do so much more. Cherries are an amazing way to revitalize this organ; they're the ultimate liver tonic, cleanser, and rejuvenator.

Cherries promote healthy hemoglobin and are also anti-cancerous, specifically effective at addressing non-Hodgkin's lymphoma, melanoma, and glioblastoma (a type of brain tumor). Cherries sharpen the mind by purifying the bowels—they're better at alleviating constipation than prunes! They cleanse the bladder, too, and help alleviate spastic bladders and bladder prolapse. Plus, cherries are one of the best endocrine-system-boosting foods, stimulating or suppressing the appetite as needed. If it's weight loss you're after, cherries are your new best friend.

In the world of minerals, we're familiar with the concept of macrominerals, which our bodies rely on in higher amounts, and trace minerals, which are just as critical to our functioning, though we need them in smaller doses. Cherries, for example, are a wonderful source of trace minerals such as zinc and iron. As anyone with anemia can tell you, a deficiency in iron is not small potatoes just because iron is a trace mineral—it's vital no matter what.

The same concept is true with amino acids, though science has yet to focus on this. In addition to the amino acids we're familiar with, there are minute, trace forms of amino acids that become cofactors to their macro forms—and cherries are rich in both macro and trace amino acids (including threonine, tryptophan, and lysine) that specifically work in tandem with the hormone melatonin to give your brain and body amazing stress relief. When enhanced like this, melatonin also acts as an antioxidant to help protect the brain from Alzheimer's, dementia, and brain tumors.

Phytochemical compounds and agents in cherries are amazing for removing radiation and repairing myelin nerve damage. Women receive particular benefit from cherries' cleansing properties: cherries remove toxins from the uterus and the rest of the reproductive system and help to reduce fibroids and ovarian cysts.

CONDITIONS

If you have any of the following conditions, try bringing cherries into your life:

Polycystic ovarian syndrome (PCOS), Alzheimer's disease, bladder cancer, lymphoma (including non-Hodgkin's), melanoma, bladder prolapse, fatty liver, breast cancer, autism, brain tumors, cardiovascular disease, diabetes, pelvic inflammatory disease (PID), ear infections, fibromyalgia, depression, infertility, obsessive-compulsive disorder (OCD), kidney stones, low reproductive system battery, anorexia, alopecia, dementia, Hashimoto's thyroiditis, adrenal fatigue, acne, anemia, fibroids, bursitis, urinary tract infections (UTIs) such as kidney infections and bladder infections, anxiety, connective-tissue damage, prostatitis, Graves' disease, insomnia, dysautonomia, vertigo, blood disorders, nodules on bones and glands

SYMPTOMS

If you have any of the following symptoms, try bringing cherries into your life:

Nosebleeds, sprains, tooth decay, hypothyroid, lightheadedness, constipation, lack of appetite, overactive appetite, cravings, fever, scratching and itching, dry mouth, malaise, bruising, dizziness, chest pain, hyperthyroid, impotence, cough, phobias, sluggish liver, food allergies, myelin nerve damage, fatigue, memory loss, back pain, bad breath, blood toxicity, confusion, high cortisol, inflammation, ovarian cysts

EMOTIONAL SUPPORT

If you want to cheer up friends or family members, take them some cherries and you'll notice they'll be tickled pink. If you or someone you know never feels satisfied with circumstances, let cherries work their magic of contentment. If you ever worry about being speechless, add cherries to your diet and you'll feel the conversation flow. And if you're feeling empty and deserted, cherries can point your feelings in a new direction. Simply from looking at a bowl of cherries, joy instantly enters into a person's being. Cherries ignite enthusiasm and create positive excitement. They're an amazing fruit to keep someone lighthearted.

SPIRITUAL LESSON

Cherries teach us patience. If you rush while eating a cherry—if you don't take care to bite into it carefully—you may find that you injure yourself on the stone inside. In this way, cherries teach us to take our time, to be mindful and considered in our actions so we minimize mistakes and pain.

TIPS

- Cherries are so cleansing, detoxifying so many impurities, that they serve us best in limited quantities. When eating this fruit, don't be so distracted by the delicious flavor that you forget to listen to your cutoff signal. Consume cherries in small servings portioned out daily, rather than in a large serving at one sitting.
- When selecting red cherries at the market or grocery store, look for the darkest ones. These deeper shades have the most healing benefits. If the red cherries you're looking at are colored too lightly, it means the soil of the cherry tree didn't have the optimal level of minerals.

SWEET CHERRY SMOOTHIE

Makes 2 servings

In this smoothie, the sweetness of the cherries combines with the creaminess of the bananas and a pop of tart lemon to surprise and delight you.

1 frozen banana
2 ripe bananas
1 cup frozen cherries
½ lemon, peeled
½ cup water

Place all the ingredients in a blender and blend until smooth. Pour into glasses and enjoy! (Note that this mixture will gel if left to sit, so drink immediately if you'd like it fluid or refrigerate for half an hour if you prefer a pudding consistency.)

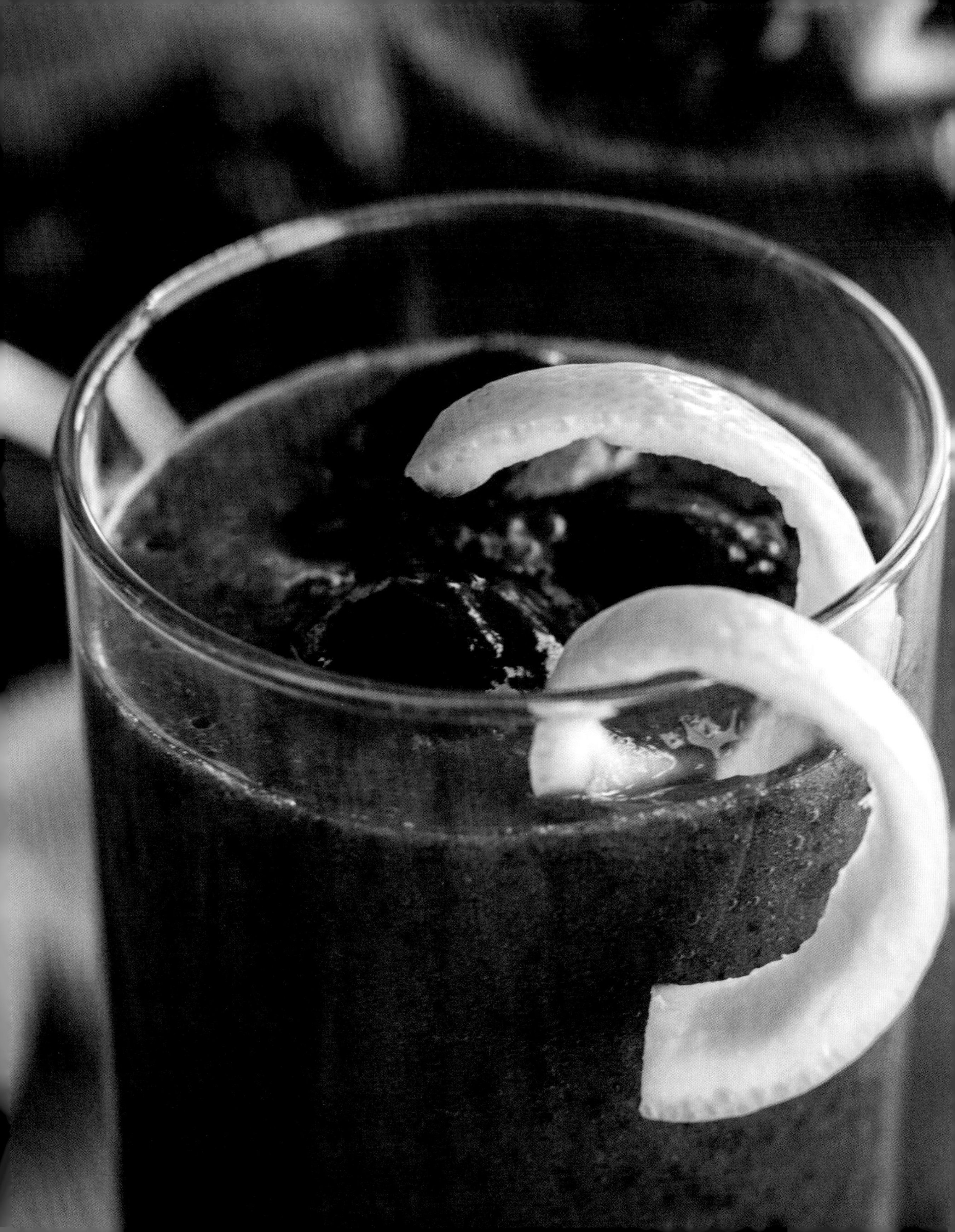

Cranberries

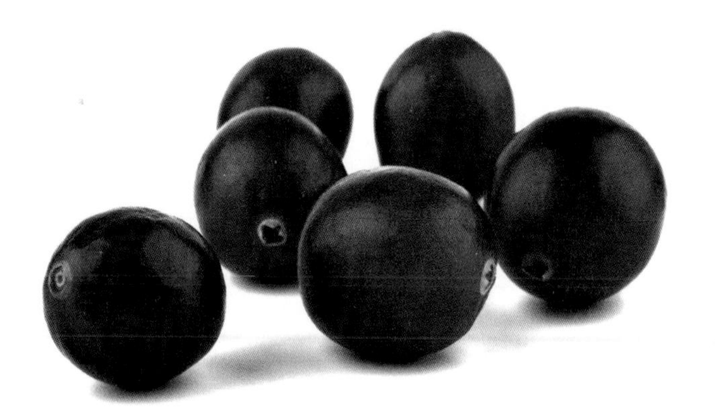

Cranberries are well known for their profound antiseptic role in healing urinary tract infections and yeast infections. That power comes from cranberries' ability to fight *Streptococcus* bacteria—because most of the time, chronic strep infections are behind these conditions. (Even though in yeast infections, the origin of the problem is misdiagnosed as fungal, really, the yeast is secondary.) And that's the least of what these powerful little berries do. Out of all the foods on the table at Thanksgiving, that dish of cranberries is by far the most nutritious. Even if your cranberry sauce is canned and saturated with syrup, the medicinal factor of the cranberries overrides the downsides of the added ingredients.

Cranberries are one of the ultimate foods for reversing gallbladder disease. If you're dealing with gallstones, there's nothing more powerful for dissolving them. Cranberries are also one of the most powerful liver cleansers on earth, and they're extremely helpful when you're trying to pass kidney stones with ease. They can even dislodge earwax buildup and help bring back hearing.

Not to mention, cranberries are high in the antioxidants (such as anthocyanins) that help heal cardiovascular disease and arteriosclerosis. They also hold phytoestrogen compounds that disarm invading estrogens from outside sources such as plastics, environmental pollutants, pesticides, and other synthetic chemicals. Cranberries destroy these toxic hormones that are responsible for so many of women's health conditions.

Filled with compounds and agents that draw radiation out of your body, amino acids that protect connective tissue, enzymes that specifically detoxify your organs, and more than 50 trace minerals to address deficiencies you may not even know you have, cranberries also have anti-proliferative compounds that help halt the growth of bacteria, viruses, and anything else harmful that may be growing inside of you. At the same time, cranberries provide potent stress assistance during your times of need.

And if you're trying to lose weight, cranberries are another of your strongest allies. Consuming a bowl of cranberries daily will suppress your appetite and help you shed those extra pounds.

CONDITIONS

If you have any of the following conditions, try bringing cranberries into your life:

Seasonal allergies, migraines, hiatal hernia, human immunodeficiency virus (HIV), hypertension, cervical cancer, yeast infections, carpal tunnel syndrome, arteriosclerosis, cardiovascular disease, miscarriage, leukemia, ovarian cancer, *Streptococcus* infection, bladder infections, obesity, pneumonia (all varieties), conjunctivitis, renal failure, staph infections, gallbladder disease, gallstones, kidney infections, kidney stones, anemia, anxiety, shingles, diabetes, gout, HHV-6, cytomegalovirus (CMV), nodules, Lyme disease

SYMPTOMS

If you have any of the following symptoms, try bringing cranberries into your life:

Memory loss, muscle cramps, nail biting, hypothyroid, premenstrual syndrome (PMS) symptoms, weight gain, bloating, flatulence, dyspepsia, jaundice, mania, confusion, intermittent vaginal bleeding, tremors, hearing loss, calcifications, bruising, cravings, dizzy spells, earwax buildup, blisters, hyperthyroid, inflammation, blurred vision, anxiousness, foot pain, scar tissue

EMOTIONAL SUPPORT

Cranberries promote a cheery disposition. Whenever you're feeling foggy on an emotional level—unclear about what decisions to make, confused about your direction in life—eating cranberries can light your path. When disorganization flusters you, colors how others see you, and impedes the way, cranberries (which grow in a very orderly fashion) can help you sort matters out and move on.

Cranberries also help when neurons and receptors are stuck in a pattern of criticism. Whether you're criticizing others too much or on the receiving end of reproach, cranberries will help. Regular consumption of cranberries can relieve feelings of rejection and humiliation. And if you're ever experiencing a sense of alienation, cranberries can help you change course and get reconnected with community.

SPIRITUAL LESSON

As we settle into adult life, we learn that it isn't always safe to come out and play. Sometimes responsibility requires our full attention and seriousness—or we're in company that will take advantage of us if we open up and expose our true selves. In much the same way, the cranberry vine has an instinct to stay low to the ground, protecting itself from cold and windy conditions. It can be difficult to even see the small red berries when it's in this self-shielding mode.

Sometimes we get stuck in this mentality, afraid that taking a moment for delight makes us vulnerable and means we aren't working hard enough. Yet growing up doesn't mean that we're supposed to suppress our joy all the time. Joy is essential to who we are. Just as the cranberry plant takes advantage of the right warm and sunny moments during ripening season to perk up, play in the wind, and dazzle in the light, we can learn to recognize moments that are safe for us to express our true vitality, essence, and glory. We do get our days to stand up and shine, to dance in the sun. It's just a matter of balance—and there's no better teacher on the subject than the cranberry.

TIPS

- Frozen cranberries can be a great way to get your hands on this fruit. Try cooking them into your oatmeal or incorporating them into smoothies.
- If you're not making your own fresh cranberry juice, look for juice that's made 100 percent from cranberries—with no added sugars, preservatives, or other additives.
- If you don't like the tart nature of cranberries, eat them with a handful of walnuts.
- If you really dislike cranberries, it doesn't mean they can't help you. Weekly, set out a bowl of cranberries in your house. Just having them out on the kitchen counter to look at will help you (and anyone else passing through) reap their emotional benefits as the berries' properties enter into you metaphysically. And if you take a moment each day to touch the cranberries, running your fingers over them or resting a few in your palm, you'll also receive the fruit's physical benefits.

RAW CRANBERRY RELISH

Makes 2 to 4 servings

When you think of cranberries, you may envision a gelatinous blob on the table at Thanksgiving dinner. This raw cranberry relish is anything but boring. The fresh cranberries are chopped with bits of apple, orange, and coconut sugar that offset the cranberries' natural tartness. This simple side dish is a great accompaniment to any holiday meal, or is perfect on top of a salad any time.

1 cup cranberries
2 cups roughly diced apple
½ cup orange sections
¼ teaspoon orange zest
4 tablespoons coconut sugar
3 mint leaves

Pulse-blend all the ingredients in a food processor until roughly combined. Store in the refrigerator for at least 30 minutes before serving.

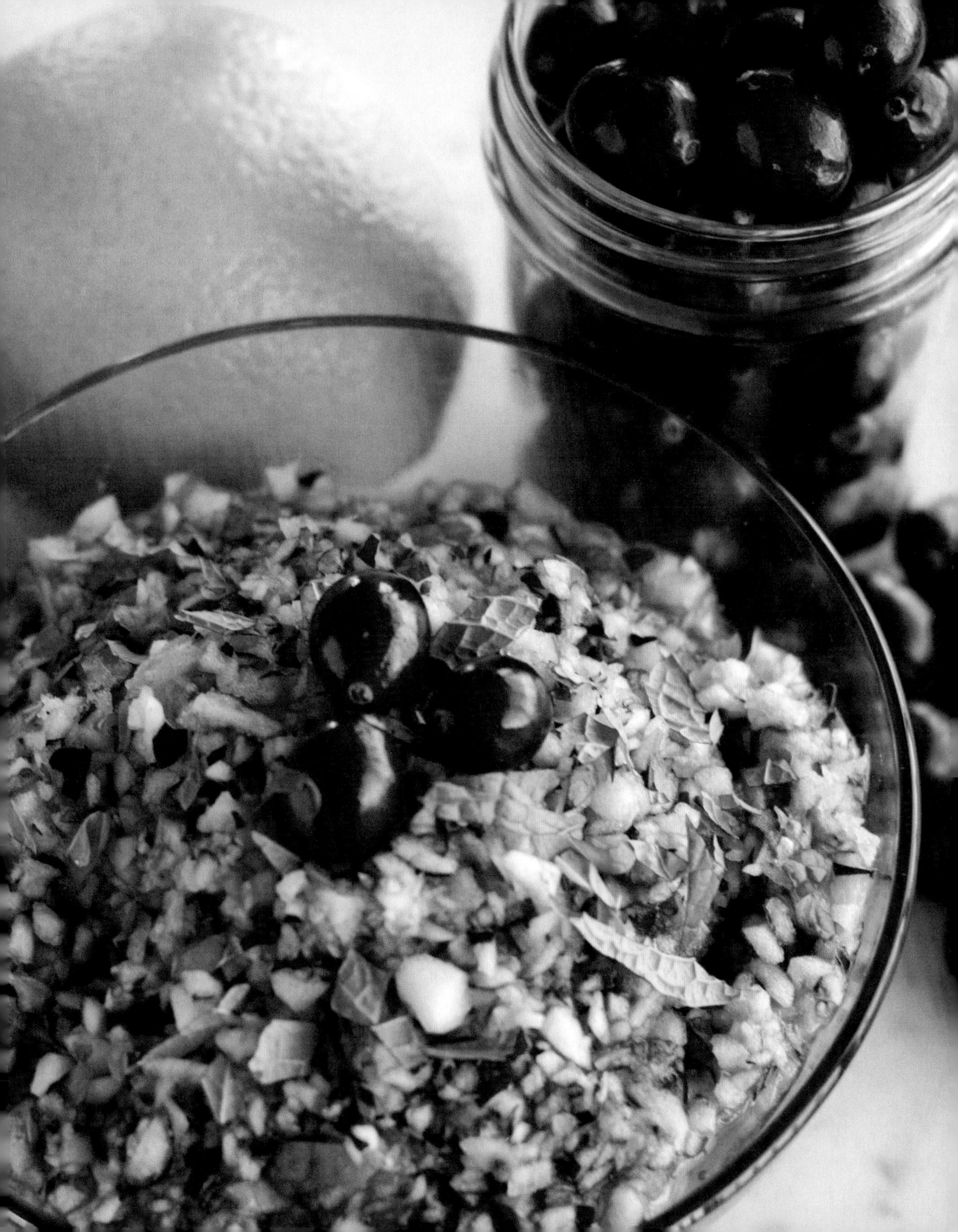

Dates

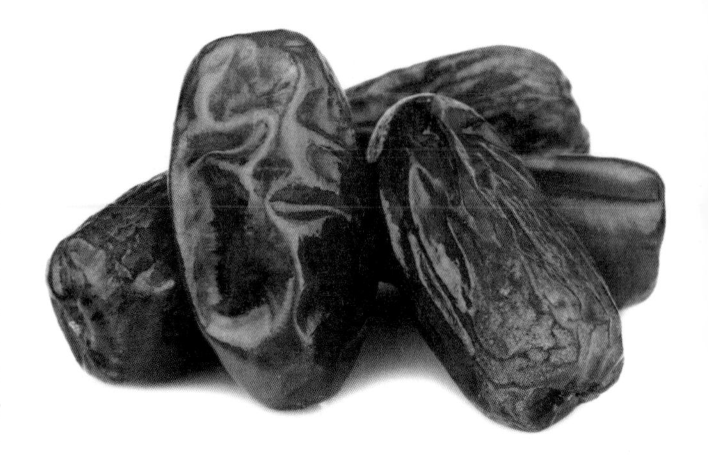

Dates are amazing for the digestive system. As one of the most anti-parasitical foods on the planet, dates bind onto, destroy, and sweep away parasites; yeast, mold, and other fungus; heavy metals; unproductive bacteria; viruses; and other poisonous pathogens from the gut. It makes them one of the most beneficial *Candida* killers known to humankind—despite the misinformation out there about dates feeding *Candida*. (For more on the truth about this condition, see the entire chapter devoted to it in my first book, *Medical Medium*.) Dates also help restore peristaltic function in the intestines, retraining the intestinal tract after paralysis or dysfunction to move properly and expel any rotting food.

Contrary to popular belief, dates are also an ideal food for people dealing with diabetes and hypoglycemia, because they deliver vital glucose to the liver—addressing the very glucose loss that's responsible for blood sugar issues. They're also ideal for athletes and other adventurous and active people, as the high potassium and fruit sugar content is perfect for refueling the brain and muscles, which rely on glucose to power you through exercise.

Dates are rich in nearly 70 bioactive minerals (much higher than is documented) that support the adrenal glands to help you handle life's daily challenges. One of the most heart-healthy foods available, dates also contain a record-breaking, undiscovered amount of amino acids. Similar to what happens with bananas, the amino acids in dates, such as leucine, help elevate the fruit's potassium to its highest potential in sustaining and fortifying muscles and nerves. This process also stops lactic acid from taking over the body when it's under stress.

Dates are a warming food that expels dampness from organs such as the spleen and liver, though not to the point of creating unproductive dryness. Dates are also abundant in anti-cancerous properties, making them a must for anyone seeking disease prevention and optimal health.

CONDITIONS

If you have any of the following conditions, try bringing dates into your life:

Diabetes, hypoglycemia, small intestinal bacterial overgrowth (SIBO), cardiovascular disease, fungal infections, gastroesophageal reflux disease (GERD), hypertension, lung cancer, obesity, thyroid disease, aneurysm, post-traumatic stress disorder (PTSD), narcissistic personality disorder, obsessive-compulsive disorder (OCD), adrenal fatigue, phobias, chronic sinusitis, rosacea, schizophrenia, social anxiety disorder, autism, attention-deficit/hyperactivity disorder (ADHD), tuberculosis, vertigo, eating disorders, insomnia, gum disease, edema

SYMPTOMS

If you have any of the following symptoms, try bringing dates into your life:

Blood sugar imbalances, mucus in the stool, *Candida* overgrowth, constipation, muscle fatigue, earache, dizziness, shortness of breath, vaginal pain, heart palpitations, anxiousness, sweats, urinary urgency, lack of focus and concentration, tremors, food allergies, sleep disturbances, panic attacks, ringing or buzzing in the ears, spasms, tics, head pain, headaches, gum pain, ear pain, cough, confusion, brain fog

EMOTIONAL SUPPORT

Eating dates can put up a shield around you, providing protection from people who feel jealousy toward you. And while you sleep, they help to release your own stored-up toxic emotions—such as fearfulness, shame, demoralization, and the sense of being judged, wronged, or bullied. Ultimately, dates strengthen your sense of purpose so you can be your most productive and enthusiastic.

SPIRITUAL LESSON

Dates teach us to shift from selfishness to selflessness. Their sweet, nourishing nature can be positively addicting—their delicious flavor so enjoyable that we tend to want to keep them all to ourselves. The lesson is in holding back from hoarding your supply of dates. Eat only a few at a time, so you can share your bounty with others. Watching friends and family smile as they take the dates' sustenance into their bodies will help you cleanse yourself of greed, reorient toward giving, and ultimately recognize the truth that connecting to your inherent selflessness is an essential component of spiritual success.

TIPS

- To experience dates' maximum benefits, eat four to six daily.
- If you're in need of a better night's sleep, eat one date two hours before you retire for bed.
- For a more profound experience from whichever form of meditation you choose, eat three dates before you begin your session.
- When you're packing for a trip that involves uncertainty about when, where, or how you'll find food along the way, seal one date in plastic wrap and stow it in your pocket or baggage. You don't have to actually eat the date on your journey (although it's great for an emergency)—rather, this traveling date will be your good luck charm to help ensure you never go hungry.

RAW DATE GRANOLA

Makes 1 to 2 servings

This recipe is perfect for anyone on the go. Make a big batch and store it in a jar in the fridge for anytime snacking. The sweet and salty combo will be a major hit with the whole family. It can be eaten by itself as a snack, or on top of any fruit or smoothie bowl.

2 cups dates, pitted
¼ cup coconut flakes
¼ cup almonds
¼ teaspoon sea salt

Process all the ingredients in a food processor until roughly combined. Store the granola in a jar in the refrigerator for up to 2 weeks.

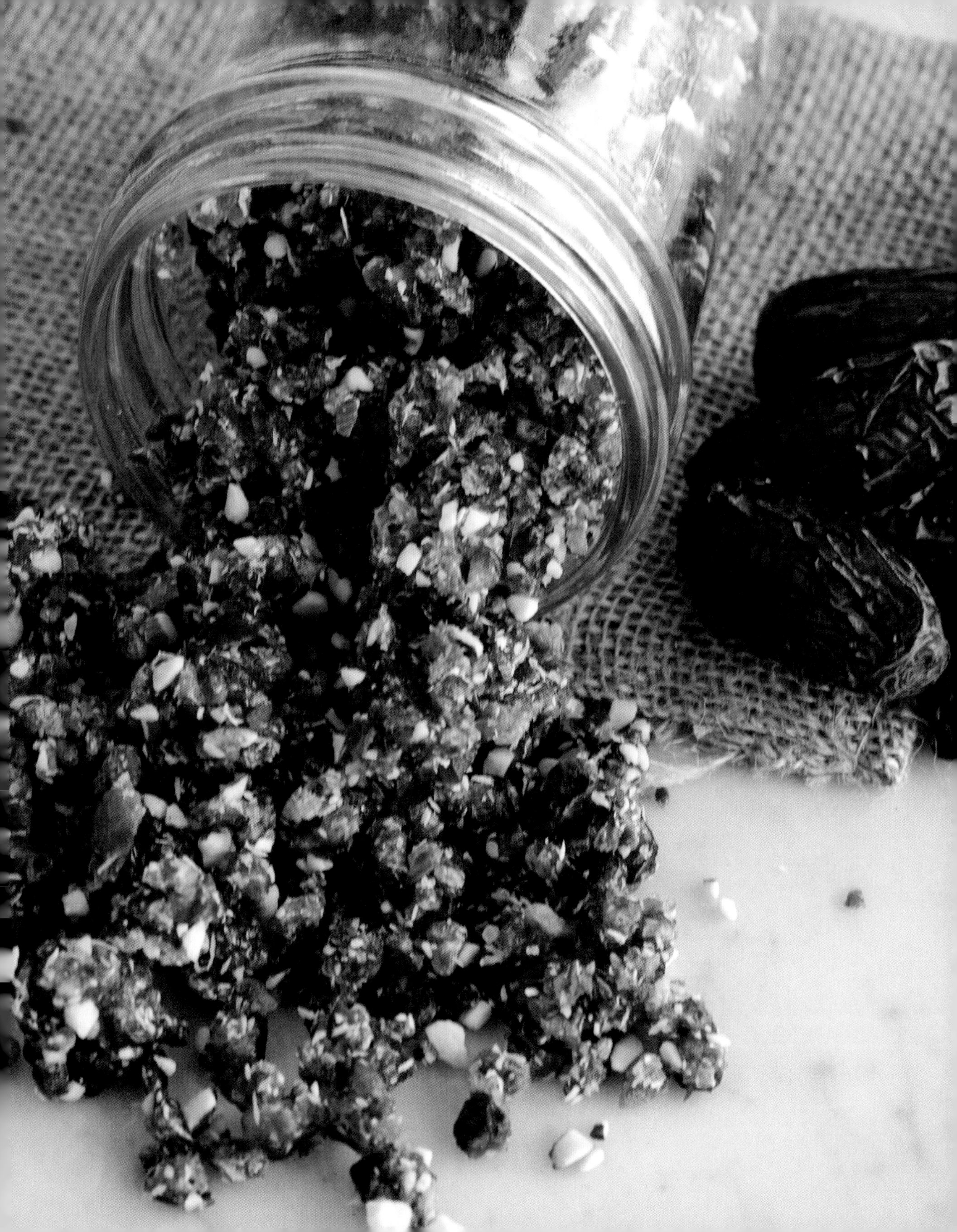

Figs

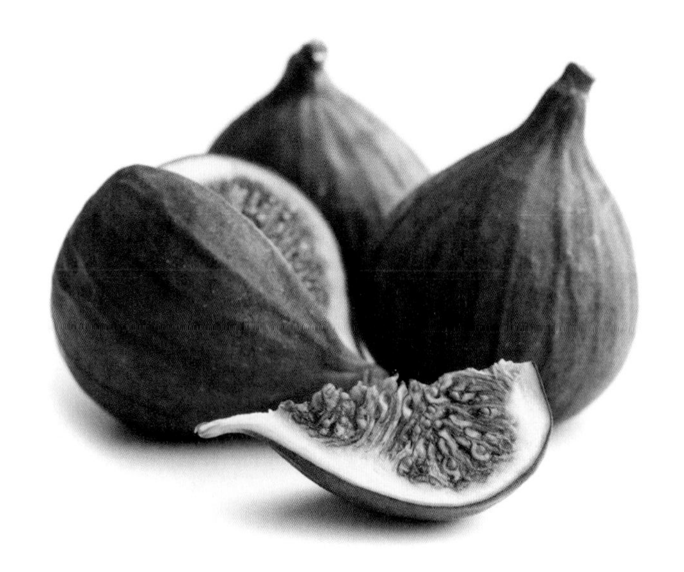

If you're seeking answers for brain and gut health, look no further than the fig. It's the ultimate tool for balancing these two intertwined aspects of well-being. Figs have unique phytochemicals that are bonded to minerals such as bioavailable potassium and sodium that specifically nourish and build neurotransmitters while also supporting neurons and synapses in the brain. It's a powerful fruit for preventing Alzheimer's, Parkinson's, dementia, and other neurological diseases, including ALS.

On the intestinal side, figs are, like dates, one of the most effective bowel-cleansing foods on the planet. The skins feed good gut bacteria and are also antiseptic, killing unproductive gut bacteria, parasites, mold, and toxic heavy metals, while the seeds get into intestinal crevices and destroy disease-causing bacteria, viruses, and fungus that hide in those pockets. The fruit's pulp and fiber massage the intestinal lining and build up the digestive immune system to help you stop struggling with stomach pain and bloating. Figs are effective in alleviating all types of gut problems, including diverticulitis, appendix inflammation, constipation, inflamed colon, and complications from *C. difficile*.

Figs are high in vitamins such as the B vitamins, which are specifically bonded to phytochemicals to reduce radiation in the body. Also abundant in trace minerals, micronutrients, antioxidants, and more, figs are a wonder food for all manner of ills; they should never be overlooked. The next time you're dealing with any health issue, think of figs as your secret weapon.

CONDITIONS

If you have any of the following conditions, try bringing figs into your life:

Alzheimer's disease, Parkinson's disease, dementia, amyotrophic lateral sclerosis (ALS), diverticulitis, Wilson's disease, attention-deficit/hyperactivity disorder (ADHD), epilepsy, *Salmonella* poisoning, stroke, posttraumatic stress disorder (PTSD), multiple myeloma, lymphoma (including non-Hodgkin's), ovarian cancer, colon cancer, heart disease, bone cancer, chronic diarrhea, appendix inflammation, dyslexia, gallstones, urinary tract infections (UTIs), postural tachycardia syndrome (POTS), neuropathy, *E. coli* infection, celiac disease, Crohn's disease, eczema, psoriasis, hepatitis A, hepatitis B, hepatitis C, hepatitis D, megacolon, small intestinal bacterial overgrowth (SIBO), Morton's neuroma

SYMPTOMS

If you have any of the following symptoms, try bringing figs into your life:

Chest pain, sciatica, sacroiliac (SI) joint pain, rectal pain, lightheadedness, nausea, shortness of breath, torn knee cartilage, hearing loss, blurred vision, enlarged spleen, hemorrhaging, clogged veins and/or arteries, constipation, itching, trigeminal neuralgia, scar tissue in the liver, nerve inflammation, appendix inflammation, liver adhesions, sinus issues, sinus pain, blood toxicity, brain fog

EMOTIONAL SUPPORT

Figs are beneficial to relieve emotional wounds formed from feelings of being excluded. On the flip side, they help you make wise choices about whom to exclude from your own life. They also reduce feelings of animosity; when you're approaching someone you suspect will be hostile toward you, bring figs as a peace offering. And when you've just heard shocking news or experienced upheaval, figs can support your body through the trauma and reduce the upset's aftereffects. If you struggle with moodiness, gloom, disappointment, or you go in and out of funks, turn to figs to help lighten your emotional load.

SPIRITUAL LESSON

Have you ever known someone who was quick to fly off the handle, to react with emotions in challenging situations, then later regretted her or his words and actions? Have you ever known someone who didn't speak up at the right times because she or he was overwhelmed by doubt and fear? Have you ever experienced these scenarios yourself? The key to overcoming these states—this spiritual disconnect between head and gut—is to connect with the equilibrium of the fig tree, whose roots are just as strong and far-reaching as her boughs.

The fig tree is a landmark of wisdom. Unlike other trees, which are governed by the chance nature of pollination and nutrient uptake—and can therefore underproduce or overproduce fruit—each fig tree has a built-in intelligence that decides how many figs the tree will yield and the order in which the tree will bear them. Fig trees are wise enough to grow tall and wide, producing an abundance of food so that plenty of people can nourish themselves from the bounty. And under the surface, fig trees possess deep-reaching roots surrounded by powerful and protective beneficial microorganisms that balance the pH of the clays at that level in the earth, allowing the root hairs to absorb nutrients that other trees can't.

In other words, figs don't just balance the physical health of our brains and digestive systems; they're also a model of balance themselves. When we take their fruit into our bodies, they promote metaphysical balance between our heads and guts. Those of us who react only with our heads, who don't think before words we can't take back come out of our mouths, gain grounding. Those of us who react only with our guts, who overthink ourselves out of having a voice, learn to express ourselves at the right time.

TIPS

- To connect with everything figs can offer you, both nutrient-wise and metaphysically, count the number of figs you eat—just as the fig tree counts each of its fruits. Try to end the day on a nine (or one of its multiples). Nine is the number of completion, signaling that you've completed maximum absorption of the figs' nutrients—and also received a full transmission of spiritual knowledge from the fig tree.
- Munching on a celery stick (rich in mineral salts) with each fig you eat is a perfect nutritional combination.
- When eating a fig, imagine the tree it came from standing in front of you. This will amplify its healing, grounding power.

FIG AND "GOAT CHEESE" SALAD

Makes 2 servings

It's hard to improve upon the perfection of a fig that is bursting with ripeness. This salad is a great option when you're ready to change things up. The classic pairing of figs and goat cheese is given a new twist with a raw macadamia "cheese" and the brightness of fresh lemon juice. Enjoy this timeless salad over long summer evenings as you relax with friends and family.

4 cups arugula
½ pound fresh figs
½ cup raw macadamia nuts
1 lemon, juiced
½ teaspoon olive oil
1 dime-size sliver of garlic
2 teaspoons raw honey (optional)

Divide the arugula onto 2 plates. Slice the figs and arrange on the plates atop the arugula. Blend the macadamia nuts, half of the lemon juice, the olive oil, and the garlic until smooth. Add water, if needed (as little as possible). Crumble the macadamia "cheese" over the salad plates. Serve topped with a squeeze of fresh lemon juice and a drizzle of raw honey, if desired.

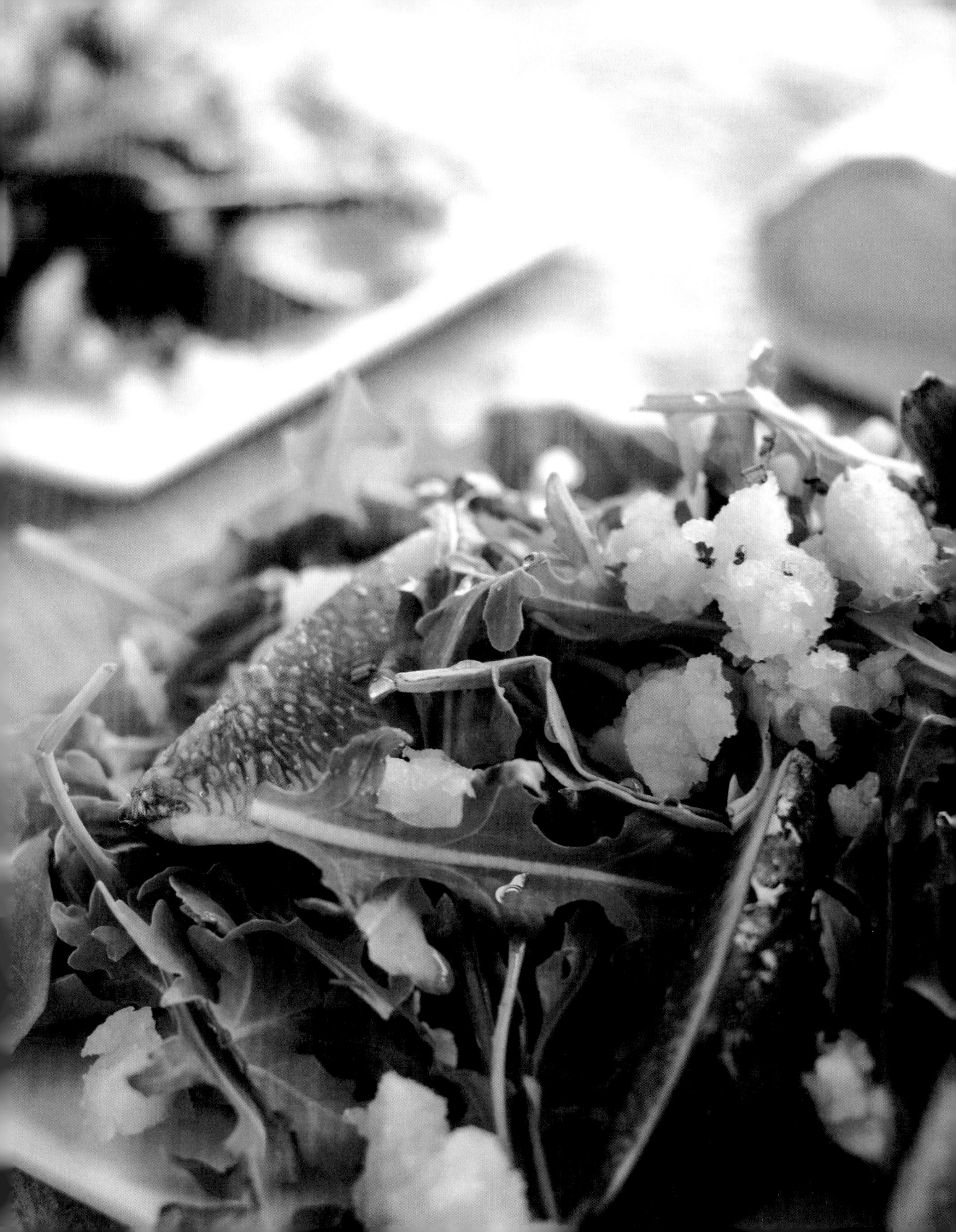

Grapes

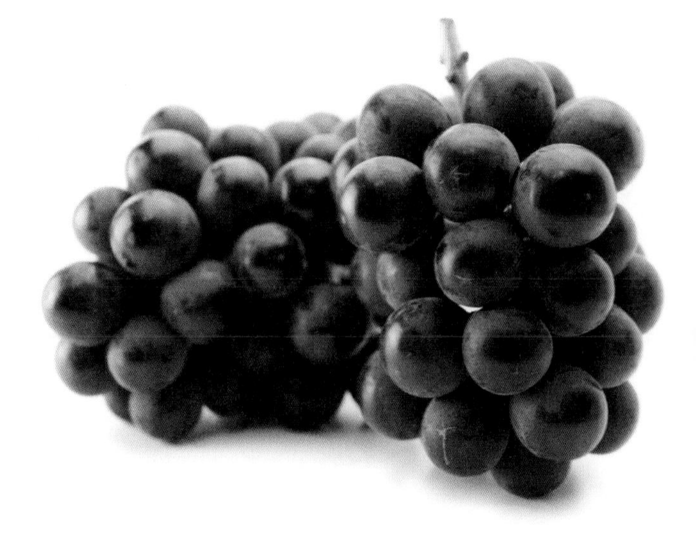

Grapes should not be misunderstood as being too high in carbs, sugar, or calories to be good for us. It's just the opposite. Like bananas, grapes are a first-rate fruit that promotes wellness of the highest level. And grapes are less sweet than we think; they are more defined by tartness, which is a key medicinal quality. That sourness indicates the presence of phytochemicals critical to kidney function. If you've ever heard that you have elevated creatinine levels, this means your kidneys have become compromised in their ability to remove and excrete waste products from the bloodstream. Grapes are the ultimate kidney tonic—their phytochemicals bind onto waste that the kidneys have trouble filtering.

Many people are also concerned about liver health. Like cherries, grapes are an amazing liver-cleansing food. Their phytochemicals are able to dislodge debris, processed food, and by-products that can clog up lobules in the liver. And for those looking for digestive benefits, grape skins hold powerful micronutrients that expel parasites, mold, and other unproductive fungus from the intestinal tract. Further, antioxidants such as malvidin and other anthocyanins (which explain grapes' blue, black, dark red, and purple shades) give grapes the power to help fight and prevent most types of cancer.

Grapes are an amazing food to fight the Unforgiving Four: they expel radiation from the body; their amino acids such as histidine, methionine, and cysteine work together with their anthocyanins to become a magnet that draws DDT and toxic heavy metals out of the liver, kidneys, spleen, and other organs; plus they're a potent antiviral for autoimmune disease, which is caused by the viral explosion.

Finally, grapes are an outstanding energy food. They offer a critical boost, whether you're an athlete, constantly on the go, or you're a thinker—that is, engaging your brain all day with cognitive tasks (and multitasking), trying to excel at a given project, or in need of fuel to come up with your next big idea.

CONDITIONS

If you have any of the following conditions, try bringing grapes into your life:

Bacterial gastroenteritis, mold exposure, macular degeneration, hypertension, hypertension-related kidney disease, creatinine issues with the kidneys, kidney stones, gallstones, hypoglycemia, attention-deficit/hyperactivity disorder (ADHD), autism, breast cancer, diabetes, metastatic brain tumors, sepsis, pancreatic cancer, endometriosis, bronchitis, *E. coli* infection, mystery infertility, fatty liver, hepatitis C, nodules, depression, colon cancer, edema, anemia, sleep disorders, fibromyalgia, chronic fatigue syndrome (CFS), multiple sclerosis (MS), neurological disorders, autonomic neuropathy, hemorrhoids, herpes simplex 1 (HSV-1), herpes simplex 2 (HSV-2), hepatitis C, hepatitis B, *H. pylori* infection, fibroids, common colds, vertigo, low reproductive system battery, all autoimmune diseases and disorders, bacterial infections

SYMPTOMS

If you have any of the following symptoms, try bringing grapes into your life:

Food allergies, palm sweats, emotional eating, dizziness, nausea, Bell's palsy, shortness of breath, hearing loss, tremors, body odor, chest pain, premenstrual syndrome (PMS) symptoms, confusion, brain fog, cough, backache, inflammation, myelin nerve damage, scar tissue in the liver, blood toxicity, fatigue, brain lesions, hot flashes, hair loss, congestion, brittle nails, blurry eyes, ringing or buzzing in the ears, food allergies, food sensitivities, sensations of humming or vibration in the body

EMOTIONAL SUPPORT

Grapes help when you're feeling emotionally broken, lifting your spirits and encouraging a jovial, lighthearted outlook on life. They can prevent you from becoming wounded if you're ever falsely accused of a misdeed and promote healing when you feel excluded in social situations. If you ever feel disappointed that you weren't chosen for a certain project or job, go out and buy some grapes—they can help you forge ahead and create new opportunities.

And if you're someone who's reluctant about change, passing up opportunities and later regretting it, embrace grapes in your diet and feel the transformation as you're able to be braver and take advantage of the special moments life presents. Finally, offer grapes to friends and family members who seem aloof, adrift, or complacent; over time, this fruit can help alter their direction and improve their behavior.

SPIRITUAL LESSON

When you feel isolated—living your life with little interaction or coping with shyness and yet yearning for a sense of belonging with a group that accepts you—make grapes a part of your life. Remember, grapes are bunched together. As each cluster grows on the vine, the little globes stay close to each other, connecting on both a physical and metaphysical level. Each grape adjusts to fit perfectly into place with those around it. Focus on this wonder when you select and eat grapes. It will create a sacred intention, prepare you consciously and subconsciously to find your people, and point you toward your true home.

TIPS

- We tend to overlook raisins. Don't let their humble status fool you. Raisins are more powerful for your health than goji berries!
- Try this recipe for fresh grape jelly: In the food processor, combine Concord grapes, raw honey to taste, and a squeeze of lemon as preservative. The sugar from the honey extracts healing phytochemicals from the tart, medicinal skin of the grapes, making these nutrients bioavailable and delivering them deep into your vital organs.
- When preparing organic grapes to eat, simply give them a gentle rinse. The residue on organic grapes is actually beneficial, because it's filled with the elevated biotics we looked at in the "Adaptation" chapter.

GRAPE SLUSHY

Makes 2 servings

Easy to make and incredibly delicious, this ice-cold slushy is the perfect way to make use of grapes and coconut water when you have them. You'll want to come back to this recipe over and over again.

4 cups frozen* grapes
3 cups coconut water

Blend the frozen grapes and the coconut water in a blender until well combined. Serve and enjoy.

*Fresh grapes may be used in place of frozen if you don't want an icy drink. Reduce the coconut water to 2 cups.

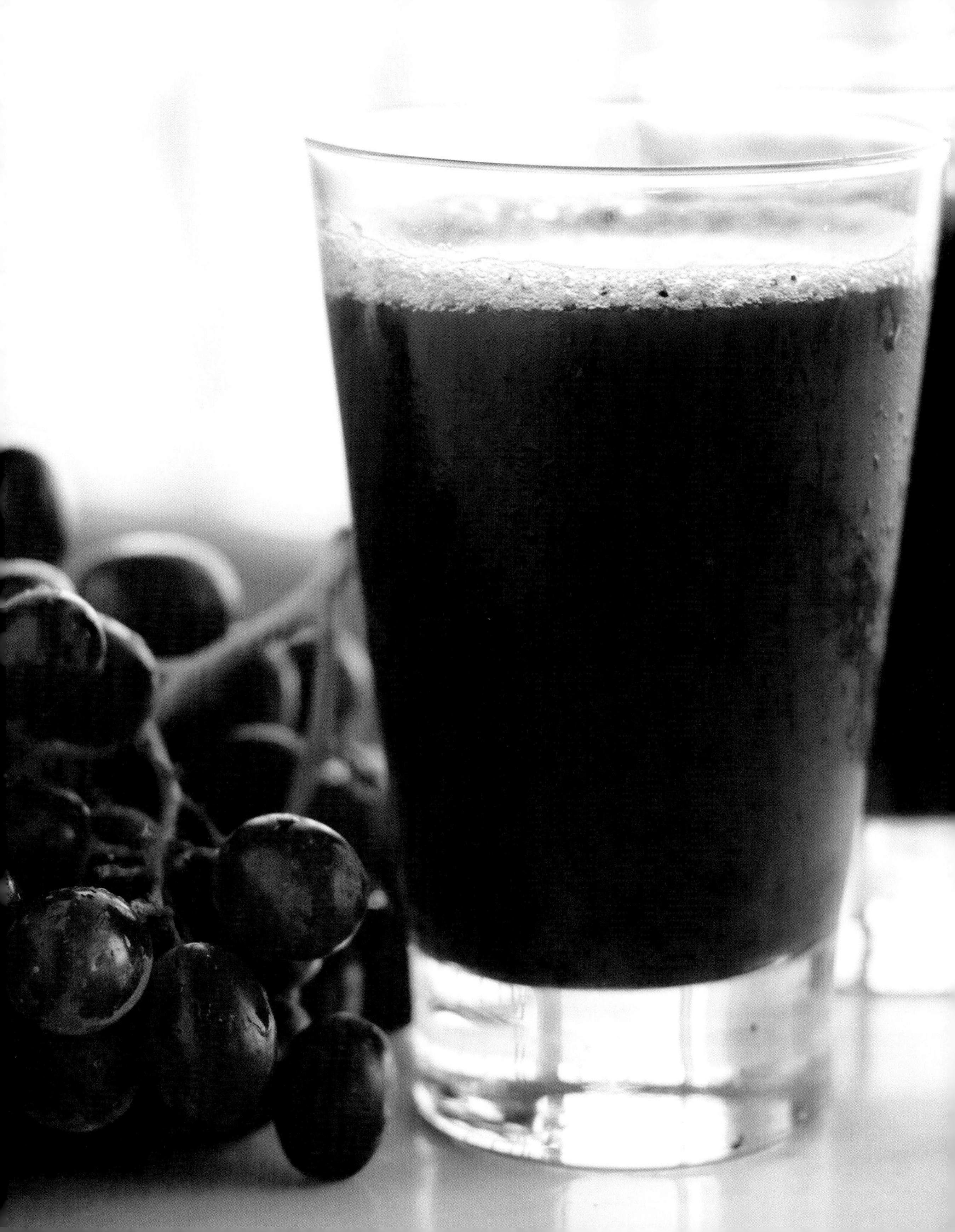

Kiwis

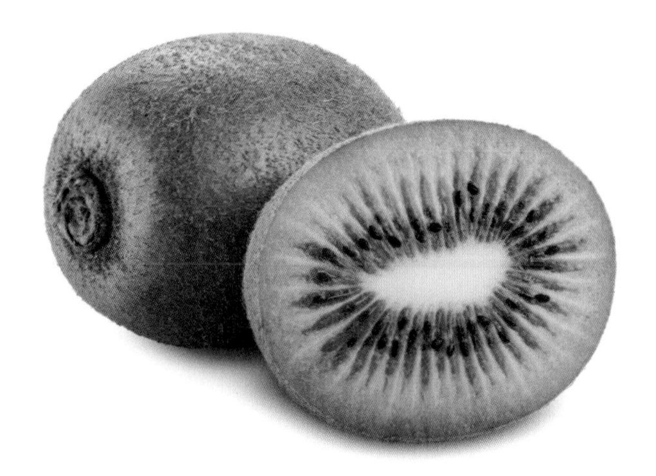

If you're concerned about regulating blood sugar, turn to kiwis for support. Kiwis are an amazing food for diabetes, hypoglycemia, and hyperglycemia. Whether your blood sugar levels are too low or too high, eating this fruit will bring you back to center as it simultaneously lowers fat in the bloodstream. Imbalanced blood sugar levels also often tie into moodiness, OCD, depression, and difficulty controlling emotions. Kiwis are the ultimate companion in these situations, because they offer a high-quality sugar source—that is, valuable bioavailable glucose to feed the neurons in your brain and alleviate your distress. Kiwis are an amazing food for stress assistance.

With over 40 trace minerals, kiwis are an excellent source of nourishment. Kiwis also possess a powerful vitamin C that's bonded to isothiocyanates and anthocyanins; this compound works in congruence with the phenolic acid compounds in kiwi seeds to remove radiation from the body and inhibit viruses.

Kiwis are also fantastic to help alleviate digestive disorders and discomfort, including acid reflux, Barrett's esophagus, gas, abdominal pain, and bloating—conditions and symptoms that are often related to low hydrochloric acid levels in the stomach. Kiwis' plethora of amino acids (including serine, leucine, and lysine) raise those hydrochloric acid levels to provide welcome relief. Further, the amino acids are bonded to enzymes and coenzymes, helping to strengthen the digestive system even more, so it can keep unproductive bacteria, viruses, parasites, yeast, mold, and other disruptive fungus at bay.

CONDITIONS

If you have any of the following conditions, try bringing kiwis into your life:

Knee bursitis, gout, rheumatoid arthritis (RA), Sjögren's syndrome, systemic lupus, athlete's foot, prostatitis, adrenal fatigue, Barrett's esophagus, obsessive-compulsive disorder (OCD), depression, mitral valve prolapse, chronic bronchitis, diabetes, hypoglycemia, hyperglycemia, endometriosis, autism, attention-deficit/hyperactivity disorder (ADHD), *Salmonella* poisoning, jaundice, human immunodeficiency virus (HIV), *H. pylori* infection, eye infections, small intestinal bacterial overgrowth (SIBO), sepsis, neuropathy

SYMPTOMS

If you have any of the following symptoms, try bringing kiwis into your life:

Anal itching, belching, bloating, abdominal pain, acid reflux, gastritis, constipation, flatulence, blood in the urine, diarrhea, tongue issues, ringing or buzzing in the ears, moodiness, pinched nerves, dandruff, fatigue, seizures, appendix inflammation, sacroiliac joint pain, pins and needles, heart palpitations, nerve inflammation, loss of libido, low cortisol, high cortisol, joint inflammation, low hydrochloric acid, intestinal spasms, inflamed spleen, inflammation, fluid retention, chronic loose stools

EMOTIONAL SUPPORT

Offer kiwis to a friend or loved one who you wish would be more appreciative and considerate. And when you're trying to bring those qualities out in yourself, kiwis are a go-to tool. When you're working with someone whose mood changes are unpredictable and problematic, bring along a few kiwis for the two of you to snack on. If you're the only one who partakes, you'll still serve the situation, as the kiwis will feed your enthusiasm and vibrancy to help influence and override your co-worker's emotions.

SPIRITUAL LESSON

It's easy to get caught up in our day-to-day lives. We put blinders on that block out a larger sense of what's around us, distance ourselves from a true sense of who we are, and our worlds become shallow. Kiwis counteract all that.

The next time you slice a kiwi in half, study what you see inside. It's like looking at an image of outer space! During growth, a mother kiwi vine (the female vine that bears the fruit) channels the universe's energy, depositing a snapshot of our greater surroundings into each growing kiwi. No other food contains a miraculous picture of the stars, planets, mysteries, and miracles of the world—of which our earth is just one tiny part.

Meditate on this when you enjoy kiwis. This fruit with the humble outward appearance that opens to reveal a galaxy opens us up, too. Consciously and subconsciously, we can disconnect from the annoyances that keep us mired down and closed off. We can remember the vastness of the universe, the depths we ourselves contain, and shock ourselves out of the shallows of our daily lives so that we can find our purpose and connect to the secrets of existence.

TIPS

- To feel the full effect of what this fruit can do for you, eat kiwi three times a day for one week. Think of it as an emotional, physical, and spiritual supplement, taking one at 9 A.M., noon, and 3 P.M. For those seven days, journal the changes that occur: the differences you feel, the epiphanies, and all the other revelations.
- Keep your kiwis in a bowl on your nightstand. This will enhance the emotional aspects that the kiwi can impart. Sleeping beside the ripening fruits will intimately connect them with your being, deepening their effects on every level so they can have the most life-changing results.

KIWI SKEWERS WITH STRAWBERRY-DATE SAUCE

Makes 2 to 4 servings

These beautiful kiwi skewers are easy to make and a hit with both kids and adults. They're fun and festive and perfect for any occasion. The strawberry-date sauce is the perfect way to take the sweet perfection of this pretty snack over the top.

6 kiwis
1 mango, cubed
1 cup raspberries
1 cup strawberries
1 cup dates, pitted
8 wooden skewers

Peel and slice the kiwis. Arrange the kiwi slices, mango cubes, and raspberries on skewers as desired. For the sauce, place the strawberries and dates in a blender and blend until smooth.

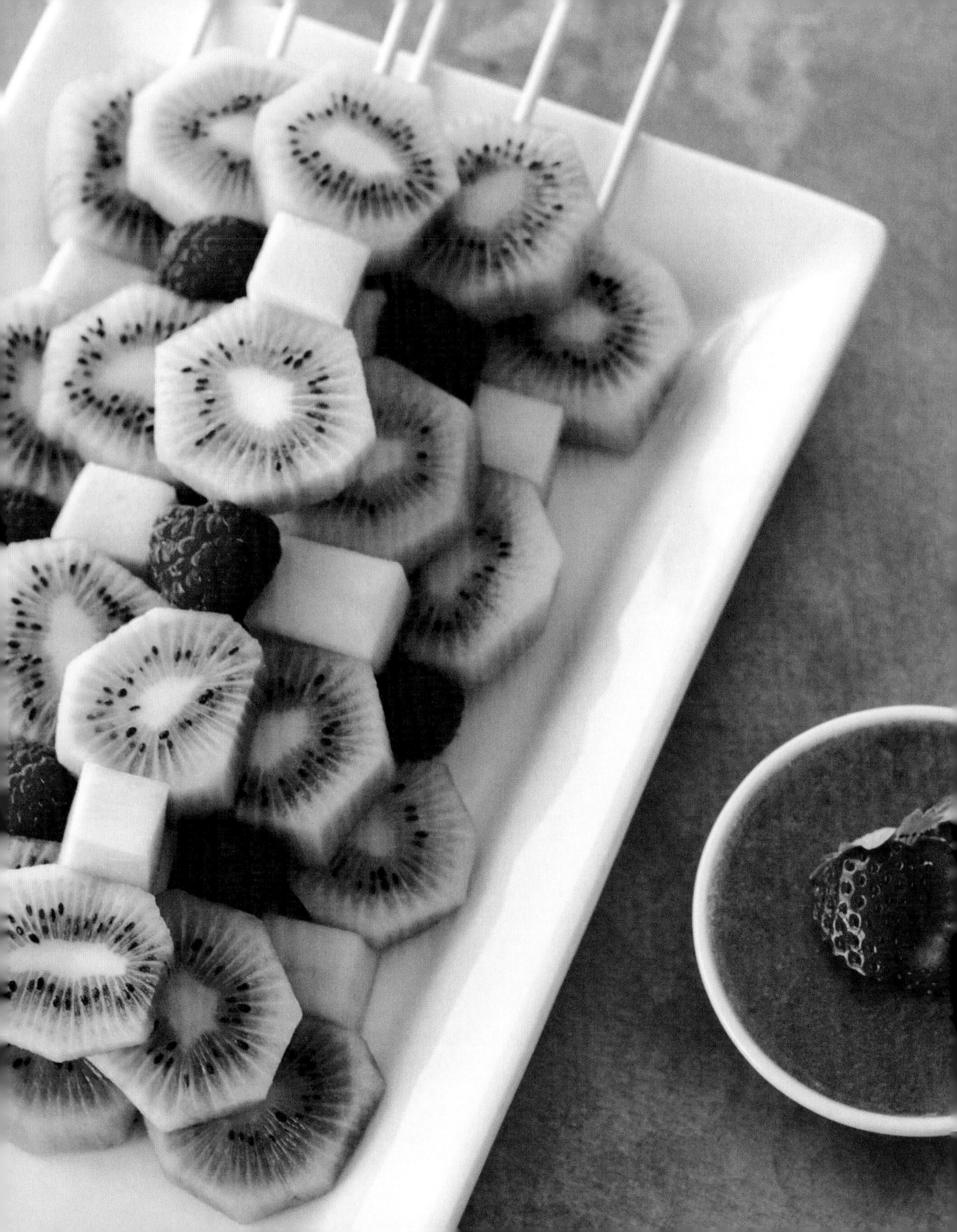

Lemons & Limes

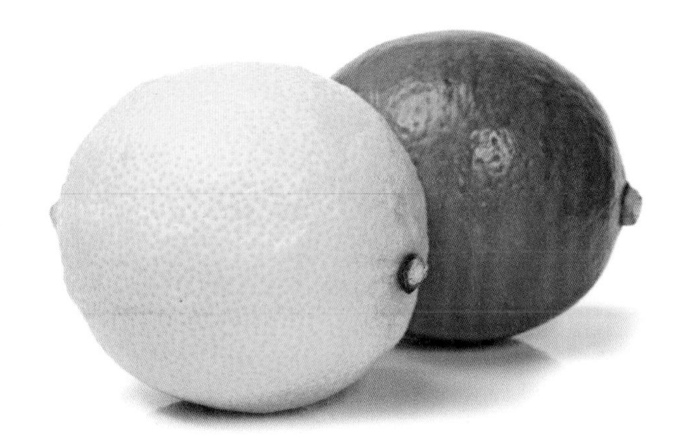

Without lemons, the world would be a completely different place. Imagine childhood without lemonade, a sore throat without lemon-honey tea, or summer without lemony baked goods. It's true for limes, too—think of life without guacamole, key lime pie, and limeade. Lemons and limes are an essential part of our human fabric, woven through from ancient to modern times. Is it just their taste that we love so much, though, or is it more than that? Could it be the remarkable healing power of lemons and limes that's drawn us to them throughout the ages?

The roots of lemon and lime trees go deep into the earth, extracting dozens of precious trace minerals that get passed onto you when you consume the fruits. Lemons and limes are ultrahydrating and electrolyte-producing, because they are a top source of mineral salts and trace mineral salts. Traces of bioavailable sodium in lemons and limes are a driving force in the value they offer our bodies.

These citrus siblings have some of the most highly absorbable vitamin C around. And you often hear people concerned about where to get their calcium. Look no further than fresh-squeezed lemon or lime, which offers bioactive calcium that your body craves. Plus, phytochemicals called limonoids in lemons and limes actually bond the vitamin C and calcium together, so that wherever one goes in the body, the other rides along. This enhances the bioavailability of each, and also creates alkalinity in the body to help prevent the growth of almost every type of cancer. The antioxidant flavonoids in lemons and limes are another ally in fighting disease. And when you're dealing with a cold, flu, bronchitis, or pneumonia, lemon is one of the most effective mucus expellers you can find. Lemons and limes are also amazing cleansers of the liver, kidneys, spleen, thyroid, and gallbladder. They purge the many toxic substances we collect from exposure to plastics, synthetic chemicals, radiation, and poor food choices.

When going through any sort of detox process, even if it's just increasing the amount of fruits and vegetables in your diet, it's a good idea to drink lemon or lime water first thing in the morning. Going through detox without drinking enough water is like taking the trash to the curb with no waste-management service to pick it up. Once detoxification has drawn the gunk out of your cells and tissues (your liver does much of its work overnight), it needs to be flushed out when you wake up—otherwise, those toxins settle back in. Lemon or lime water is more beneficial for this process than plain water, because filtration has often taken the life out of drinking water, and these citrus stars reawaken its healing abilities.

CONDITIONS

If you have any of the following conditions, try bringing lemons and/or limes into your life:

Urinary tract infections (UTIs), staph infections, kidney disease, kidney stones, gallstones, pancreatitis, rosacea, conjunctivitis, pneumonia, bronchitis, obesity, multiple sclerosis (MS), rheumatoid arthritis (RA), mystery infertility, diabetes, adrenal fatigue, influenza, nutrient absorption issues, human immunodeficiency virus (HIV), head colds, herpes, acne, all types of cancer, strep throat, low reproductive system battery, atrial fibrillation, chronic ear infections, hepatitis C, anxiety, migraines, insomnia, hypertension

SYMPTOMS

If you have any of the following symptoms, try bringing lemons and/or limes into your life:

Muscle pain, postnasal drip, earache, *Candida* overgrowth, digestive discomfort, acid reflux, toothache, fever, dry mouth, excess mucus, nausea, unquenchable thirst, arrhythmia, food allergies, vaginal discharge, sinus discharge, low hydrochloric acid, vomiting, weight gain, cough, headaches, tremors, heartburn, belching, blood sugar imbalances, blurred vision, fluid retention, head pain, high cortisol, appendix inflammation, nervousness, dehydration

EMOTIONAL SUPPORT

Lemon or lime is the ideal soother when you've been rattled by difficult news. These wonder fruits can alter feelings of sadness, distress, and worry, helping to lift the spirits, lighten the heart, and reverse melancholy during troubled times.

SPIRITUAL LESSON

If you look at the branches of a lemon or lime tree, you'll see thorns. This is because these trees are extremely protective and want to ensure that only the most deserving and careful people harvest their fruit—and only slowly, over time. You can't just go mindlessly picking a lemon or lime tree bare; it takes mindful appreciation to gather each fruit.

The same is true of human relationships. You may have observed that some people have their guards up—they're prickly—or you may have heard this about yourself. Like thorns on a lemon or lime tree, this self-protectiveness is a natural defense mechanism we use to prevent others from coming in and only taking. What we really want, just like lemon and lime trees, is a fruitful relationship of mutual respect, admiration, and symbiosis with those around us. Sometimes it takes a little poke to remind us to take care with each other.

TIPS

- If there's someone important in your life and you'd like to see your relationship continue to develop, sit down together and drink tea with lemon. This will enhance conversation, allowing you both to open up and further your involvement.
- Try drinking two 16-ounce glasses of water (with half a lemon or lime squeezed into each) just after waking up, then give your liver half an hour to clean up before eating breakfast.
- Though you may think you should avoid getting citrus in a cut, fresh lemon or lime juice squeezed on a small cut or abrasion is a powerful disinfecting, antibacterial aid; it can even prevent staph infections.
- Contrary to popular belief, lemon and lime juice is excellent for oral health. Dilute the juice with some water to make the best antibacterial mouthwash and gum cleanser.
- If you have difficulty sleeping, a cup of warm water with raw honey and lemon or lime juice squeezed into it can calm busy electrical impulses and neurotransmitters, and aid in a restful sleep.

LEMON SORBET

Makes 3 to 4 servings

It doesn't get any more refreshing than a lemon sorbet with a hint of honey and sage. This sorbet is so easy to bring together and keeps well in the freezer for up to three weeks. Enjoy it as an after-dinner treat or a sweet palate cleanser any time of day.

¾ cup honey

3 sage leaves

1½ cups water

1 cup fresh-squeezed lemon juice (from about 6 lemons)

1 tablespoon lemon zest

Combine the honey, sage leaves, and 1½ cups water in a small saucepan. Warm over medium heat until the honey dissolves completely. Add the lemon juice and zest. Stir well and cool in the refrigerator. Remove the sage leaves and discard. Place the remaining mixture in an ice cream machine and process according to the manufacturer's instructions. If you don't have an ice cream machine, place the mixture in a bowl and set in the freezer; stir well every 30 minutes until the desired consistency is reached.

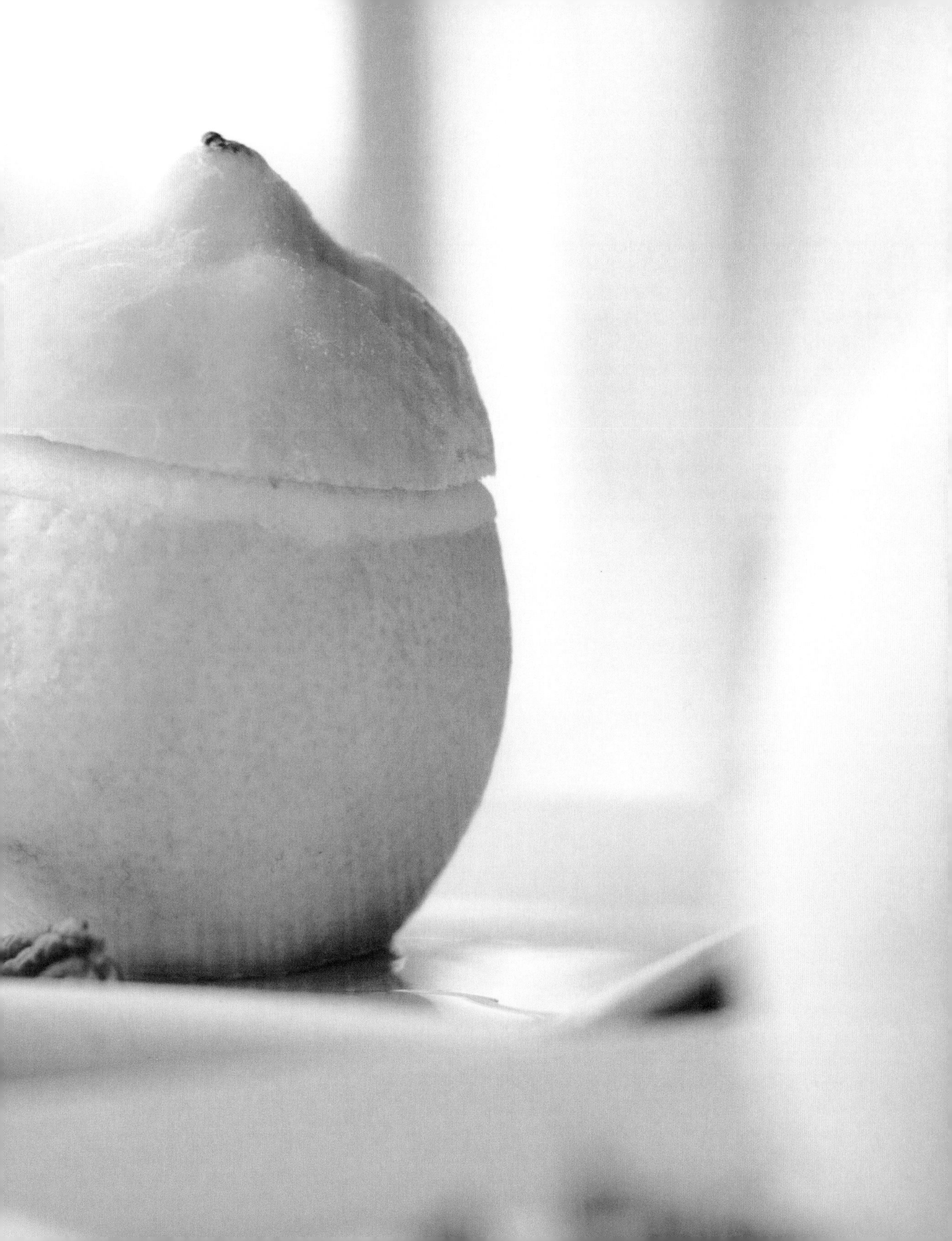

Mangoes

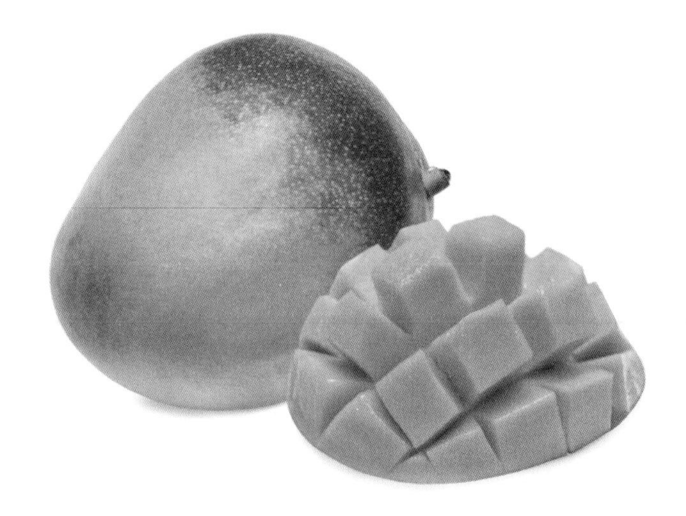

While we often think of a glass of warm milk as the go-to sleep aid, it's not a magical remedy. In reality, the combination of fat plus lactose (a form of sugar) in the milk stresses the pancreas, triggering insulin resistance, which in turn causes a false sense of sleepiness. It's just like the reaction you'll have after Thanksgiving dinner: the combination of high fat from the turkey plus processed sugar from the pumpkin pie—not the turkey's tryptophan—is what makes people's eyelids heavy after the holiday meal.

The real miracle sleep aid is mango. When you eat mango before bed, phytochemicals from the fruit, along with amino acids such as glycine, glutamine, and cysteine combined with fructose and glucose, travel to the brain and quickly restore depleted neurotransmitters. This allows most insomniacs a chance to finally get some true rest during the night.

Mangoes are also beneficial for a whole slew of other aspects of health. Wonderful for stress assistance and viral protection, mangoes are also rich in beta-carotene to strengthen and support the skin; they even help prevent all varieties of skin cancers. Mangoes are a powerful tool to help reverse hypoglycemia, prediabetes, and type 2 diabetes. Their highly bioavailable trace magnesium coupled with phytochemical phenolic acids calms the central nervous system, which aids in staving off strokes, seizures, and heart attacks. The fruit's pulp soothes the stomach and intestinal lining to alleviate constipation. And finally, mango is an amazing exercise food, because it provides your muscles with traces of sodium, preciously needed glucose, and magnesium, which translates to longer, harder workouts while feeling less of "the burn."

CONDITIONS

If you have any of the following conditions, try bringing mangoes into your life:

Gastroesophageal reflux disease (GERD), attention-deficit/hyperactivity disorder (ADHD), Alzheimer's disease, dementia, ulcers, skin cancers, insomnia, stomach cancer, renal failure, peptic ulcers, diabetes, Parkinson's disease, kidney stones, epilepsy, Graves' disease, Hashimoto's thyroiditis, glaucoma, macular degeneration, hypoglycemia, Crohn's disease, posttraumatic stress disorder (PTSD), urinary tract infections (UTIs), depression, personality disorders, anxiety, eating disorders, seasonal affective disorder (SAD), adrenal fatigue, chronic fatigue syndrome (CFS), cognitive issues, colitis, Cushing's syndrome, fibroids, fatty liver, sunburn, mystery infertility

SYMPTOMS

If you have any of the following symptoms, try bringing mangoes into your life:

Trouble sleeping, mood swings, snoring, fatigue, sluggishness, hypothyroid, hyperthyroid, blurry eyes, muscle fatigue, muscle pain, muscle cramps, anxiousness, cognitive issues, brain fog, memory loss, melancholy, listlessness, abdominal pressure, *Candida* overgrowth, Bell's palsy, colon spasms, confusion, constipation, digestive distress, brain inflammation, sluggish liver, frozen shoulder, high cholesterol, high blood pressure

EMOTIONAL SUPPORT

Mangoes are life-changing when it comes to our emotional health. Not only do they uplift the mood, they can alleviate depression and seasonal affective disorder. Mangoes are exceptionally healing for anyone who feels abandoned, cut off, forsaken, outcast, shunned, detached, lonely, hurt, left out, or let down. That's because mangoes have the power of manifestation. When we eat them, the fruit reorients us, changing our direction and opening us up to more opportunities to experience joy—which ultimately helps us connect to our destiny.

SPIRITUAL LESSON

Mangoes handle the heat like no other fruit. Even with the sun beating down on them at extreme temperatures, mangoes know how to shield themselves. When we incorporate mangoes into our lives, we internalize their inner cool. They teach us that it's possible to handle extreme situations without burning up inside. We learn how to keep calm and collected when we're up against immense stress—how to stop ourselves from becoming hotheaded and angry when the heat is on. The next time you're facing an intense situation, find a mango to snack on, or add frozen mango to a smoothie. As you take it into your body, remind yourself that this powerful tool will help you face the tough circumstance like never before.

TIPS

- For noticeable results, eat two mangoes a day.
- If you want a deeper sleep with spiritually enhanced dreams, eat mango before bed. It's the best way to prime yourself for a revelation come morning.
- While mangoes on their own can help you sleep, if you eat them with celery sticks or on a salad, it shifts their energy to do the opposite for you. The combination of mango plus greens eaten later in the day can give you a second wind when you need to stay up late working on a project.
- For a longer-lasting workout and better recovery, have mango before any type of exercise.
- If you're meditating to resolve an issue, try eating mango beforehand. It will help connect you to the insights you need.

MANGO LASSI

Makes 1 to 2 servings

This mango lassi is the perfect way to treat your taste buds. The version here uses coconut milk and mango together in a silky, rich combination. The cardamom gives an authentic twist to the classic drink, though use it sparingly if you're not used to the complex flavor of the spice.

4 cups diced mango
½ cup coconut milk
2 mint leaves
1 frozen banana
Pinch of cardamom (optional)*

Place all the ingredients in a blender and blend until smooth. Serve and enjoy!

*Cardamom has a very distinctive and strong flavor; use sparingly or omit if desired.

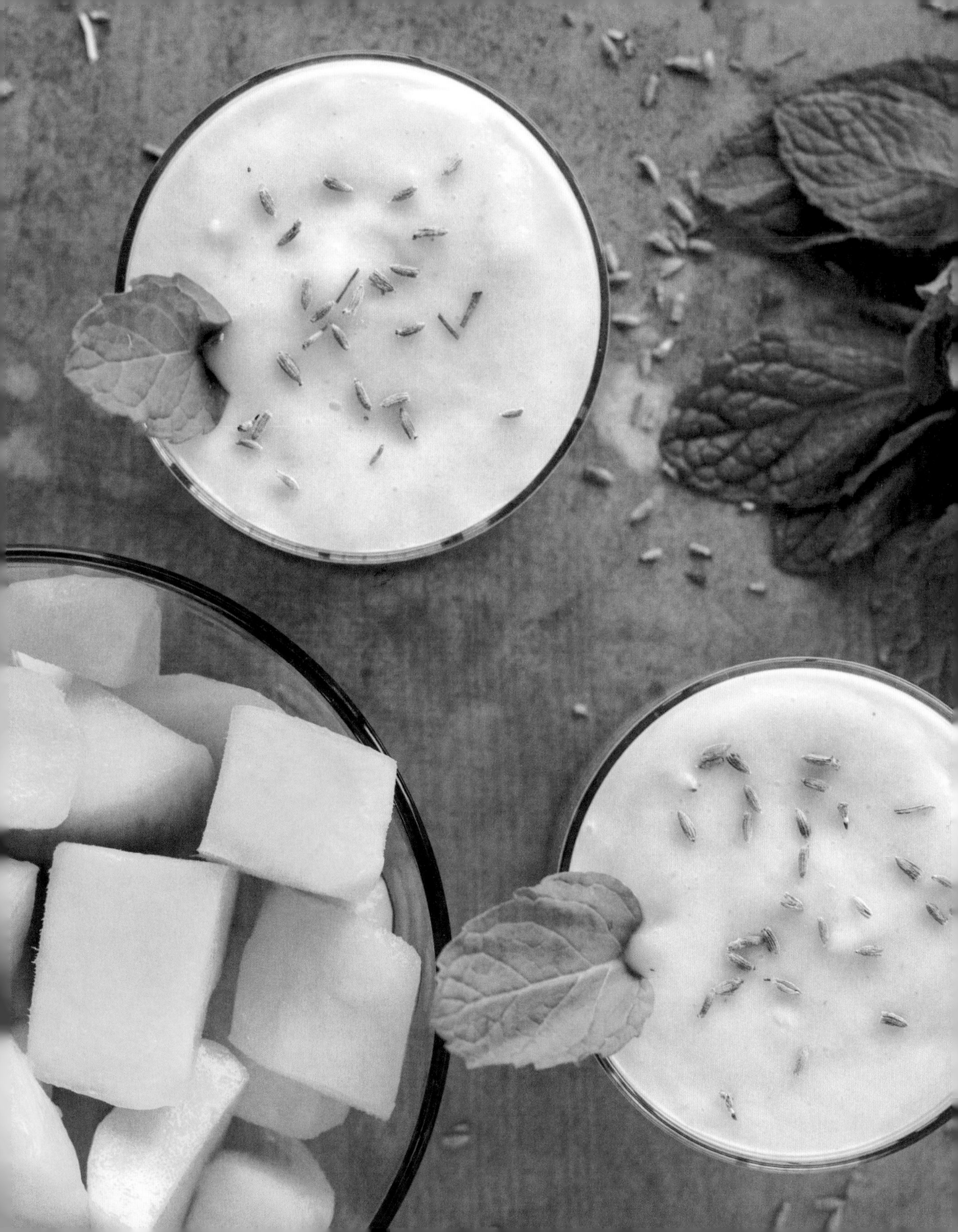

Melons

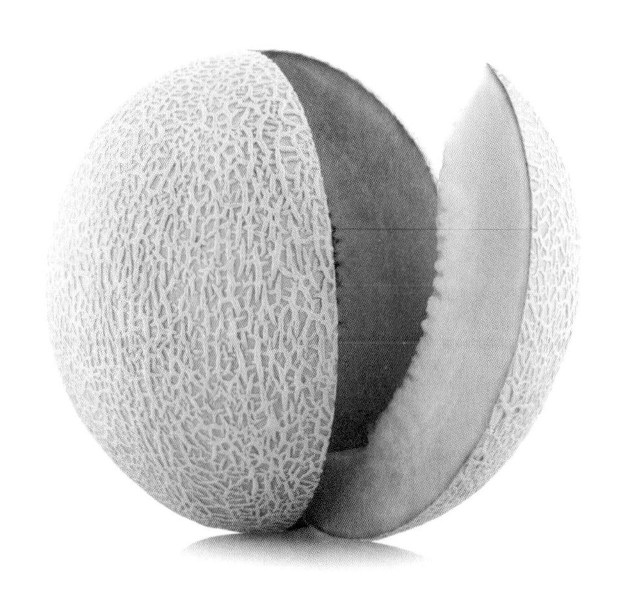

Melons are so critical to the healing process that when someone is struggling with a health condition and can't get better, the outcome may very well hinge on whether or not melon is part of her or his diet. Watermelon, honeydew, cantaloupe, crenshaw, canary, Santa Claus, galia, charentais, casaba—they are all keys to the palace of health. Ask yourself how many melons you've consumed in the past year. It may be hard to figure out, because you're probably used to having a slice here, a bite there, often alongside other food. For most people, the answer is that over the past 12 months, they've only eaten one melon in total, if that.

This is a major loss. Why? Because melons are made just for us by God and the Earthly Mother. They are like mother's milk, only one step further, because melons are predigested—meaning that melon flesh is so assimilable that our digestive systems barely need to process it when it enters the body, because it is so high in enzymes and certain coenzymes as yet undiscovered by science that strengthen them. The fructose in melon leaves the stomach in less than one minute, then the rest of the fruit drops directly into the intestinal tract, immediately fortifying and replenishing the body. Eating melon is like getting intravenous nutrient therapy.

On every level, including biochemically, melon is exactly what our bodies need. Melons are essentially balls of purified water. This highly active fluid binds onto poisons of all kinds in the body, including mold, mycotoxins, viral neurotoxins, undigested protein toxins, ammonia gas, and bacterial toxins, flushing them out to allow the immune system to restore itself. Further, the fruit's high electrolyte content helps protect the brain and the rest of the nervous system from stress-related strokes, aneurysms, and embolisms. Melon thins the blood and reduces heart attack risk, helps prevent heart disease and vascular issues, and can even reduce liver and kidney disease—if someone is suffering from liver or kidney malfunction, melon can mean the difference between life and death. The water in melon is nearly identical to our blood, and its sodium, potassium, and glucose are also abundant and bioavailable, making melon one of the most hydrating foods you can eat. This hydration is critical, as it helps to lower high blood pressure, among other benefits.

Melon is one of the most alkalizing foods. The fruit's highly bioavailable and bioactive trace mineral count is responsible for driving electrolytes higher than normal, making them easily usable by the body. In return, the body's detoxification processes become amplified, driving out traces of DDT, other pesticides, herbicides, and heavy metals from deep within the organs. High in silica, melon is an excellent food to restore ligaments, joints, bones, teeth, connective tissue, and tendons. Melon is also one of the most powerful glucose balancers, working to prevent insulin resistance and lower elevated A1C levels.

CONDITIONS

If you have any of the following conditions, try bringing melons into your life:

Mystery infertility, Crohn's disease, colitis, peptic ulcers, Barrett's esophagus, irritable bowel syndrome (IBS), low reproductive system battery, aneurysm, embolism, stroke, heart attack, heart disease, liver disease, cirrhosis of the liver, liver cancer, kidney disease, breast cancer, pancreatic cancer, pancreatitis, tendonitis, epilepsy, sepsis, osteoporosis, *H. pylori* infection, multiple sclerosis (MS), amyotrophic lateral sclerosis (ALS), Sjögren's syndrome, Addison's disease, Parkinson's disease, obsessive-compulsive disorder (OCD), attention-deficit/hyperactivity disorder (ADHD), posttraumatic stress disorder (PTSD), diabetes, hypoglycemia, acne, depression, anxiety, herpes infection, urinary tract infections (UTIs), transient ischemic attack (TIA), heavy metal toxicity, *E. coli* infection, yeast infections, mold exposure

SYMPTOMS

If you have any of the following symptoms, try bringing melons into your life:

Constipation, low hydrochloric acid, stomach pain, upset stomach, poor circulation, accelerated aging, dental issues, food allergies, connective tissue inflammation, tremors, shakes, seizures, weakness, blood sugar imbalances, chronic dehydration, acidosis, joint pain, bone density issues, kidney pain, back pain, spasms, twitches, slurred speech, blurry eyes, inflammation, food sensitivities, anal itching, blisters, blood toxicity, insulin resistance, brain fog, body stiffness, brittle nails, chronic nausea, fever, itchy skin, leg cramps

EMOTIONAL SUPPORT

If you are easily frightened, having a difficult time bearing bad news, or dealing with a heavy load due to emotional sensitivities or PTSD, melons can come to your aid by shifting you out of any nervousness, skittishness, anxiety, or uneasiness. And if you're eagerly awaiting news, melons can give you the extra support and patience you need during the process. Offer melon to a friend or family member who you feel has no patience, or whose judgments and opinions are stumbling blocks. Your gift could ease that person's energy and open up a channel so that she or he becomes more accepting.

SPIRITUAL LESSON

The predigestion miracle of melon teaches us that powerful processes can be in play without us even realizing. We don't have to fight tooth and nail for every good thing in life. Sometimes good comes to us without our labor: Powerful healing takes place in our bodies, spirits, and souls, and all we have to do is let it happen. Situations made for us present themselves, and all we have to do is grab the opportunities. Allow for this type of grace in your daily life.

TIPS

- To reap melon's benefits, try eating at least half of a small melon per day.
- Predigestion is the reason that you may associate eating melon with getting a stomachache. Since melon moves so quickly through the digestive tract, it can get held up and start to ferment in the gut if eaten with denser foods, or on the same day that you've eaten a heavy meal. Melon is best eaten as the first meal of the day, either on its own or accompanied by fresh vegetable juice.
- Different melons take varying amounts of time to ripen. A sweet aroma and a little bit of give on the blossom end are good indications that most melons are ripe.

WATERMELON WITH MINT AND LIME

Makes 2 servings

While this watermelon salad may seem simple, the combination of flavors couldn't be more perfect. The light sweetness of watermelon sings with a burst of lime juice and a pop of fresh mint. Your mouth will be watering for this one all summer long.

8 cups diced watermelon

Lime juice (from about 2 limes)

¼ cup finely chopped mint leaves

Place the watermelon in a serving bowl. Squeeze the lime juice generously over the top. Sprinkle with finely chopped mint leaves and serve.

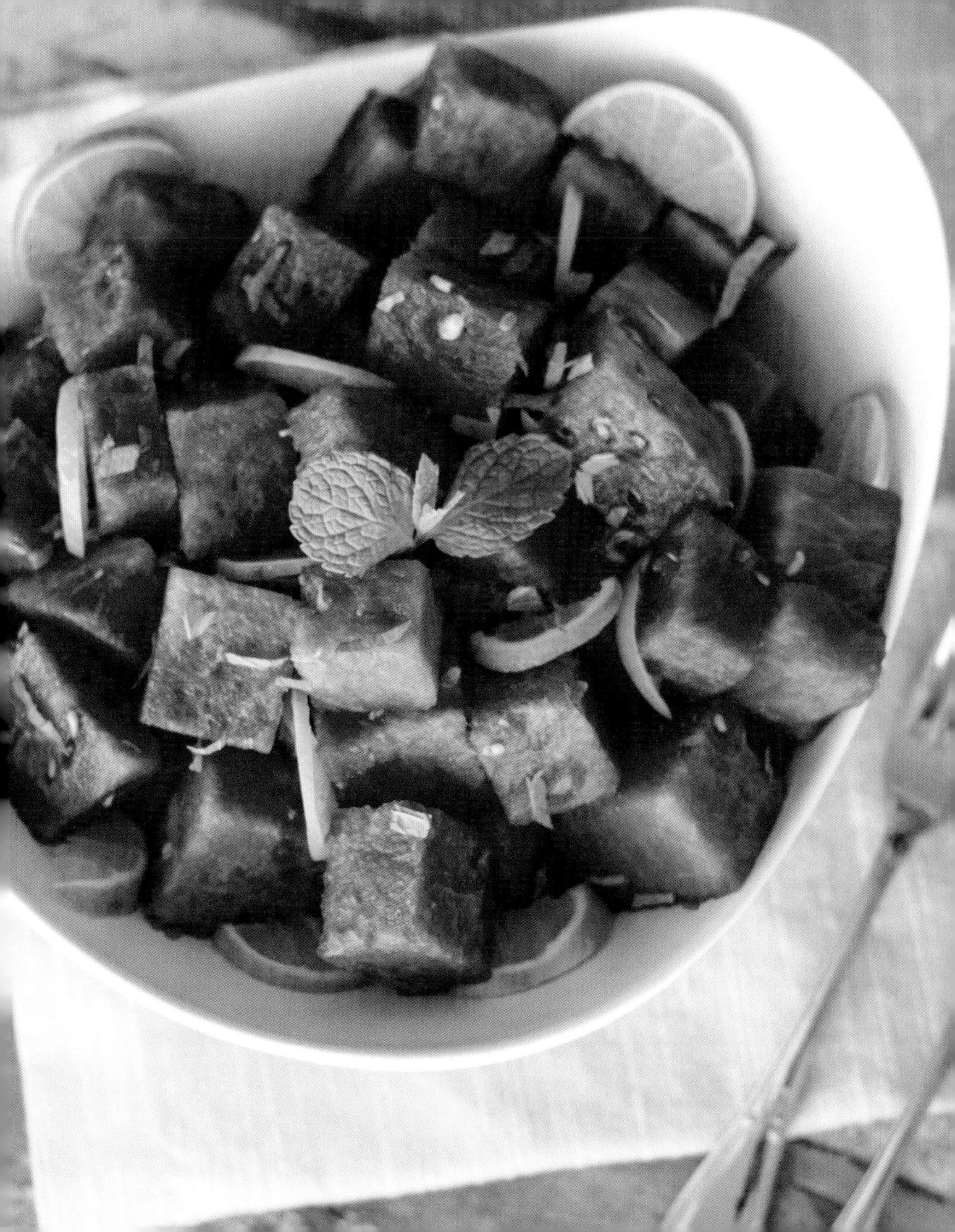

Oranges & Tangerines

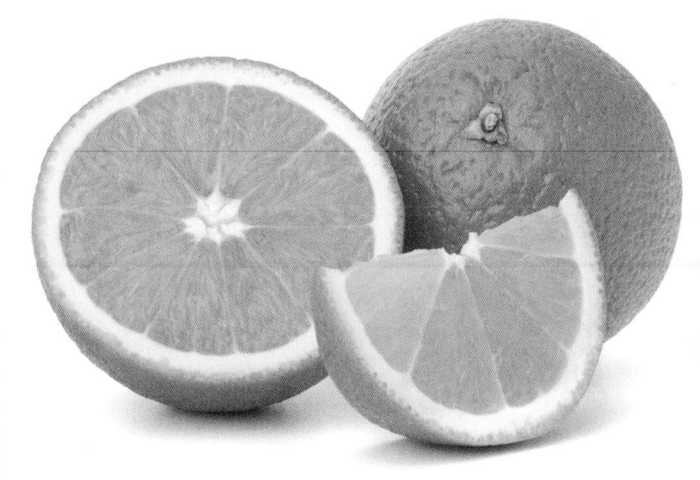

Historically, people who lived in northern climates became extremely deficient in vitamin C, magnesium, and potassium during the winter. That's because all they had to eat after a certain point in the year were dairy, eggs, grains, and some meat—with a paltry amount of vegetables remaining and even less fruit. Before truck deliveries of produce became a mainstay of modern life, townspeople would crowd around trains that were rumored to carry the rare crate of oranges from a southern land—although when citrus was on board, most of it would go to wealthy families and town selectmen. If a stray orange did get into the hands of a less fortunate townsperson, it would be worth its weight in gold. That's because people of the time valued oranges for what they were: miracle fruits.

Today, oranges have lost their luster in the public eye. Now people worry about citrus allergies, and dentists warn that the acid is bad for tooth enamel. Don't get caught up in the orange outrage. The truth is that oranges (and their cousins, tangerines) are full of the coenzyme glutathione, which goes into activation because of their high content of flavonoids and limonoids. This is a relationship medical research has not yet tapped into, and one that makes oranges and tangerines a key to healing the 21st-century epidemic of chronic illness. Together, glutathione, flavonoids, and limonoids fight off viruses, protect the body from radiation damage, and deactivate toxic heavy metals in the system.

Oranges and tangerines are also abundant in a form of bioactive calcium you can't get anywhere else. The body instantly absorbs this calcium, which means that these citrus beauties actually help regrow teeth, not destroy them. Their acid content is not destructive; rather, it works for you by dissolving kidney stones and gallstones.

It's time to reconnect to that period when we appreciated oranges' and tangerines' true value. These citrus fruits are life-giving, and they should be a foundation in the diet. The next time you walk by a navel, blood orange, Valencia, mandarin, honey Murcott, clementine, or Minneola tangelo, think about what it might have meant to an ancestor in the early 1900s and rejoice that progress has given you the opportunity to bring its sweet nectar into your life.

CONDITIONS

If you have any of the following conditions, try bringing oranges and/or tangerines into your life:

Gum disease; kidney stones; strep throat; gallstones; osteoporosis; diabetes; hypoglycemia; mold exposure; adrenal fatigue; mystery infertility; posttraumatic stress disorder (PTSD); anxiety; depression; urinary tract infections (UTIs); arteriosclerosis; stomach and intestinal cancers; acne; hypertension; low reproductive system battery; HHV-6; cytomegalovirus (CMV); shingles; HHV-7; the undiscovered HHV-10, HHV-11, and HHV-12; chronic fatigue syndrome (CFS); fibromyalgia; multiple sclerosis (MS); lupus; Graves' disease; amyotrophic lateral sclerosis (ALS); vertigo; lymphoma (including non-Hodgkin's); Epstein-Barr virus (EBV)/mononucleosis; Hashimoto's thyroiditis; human papilloma virus (HPV); Huntington's disease; herpes simplex 1 (HSV-1); herpes simplex 2 (HSV-2); bursitis; carpal tunnel syndrome; tendonitis; colds; nodules

SYMPTOMS

If you have any of the following symptoms, try bringing oranges and/or tangerines into your life:

Constipation, fatigue, roving aches and pains, blurry eyes, acid reflux, tingles and numbness, weakness, seasonal affective disorder (SAD), gastritis, listlessness, melancholy, mood swings, nervousness, jaw pain, water retention, food allergies, skin discolorations, hormonal imbalances, blood sugar issues, ringing or buzzing in the ears, sensations of humming or vibration in the body, back pain, backache, body aches, body stiffness, bruising, cold sores, dehydration, difficulty swallowing, difficulty breathing, ear pain, hot flashes, loss of energy, tremors, sore throat, hyperthyroid, hypothyroid

EMOTIONAL SUPPORT

The juice of an orange or tangerine is like liquid sunshine. If you often feel sad, weepy, glum, or down, oranges cut through the gloom and shine a light on your life. They are the perfect food to eat when you feel sun-deprived and lonely, as though there's an empty void that needs to be filled. Oranges take out all the chill and fill you with warmth instead.

SPIRITUAL LESSON

Oranges and tangerines remind us that we sometimes overlook the most important ingredients in our lives. Every now and then, we have to think about what we push aside or forsake and reevaluate whether all of it deserved to be devalued. In the case of these fruits, you may drink only the occasional orange juice (and feel guilty when you do), snack on a clementine once a year, or try an infrequent spread of orange marmalade on toast—whereas oranges and tangerines should rightfully be a centerpiece in your diet. As you make them a bigger part of your life, look around. What else is worthy of a second glance?

TIPS

- For optimum realization of the benefits of oranges and tangerines, consume four per day.
- As a snack, drizzle raw honey over slices of orange or tangerine. The honey will increase the citrus pectin's ability to kill off and eliminate mold, yeast, viruses, and unproductive bacteria in the gut by 50 percent.
- For a predigestive aid, try adding a squeeze of fresh orange or tangerine juice over your favorite salads and dishes. It will help ensure that you digest your meal at the best level possible.

SPANISH ORANGE AND OLIVE SALAD

Makes 2 to 4 servings

With juicy oranges and satisfying olives and avocado, this sweet-savory dish is perfect when you're looking for a meal that feels light and filling at the same time. Plus, it's a stunner, with vibrant colors that offer both health benefits and eye appeal. Enjoy this salad on its own, over salad greens, or in a wrap.

6 oranges, any variety
¼ cup sliced green olives
¼ cup finely chopped parsley
¼ cup thinly sliced red onion
1 avocado, diced
Black pepper (optional)

Cut off the top and bottom of each orange. Then, resting each orange flat on the cutting board, cut down and around the sides, removing all of the peel. Slice the oranges horizontally into disks and arrange on plates. Top the oranges with the remaining ingredients, serve, and enjoy!

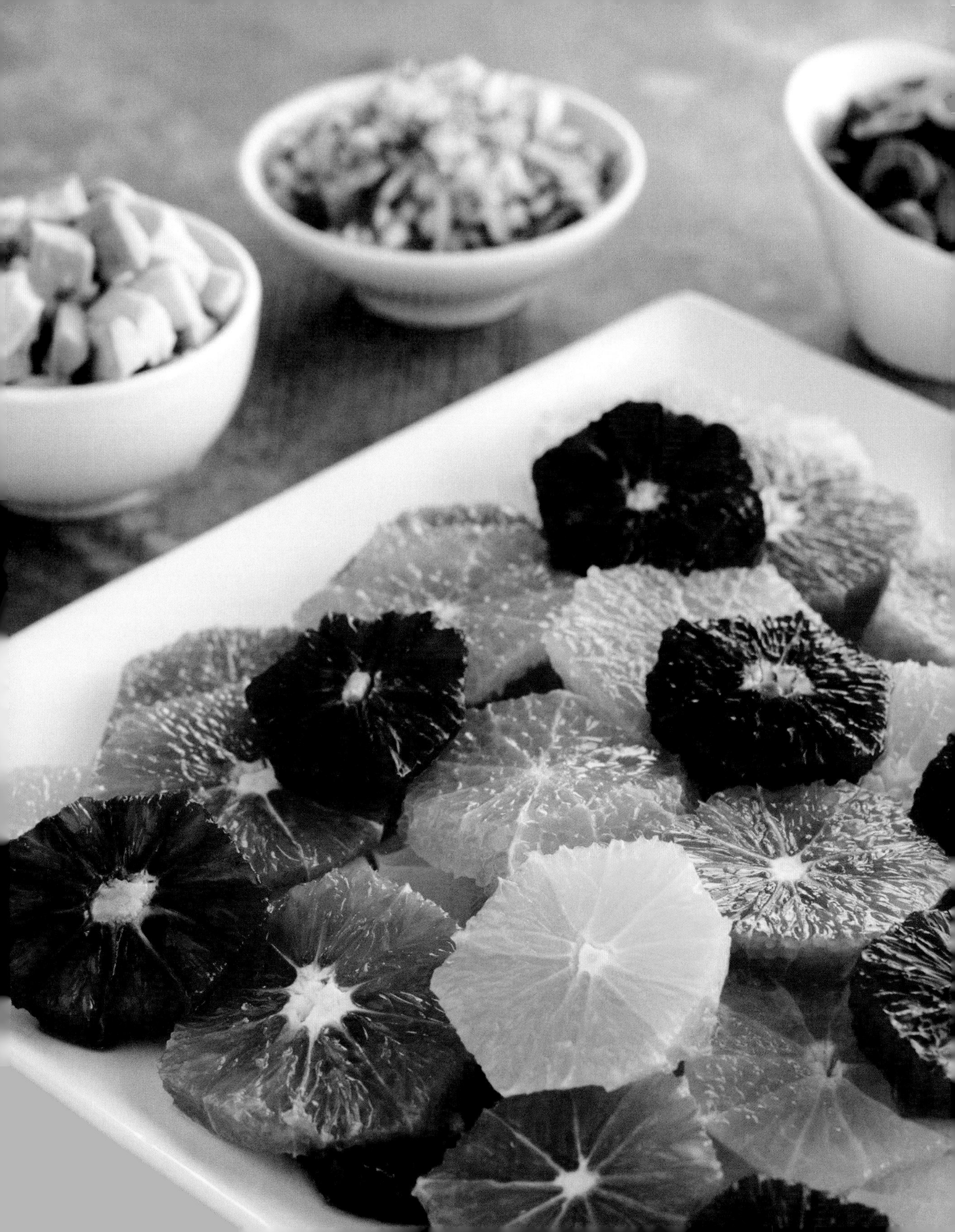

Papayas

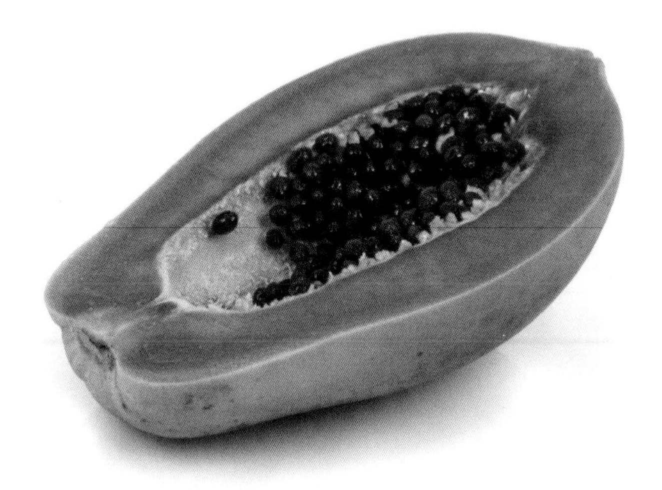

Passersby at the supermarket usually ignore the humble papaya. Little do they know that by avoiding this fruit, they're missing out on a piece of their salvation. If you're struggling with any kind of stomach or intestinal disorder, papayas cannot be beat. They can reverse colitis, Crohn's, IBS, ulcers, diverticulitis, gastritis, gastric spasms, liver disease, and pancreatitis. They also kill off *H. pylori*, *C. difficile*, and *E. coli*, plus rid the gut of other unfriendly bacteria and parasites, including worms. Papaya is an ideal food if you're dealing with SIBO.

Papaya is the number-one fruit for digestibility. Each papaya contains more than 500 undiscovered powerful digestive enzymes that support the pancreas, aid digestion, and mend the walls of the intestinal tract, reducing inflammation and preventing scar tissue from forming there. Papaya's amino acids and enzymes combined create undiscovered subcompound phytochemicals that repel viruses. Papaya also contains potent and as yet undiscovered coenzymes that enhance the alkalinity inside the intestinal tract.

If you need help relieving constipation, papaya is for you. If you suffer from stomachaches or an inflamed intestinal lining, papaya will be your ally in healing the irritated nerve endings that contribute to these ailments. Whenever someone has gone through a period of not eating, whether from fasting, anorexia, or grave illness, blended papaya is like magic for the refeeding process, because it offers ample calories, optimal nutrition, and digests so favorably.

Papaya is also a miracle worker for the skin. This fruit has anti-wrinkle, fountain-of-youth powers due to its high content of vitamins, minerals, and most important, caratenoids. Not only can it help your skin glow again, it can also clear up eczema, psoriasis, and acne.

CONDITIONS

If you have any of the following conditions, try bringing papayas into your life:

Constipation, irritable bowel syndrome (IBS), Crohn's disease, colitis, ulcers, diverticulitis, liver disease, gallbladder disease, parasites, *C. difficile* infection, *E. coli* infection, *H. pylori* infection, worms, eczema, psoriasis, acne, gastroparesis, lupus, chronic fatigue syndrome (CFS), Epstein-Barr virus (EBV)/mononucleosis, small intestinal bacterial overgrowth (SIBO), fibromyalgia, multiple sclerosis (MS), amyotrophic lateral sclerosis (ALS), shingles, Lyme disease, all autoimmune diseases and disorders, migraines, depression, urinary tract infections (UTIs), incontinence, diabetes, hypoglycemia, Graves' disease, Hashimoto's thyroiditis, blood disorders, enterocutaneous fistula, eating disorders, digestive disorders

SYMPTOMS

If you have any of the following symptoms, try bringing papayas into your life:

Stomachaches, stomach pain, bloating, gas, gastric spasms, gastritis, skin discolorations, brittle nails, central nervous system sensitivities, anxiousness, joint pain, dark under-eye circles, fatigue, weakness, chemical sensitivities, body pain, temporomandibular joint (TMJ) issues, frozen shoulder, tingles and numbness, Bell's palsy, hypothyroid, burning skin sensations, muscle stiffness, hair loss, hyperthyroid, eye floaters, eye dryness, stagnant liver, blood imbalances, bladder pain, bladder spasms, weak digestion, anal itching, brain fog, memory loss, acid reflux, diarrhea, digestive discomfort, flatulence

EMOTIONAL SUPPORT

Papaya can quickly lift you or a loved one out of grouchiness. Keep it on hand to share when feelings of crankiness, crabbiness, or impatience creep in. Papaya breathes light into everyone who consumes it, casting out negativity and darkness, purging old judgment, resentment, and stored-up frustration.

SPIRITUAL LESSON

The papaya tree is often skinny and frail, yet each holds a large crop of one of the heaviest fruits there is. This will and determination to overcome physics and balance no matter what is almost supernatural. It teaches us that we *can* overcome our seeming weaknesses—when we are working in service to a noble cause. It's not what we look like on the outside that counts for anything; the true self that's inside each of us determines what we can really accomplish.

Hidden inside each papaya are medicinal truths. When we eat them, our bodies immediately identify these elements and put them to use, redesigning us physically so that we can heal and become our strongest selves. Papaya trees and their fruit want us to understand that there are no limitations to healing, growth, and becoming. Disease and physical challenges cannot hold us back; we can transform situations that seem, at first, impossible.

TIPS

- For constipation relief, eat half a papaya daily.
- Look for the Mexican and Central American papaya variety known as Maradol. These medium-to-large papayas are preferable to Hawaiian varieties, which have suffered GMO contamination. (If you're growing papayas at home in Hawaii, that's a different story. Just be sure to look after your trees with care to avoid GMO influence.)
- If you like spice, eat a few papaya seeds along with the fruit. Eating a small portion of papaya seeds per week can be beneficial for eliminating parasites. For the ultimate in gut-health repair, drink a tonic of papaya blended with celery juice.

PAPAYA SMOOTHIE BOWL

Makes 2 servings

These papaya smoothie bowls are almost too pretty to eat. Don't let that stop you, though. Papaya and raspberry were made for each other, and the addition of banana, mango, and mint takes this treat over the top. Have fun creating your own designs and customizing this recipe however you want. The options are endless.

6 cups cubed papaya

4 dates, pitted

2 cups raspberries, divided

1 cup diced mango

1 banana, sliced

1 tablespoon shredded coconut

1 tablespoon minced fresh mint

½ lime

Blend the papaya, dates, and 1 cup of the raspberries in a blender until smooth. Pour the mixture into 2 bowls. Arrange the mango, banana slices, and remaining raspberries on top. Finish with a sprinkle of shredded coconut, fresh mint, and a squeeze of lime.

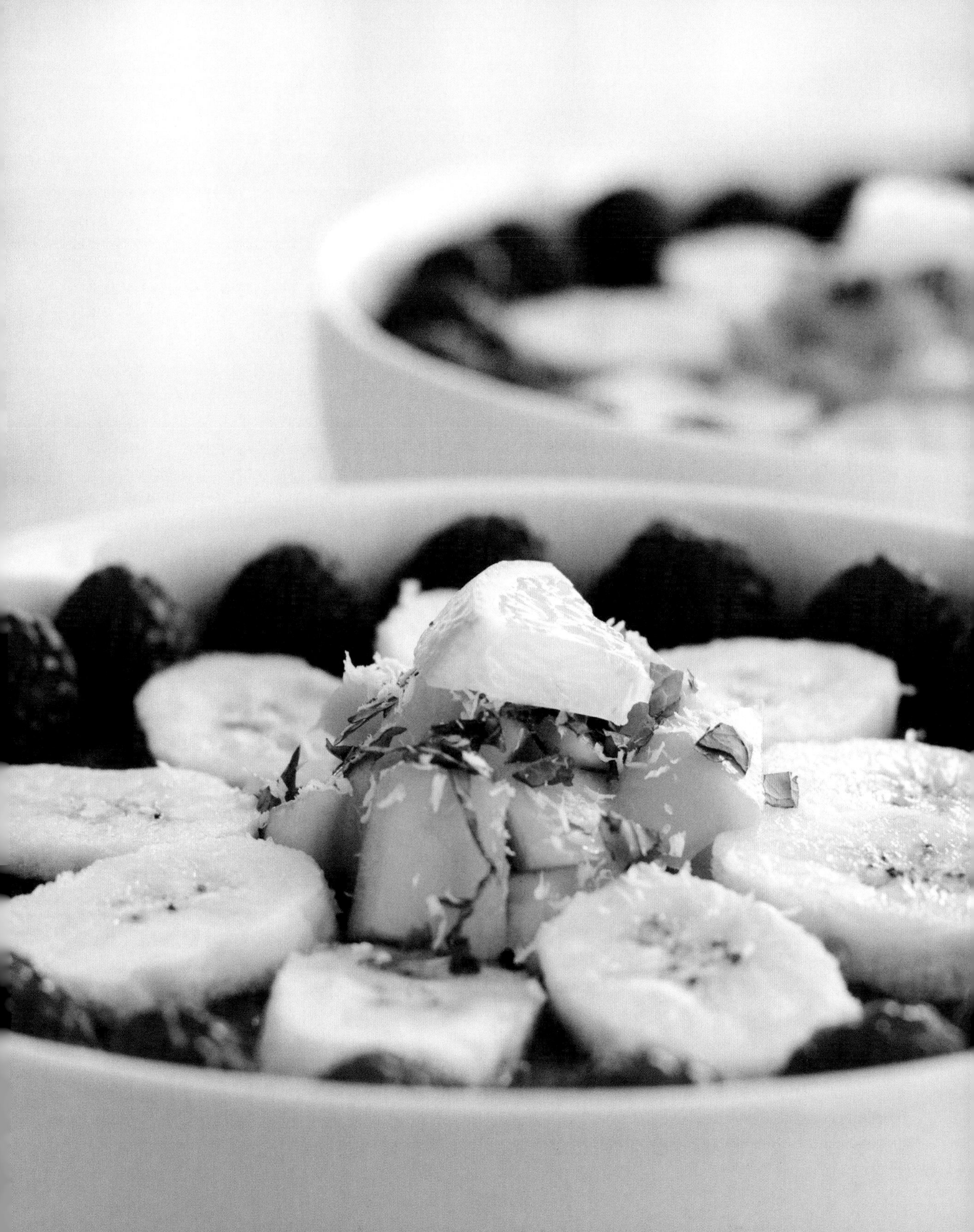

Pears

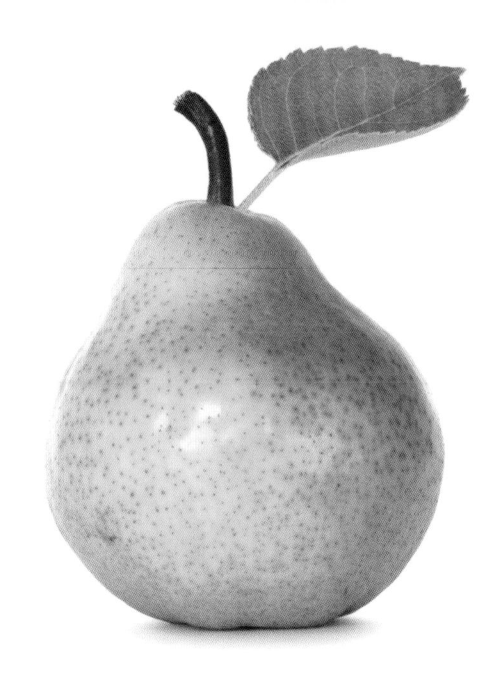

While apples are the stuff of legend, their close relatives, pears, are considered ho-hum. People often associate pears with their bland canned form, or with rare caramelized desserts; beyond that, pears don't factor into most people's daily thoughts. In the back of our minds, we know they exist, and that's about it.

Same with the pancreas: We're aware that we each have this gland, yet unless it develops an issue, we barely register that it's there. Meanwhile, the pancreas takes much of the body's stress. And sometimes we abuse the pancreas without even realizing it by eating a combination of fried foods, rich dishes, too much table sugar, or high-fat desserts. Heartbreak, letdown, betrayal, and other forms of broken trust, as well as fear of any kind, are also hard on the pancreas. For pancreas protection and stress assistance, we must turn to the pear. This neglected fruit helps rejuvenate this neglected and overtaxed gland, alleviating pancreatitis and helping to prevent pancreatic cancer.

Pears are also amazing for other aspects of digestion. They act as an antispasmodic; help to soothe the linings of the stomach and intestinal tract; feed beneficial bacteria; starve and kill unproductive bacteria, parasites, and fungus; raise hydrochloric acid in the stomach; help prevent intestinal and stomach cancers; and reduce the bad acids produced by mucus and pathogens such as *H. pylori*. They also restore linings in the gut that have become damaged and calloused from bacteria.

The little granules in a pear's flesh are loaded with phytochemicals, trace minerals, and amino acids such as valine, histidine, threonine, and lysine. The trace minerals and amino acids combine and lock onto poisons in the body such as DDT, expelling them from your system. Trace mineral salts make pear juice high in electrolytes, which stabilizes blood sugar. Plus, pears are a great weight-loss food and heaven-sent for the liver, helping to cleanse and purify the organ and stop cirrhosis. Bring pears into your life, and you'll see that they're anything but boring.

CONDITIONS

If you have any of the following conditions, try bringing pears into your life:

Pancreatitis; pancreatic cancer; liver cancer; diabetes; food poisoning; hiatal hernia; gastroesophageal reflux disease (GERD); small intestinal bacterial overgrowth (SIBO); intestinal infection of *H. pylori*, *E. coli*, *Salmonella*, *Streptococcus*, and/or mold; cirrhosis of the liver; hepatitis A; hepatitis B; hepatitis C; hepatitis D; fungal infections; stomach cancer; esophageal cancer; diverticulitis; diverticulosis; shingles; herpes; migraines; obsessive-compulsive disorder (OCD); hypoglycemia

SYMPTOMS

If you have any of the following symptoms, try bringing pears into your life:

Acid reflux, high cholesterol, sluggish liver, dysfunctional liver, liver heat, liver stagnation, gas, bloating, constipation, gastritis, gastric distress, food allergies, upset stomach, intestinal inflammation, intestinal scar tissue, adhesions, insulin resistance, intestinal spasms, pancreas inflammation, appendix inflammation, weight gain, inflamed skin, diarrhea

EMOTIONAL SUPPORT

An overburdened, overstressed, and overheated pancreas and liver are often behind someone's unsettled emotions such as frustration, irritation, uneasiness, or lack of peace. Pears are the ideal food to remedy this situation, because they are the ultimate cooling tonic, especially for the liver and pancreas.

SPIRITUAL LESSON

The pear's simplicity is a lesson for us all. Here's a fruit that's not complicated in the least, not flashy, exotic, hard to find, nor hard to eat—and that doesn't reduce its power by one ounce. Gentle, unassuming, and quietly beautiful, pears can care for your body in a particular manner that no other fruit can. They teach us that we don't have to cry out for attention or sit in resentment of not being noticed. We, too, can hold on to our true selves and fully possess our power without any need for show.

TIPS

- Each phase of a pear's ripening process has value. When a pear is hard and crunchy, that means its fiber content is high, which lowers bad cholesterol and sweeps out mucus, pathogens, and other debris from the intestinal tract. Crunchy pear slices are a great addition to salads. When a pear is soft and juicy, its glucose levels are higher, and it's very easy to digest. Blended, ripe pear is an ideal food for someone recovering from food poisoning or another circumstance that kept her or him from eating.
- Pears are best eaten between breakfast and lunch, or in the late afternoon (shortly before dinner). They act as an appetite suppressant and stomach tonic to prevent you from craving sweets or overeating at meals.
- As a substitute for apple, try ripe pear in your fresh green-juice blends.

CINNAMON-BAKED PEARS WITH TOASTED WALNUTS

Makes 2 to 4 servings

Tender pears filled with warm maple syrup and toasted walnuts—this dish is comforting and perfect for chilly winter days. The aroma of the cinnamon baking in the oven will fill the whole house with warmth, and the end result will leave everyone feeling cozy and full. These are incredibly simple to make and a big hit with kids and adults alike.

4 pears, any variety
2 tablespoons maple syrup
¼ cup chopped walnuts
½ teaspoon cinnamon

Preheat the oven to 350°F. Slice the pears in half lengthwise and remove the seeds. Arrange the pear halves face up on a baking tray. Drizzle each pear half with maple syrup, brushing over the face of the pear and leaving some inside the center. Divide the walnuts evenly into the centers of the pears and sprinkle cinnamon over the top of each. Bake for 20 to 30 minutes, until the pears are tender and cooked through. Serve warm from the oven and enjoy!

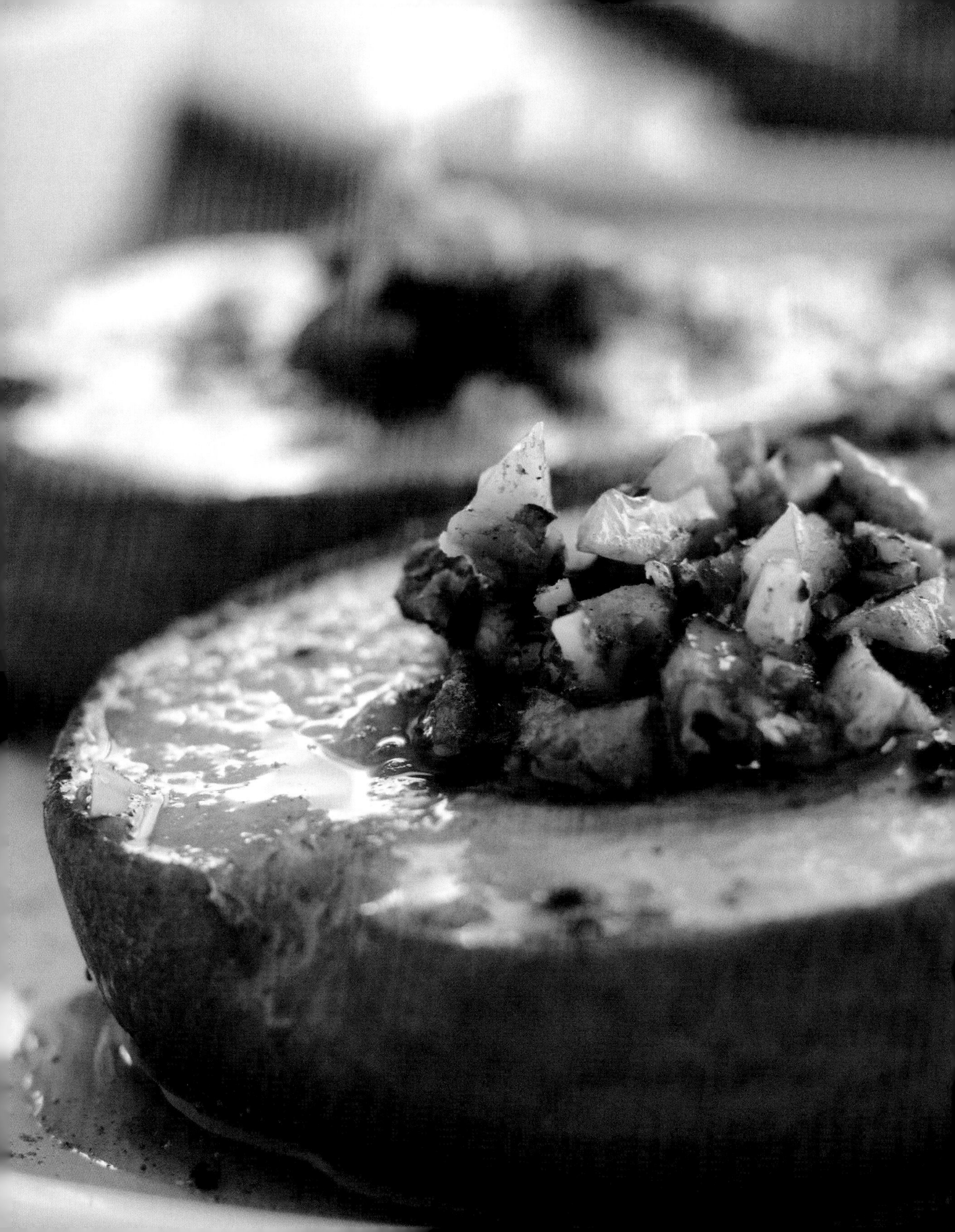

Pomegranates

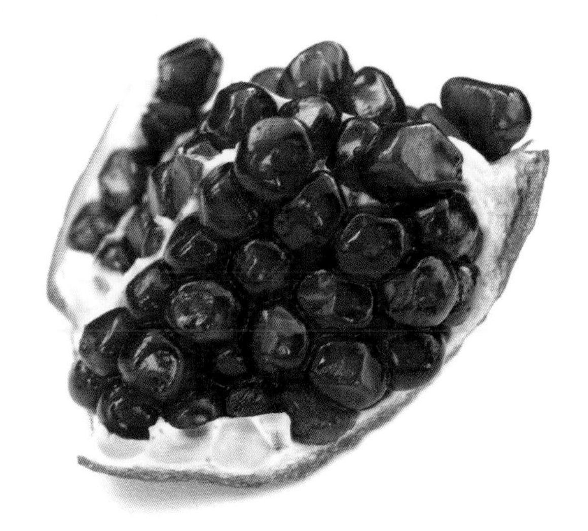

Pomegranates are popular, known especially for being high in antioxidants. What doesn't get enough attention is what a godsend this fruit is for dissolving gallstones and kidney stones, nodules, calcifications, and small cysts such as ganglia cysts. It also has anti-tumor properties. Each of the fruit's many jewellike, juicy capsules (technically called arils, though better known as seeds) inside a pomegranate contains a universe. Pomegranate seeds freshly broken open—whether between your teeth or in a juicer—release the full power of each of those tiny universes to come to your aid. When you consume fresh pomegranate, a chemical reaction occurs whenever the fruit's acids (which are filled with phytochemicals such as anthocyanins) come into contact with the types of unhealthy hardenings formed from bile, protein buildup, and toxic forms of calcium. Immediately, they start to break down. Bringing pomegranate into your life on a regular basis is especially beneficial if you suffer from PCOS.

Pomegranate is a great blood builder, as it strengthens both red and white cell counts. It serves an important role in blood sugar, too, by restoring precious glucose reserves to the liver, so that the liver can release this glucose into the bloodstream as needed. This process in turn protects the adrenal glands—because if you go for several hours without eating and your liver doesn't have glucose reserves, then your adrenals are forced to pump hormones such as cortisol into your blood to keep you going, leading to overactive adrenal glands and eventual burnout. So if you're looking for adrenal balance and blood sugar stabilization, turn to pomegranates. Pomegranates' high-quality glucose also makes them a brain food, helping with focus and concentration.

Further, pomegranates contain trace minerals such as iron, manganese, potassium, and chromium that are very bioavailable and easily assimilable. Plus, consuming pomegranates helps unclog pores and hair follicles, encouraging hair growth where it's needed and helping the skin and scalp overall. Pomegranates are amazing for regulating hormones, because they flush out toxic ones such as unproductive estrogens that contribute to cancers. This fruit also helps detoxify DDT and other pesticides, eliminate unproductive lactic acid buildup in the muscles, and clear out earwax and minimize new production of it.

CONDITIONS

If you have any of the following conditions, try bringing pomegranates into your life:

Alzheimer's disease, insomnia, dementia, adrenal fatigue, diabetes, hypoglycemia, earwax buildup, alopecia, gallstones, kidney stones, mold exposure, nodules, calcifications,

Epstein-Barr virus (EBV)/mononucleosis, Raynaud's syndrome, adenomas, autism, plantar fasciitis, Lyme disease, Morton's neuroma, tumors, polycystic ovarian syndrome (PCOS)

SYMPTOMS

If you have any of the following symptoms, try bringing pomegranates into your life:

Brain fog, memory loss, confusion, cysts, calcifications, disorientation, trouble focusing, dandruff, weight gain, persistent hunger, hair loss, muscle cramps, leg cramps, blood sugar imbalances, myelin nerve damage, trigeminal neuralgia, scar tissue in the liver, back pain, frozen shoulder, body pain, ear pain, eye floaters, foot drop, rib pain, foot pain, head pain, hives, inflammation, itchy skin, liver heat, neuralgia

EMOTIONAL SUPPORT

Pomegranates are a critical food for the person who struggles with impatience on a daily basis—and doesn't believe her or his impatience is the problem, but rather everyone else is to blame. If you know someone like this, offer her or him a pomegranate. It will shift the energy and point your companion in the direction of composure, compassion, and patience. If you feel that someone's impatience is directed at you and it's throwing you off your game, turn to pomegranates to help you keep your equanimity and focus.

SPIRITUAL LESSON

When you're dealing with a pomegranate, there's not much you can do to contain the mess. As careful as you may be, inevitably an aril bursts at just the wrong moment, and you end up with red stains on your carpet, clothes, countertop, walls, or fingers. We've all learned not to wear a silk blouse or tie when excavating a pomegranate. Opening a pomegranate requires us to put on our old jeans and a ragged sweatshirt—creative wear, the same clothes we'd wear if we were going to paint—and to approach the activity knowing it's going to get messy (and that it's well worth the reward). Consider this the next time a situation presents you with the opportunity for creativity and a rewarding outcome. Are you thinking of walking away because it could get messy? Or are you about to jump in headfirst without being prepared? Pomegranates teach us both to brace for mess and embrace it, if we want to get the most out of what comes our way.

TIPS

- Eat one or more pomegranates daily to reap the most benefits.
- Get creative with how you use pomegranates. You can sprinkle the little seeds anywhere—on salads, hummus, guacamole, or even on top of a stir-fry you've just cooked.
- If you're concerned about excessive hunger, overeating, and/or weight gain, eat pomegranate seeds before a meal as an appetite suppressant.

POMEGRANATE BARK

Makes 4 to 6 servings

Heaps of juicy pomegranate seeds and a smooth layer of creamy chocolate go together beautifully in this treat. Offer it as a gift, or make it for those moments when you're craving an indulgence you can feel good about.

10 ounces bittersweet chocolate chips (at least 60 percent cacao)

¼ cup coconut oil

¼ cup maple syrup

2 cups pomegranate seeds

Stir the chocolate chips and coconut oil in a saucepan over low heat until the mixture is melted and combined. Add the maple syrup. Spread an even layer of melted chocolate on a baking tray lined with parchment paper. Press the pomegranate seeds firmly into the chocolate layer. Place in the freezer and allow to set for at least 30 minutes. Break apart and enjoy!

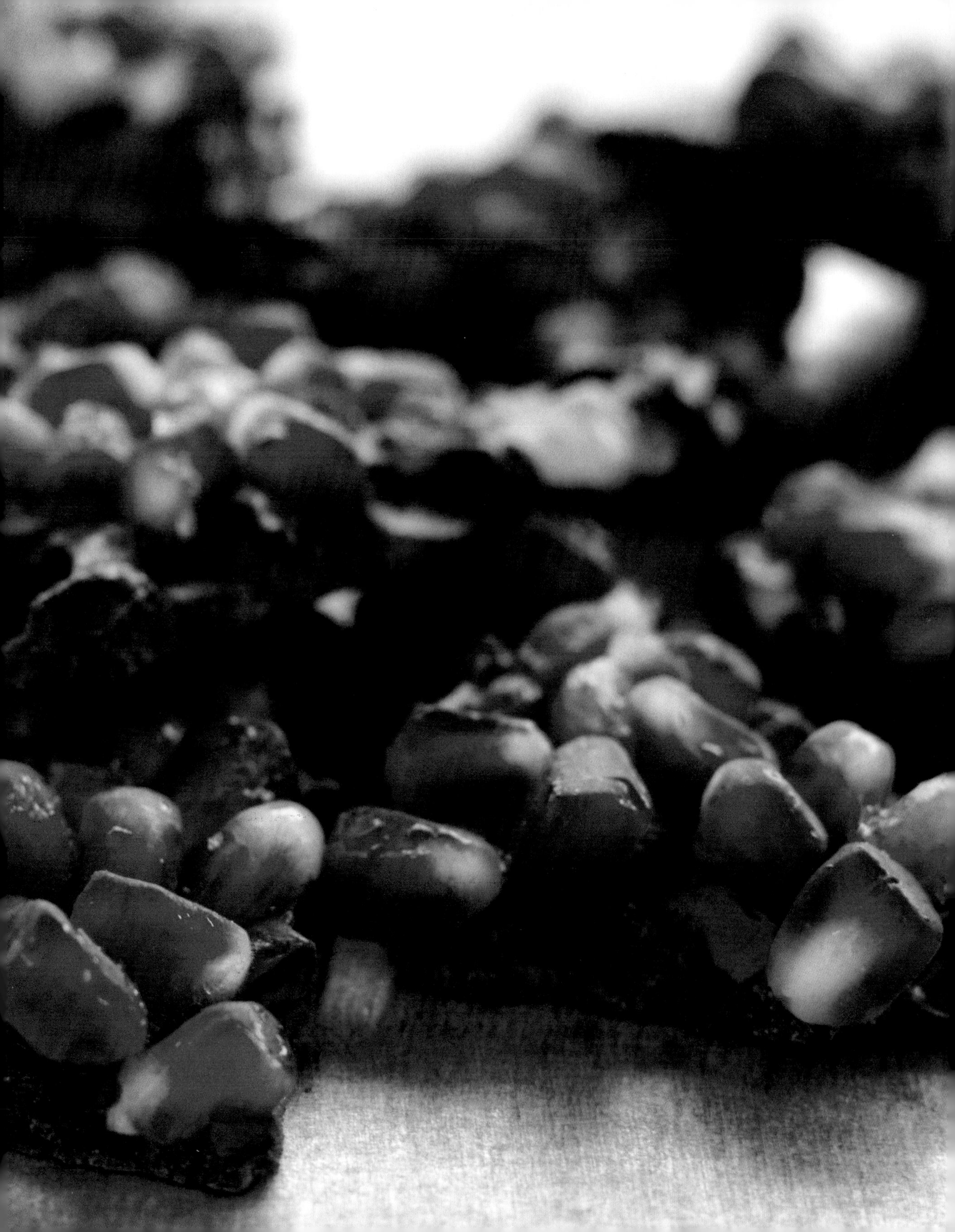

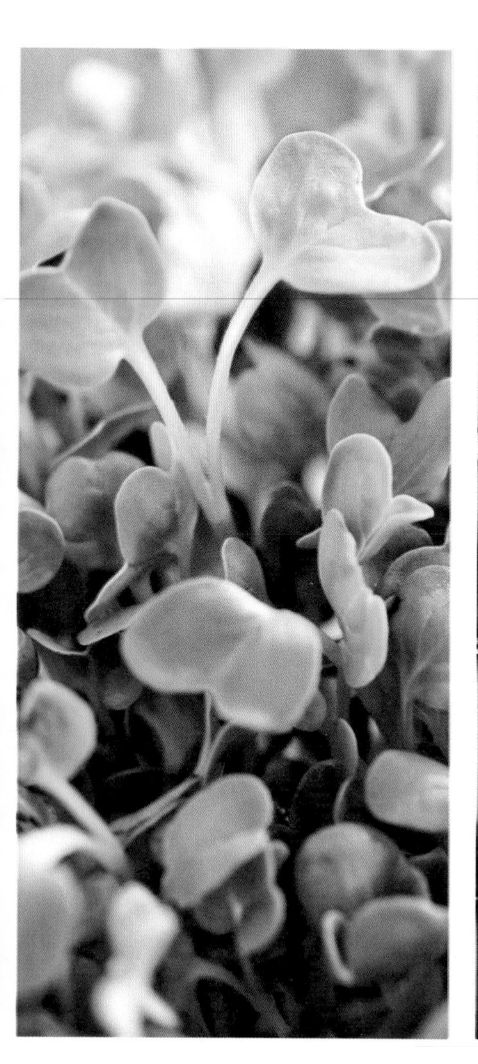
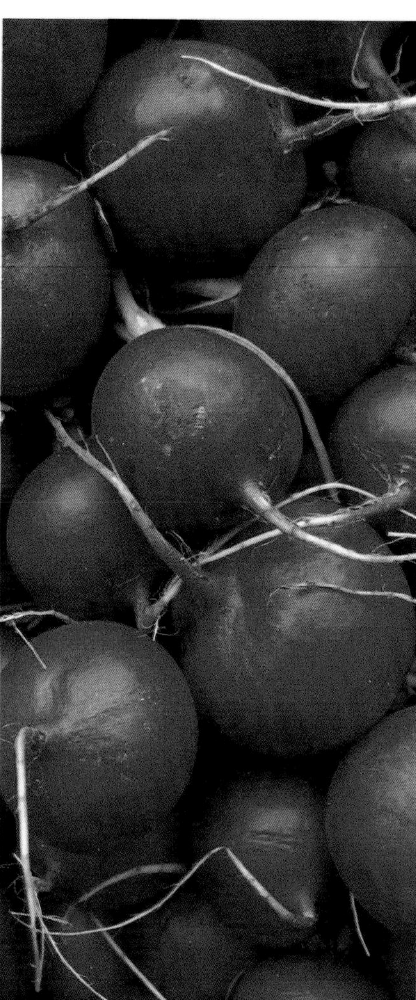
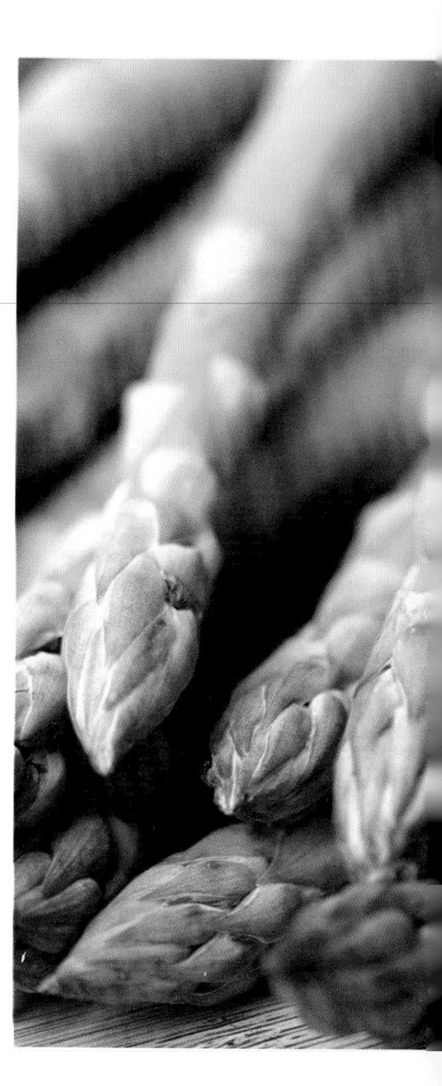

VEGETABLES

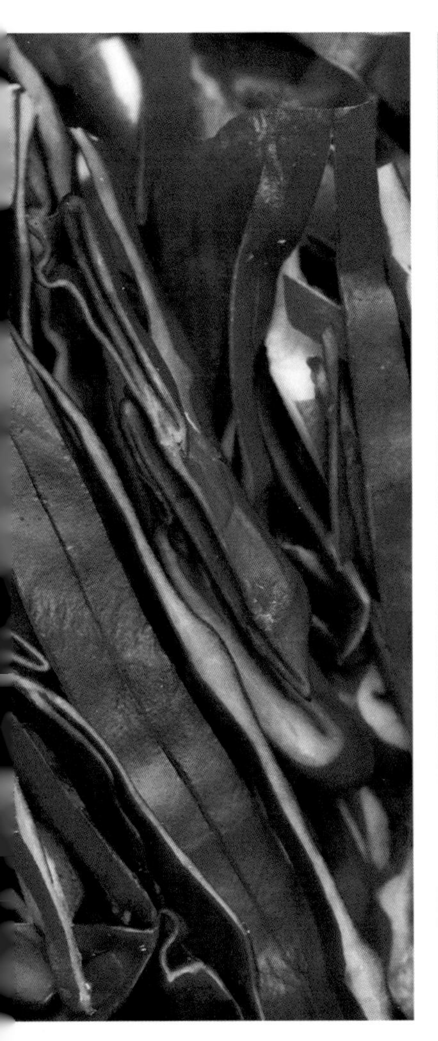

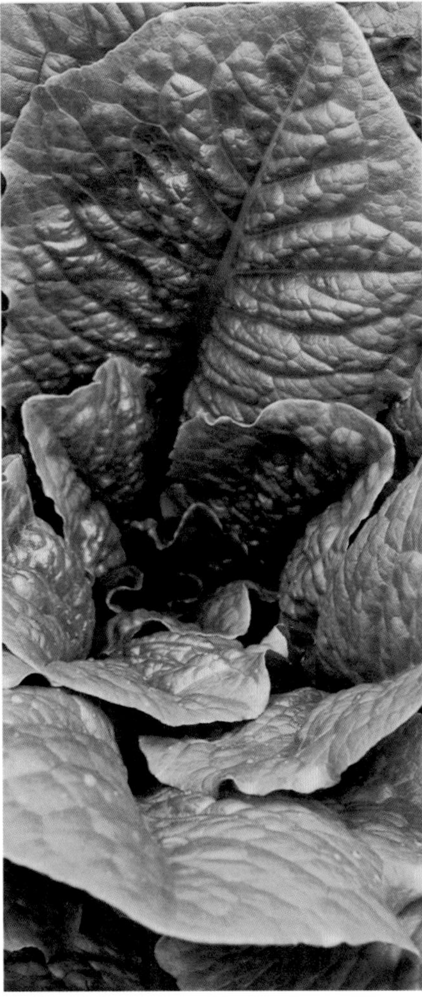

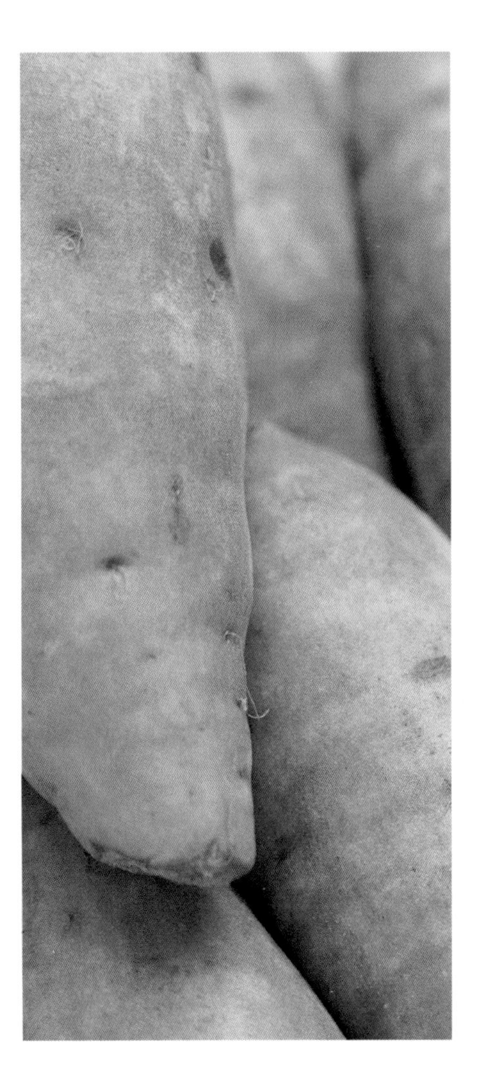

Artichokes

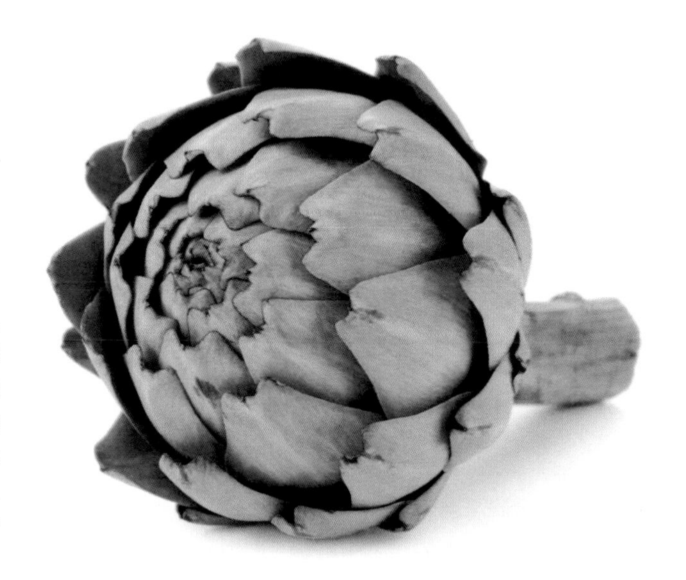

With all the superfood talk we have today, artichokes should be right there in the top 10 list. Artichokes are one of the most abundant sources of nutrition, filled with phytochemicals such as lutein and isothiocyanates; vitamins such as A, E, and K; amino acids; and enzymes. They are B_{12}-enhancing stars, wonderful for bringing balance to the gut.

Artichokes are also dense with minerals such as silica, which is one of the foundational minerals of our bodies that's critical for our existence. Artichokes' magnesium content gets attention, and rightfully so. There's a bigger picture to what gives artichokes their sedative qualities, though: In addition to magnesium, artichokes contain sedation phytochemicals that calm all body systems, as well as a compilation of calming minerals. This mineral denseness corresponds with the dense organs and glands (such as the liver, spleen, pancreas, brain, adrenals, and thyroid) that artichokes nourish. Deep within these organs, we have foundational nutrient reserves, and artichokes are one of those foods that replenish our reserves to promote longevity.

Artichokes are incredible for the pancreas, making them an ideal food for people with diabetes, hypoglycemia, and other blood sugar imbalances. They are also one of the best foods for reducing kidney stones and gallstones, as well as calcifications and scar tissue inside the body. Artichokes are remarkable for protecting the body from the radiation of X-rays, cancer treatments, dental treatment, and common exposure.

Artichokes are meant to be taken seriously in our lives, and should be considered medicine—a medicine that tastes earthy, sweet, and delicious. Many people don't bother with fresh artichokes, because they find their appearance off-putting and don't know how to deal with them. Once you learn the art of preparing and cooking an artichoke, though, you'll be bringing an amazing nutritional dish into your life.

CONDITIONS

If you have any of the following conditions, try bringing artichokes into your life:

Diabetes, hypoglycemia, kidney stones, gallstones, calcifications, internal scar tissue, shingles, osteomyelitis, thyroid disease, insomnia, carpal tunnel syndrome, bone fractures, cirrhosis of the liver, endocrine system disorders, fatty liver, hepatitis A, hepatitis B, hepatitis C, HIV, interstitial cystitis, liver cancer, Lyme disease, optic nerve conditions, pancreatic cancer, stomach ulcers, systemic lupus, low reproductive system battery, mystery infertility, Achilles tendon injury, blood cell cancers such as multiple myeloma

SYMPTOMS

If you have any of the following symptoms, try bringing artichokes into your life:

Blood sugar imbalances, food allergies, canker sores, rib pain, sleep disturbances, abnormal Pap smear results (i.e., abnormal cervical cells), food sensitivities, urinary urgency, bone density issues, bone loss, brittle nails, dysfunctional liver, electromagnetic hypersensitivity (EHS), emotional eating, inflamed colon, liver congestion, nerve pain, stomach pain, mineral deficiencies, enlarged spleen

EMOTIONAL SUPPORT

For anyone who is dealing with heart-related emotions—those who are downhearted, brokenhearted, ill-hearted, or coldhearted—artichokes are critical. Eaten on a regular basis, artichokes have the power to open up the heart chakra, and to ignite healing through this sacred channel.

SPIRITUAL LESSON

Sometimes we put up armor in order to protect ourselves. Each experience of being hurt or taken advantage of adds another layer between the core of who we are and the outside world. It's a necessary act that we learn from nature—a survival tactic. Just like the artichoke, though, if you take the time to peel back our armor, you'll find that we all have soft, sustaining hearts underneath. Artichokes teach us that while connection doesn't always come easily—sometimes it takes work to peel back the spikes—it is worth the work to get to the tender, true, and loving centers of ourselves and each other.

TIPS

- Consider having artichokes on the dinner menu four times a week for promising results.
- The most nutritious way to enjoy artichokes is to steam them. Once they've cooked and cooled, peel off the leaves, dip them in your favorite healthy dressing, and nibble the "meat" from the base of each leaf. Next, scrape off the choke and enjoy the hearts.
- If you buy prepared artichoke hearts that have a preservative such as citric acid, soak them overnight in water to get rid of this corn-derived irritant. (For more on issues with corn, see the chapter "Foods That Make Life Challenging.")
- Enjoying artichokes for dinner helps your liver purge and clean itself in the early hours of the morning, while you sleep. For best results, try eating artichokes at 7 or 8 in the evening.
- Try eating artichokes alongside romaine lettuce. Together, they help dissolve gallstones and kidney stones.

STEAMED ARTICHOKES WITH LEMON-HONEY DIPPING SAUCE

Makes 2 to 4 servings

Preparing artichokes can seem daunting. All it really requires is hot water and some patience. When steamed until tender, artichokes are just waiting for you to pull them apart and dunk them into a luscious sauce of honey, olive oil, and sage.

4 artichokes
¼ cup olive oil
¼ cup honey
¼ cup lemon juice
3 sage leaves

Prepare the artichokes by cutting off the top quarter of each and removing the stem. Using scissors, cut the remaining tips off of each of the leaves. Fill a large pot with 3 inches of water. Place the artichokes in a steamer basket inside the pot. Steam the artichokes for 30 to 45 minutes, until the leaves are tender and easily removed.

To make the dipping sauce, combine all the remaining ingredients in a small saucepan over high heat. Stir continuously until the sauce begins to thicken slightly, about 2 minutes. Remove from heat and serve immediately alongside the cooked artichokes.

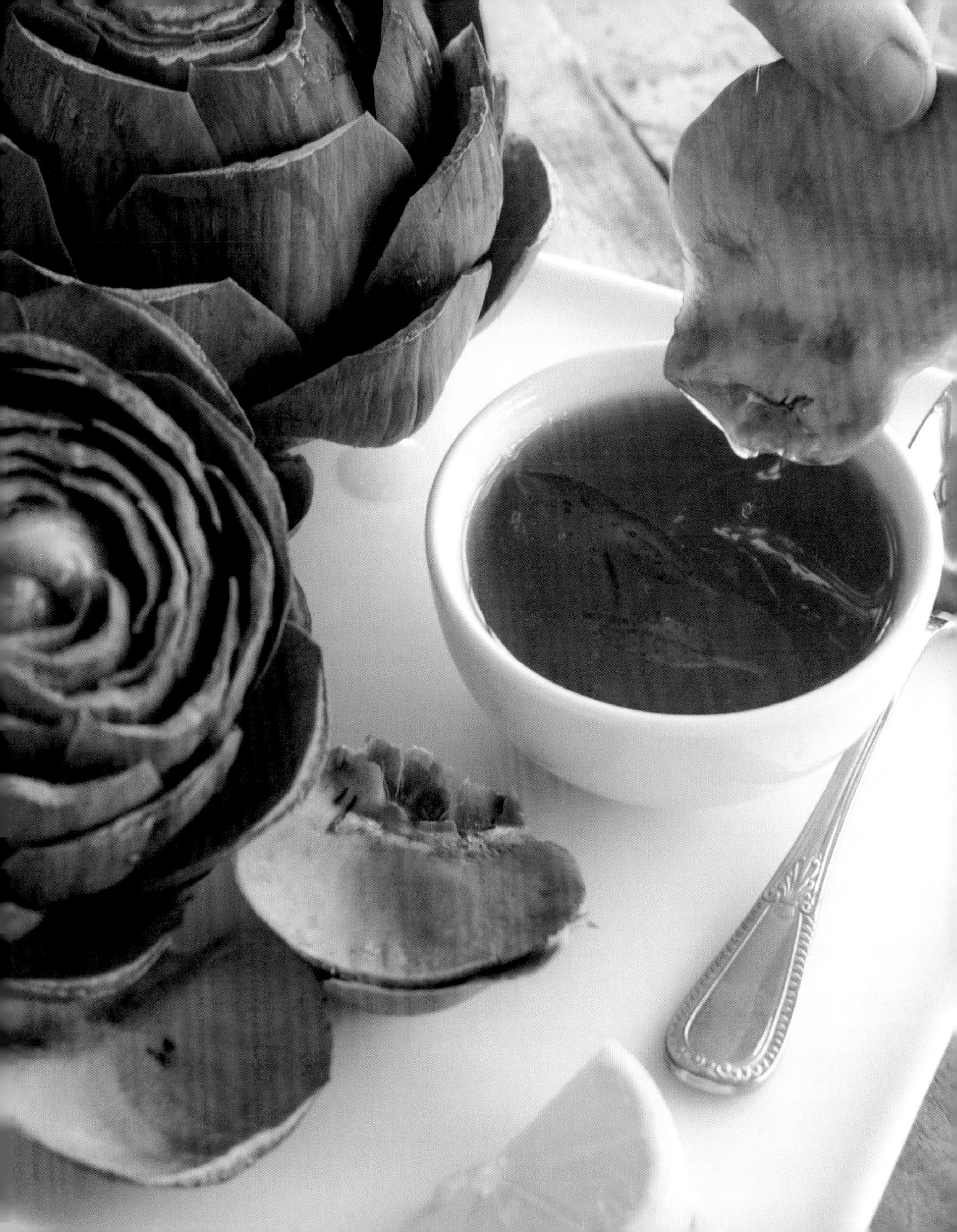

Asparagus

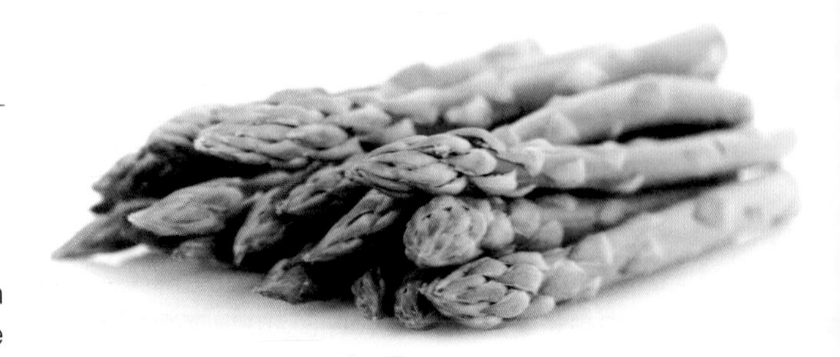

Throughout history, people have been searching for the fountain of youth. Far and wide they've traveled, seeking that magical spring flowing from the ground that will preserve good health. This source of youth is no myth, and it does come from the earth . . . it just happens to be readily available at the grocery store, too. That anti-aging wonder is asparagus.

When were you at your strongest? When could you run effortlessly, swim in the ocean without tiring? Was it 10, 20, 30 years ago, or more? Maybe it was yesterday, or this morning. Connect with your best moment, whenever it was, that time when you felt your full life force coursing through you. That's the same power that a spear of asparagus contains in its first few weeks aboveground. If you think about it, every piece of asparagus that we eat was once on its way to becoming a small tree. While every vegetable has its value, most of them can't claim that same hidden potential. When we eat young asparagus shoots, though, their propulsive energy is transferred to us. Not only does that energy keep us young, it helps with recovery and prevention of neurological disorders and symptoms.

Asparagus contains phytochemical compounds such as chlorophyll and lutein that act as critical organ cleansers. They get deep into organs such as the liver, spleen, pancreas, and kidneys, scrubbing out the toxins they find there. Chlorophyll bonded to amino acids such as glutamine, threonine, and serine provides an avenue for heavy metal detox.

What's more, some of the phytochemicals found in asparagus are toxin inhibitors (a fact as yet unknown to science). This means that once toxins such as DDT, other pesticides, and heavy metals have been driven out of the organs, these specialized phytochemicals stay behind and repel new toxins from taking up residence there. This toxin inhibition makes asparagus an amazing tool for battling virtually every variety of cancer.

When we're under immense stress, we tend to lose B vitamins very rapidly. Asparagus, which is high in very easily absorbable B vitamins, helps us reestablish our proper levels of these key nutrients. Also high in silica and trace minerals such as iron, zinc, molybdenum, chromium, phosphorus, magnesium, and selenium, asparagus is one of the most adrenal-supporting foods in existence and excellent for bringing you back to life when your adrenal glands have been pushed to the max. And we can't talk about asparagus without mentioning how valuable it is at alkalizing the body by flushing out unproductive acids. We live in a very acidic environment, and if we want to remain free from disease, we must constantly work to keep ourselves alkaline with help from trusted friends like asparagus.

CONDITIONS

If you have any of the following conditions, try bringing asparagus into your life:

Multiple sclerosis (MS), sepsis, Parkinson's disease, fibromyalgia, chronic fatigue syndrome (CFS), bladder cancer, breast cancer, bone cancer, transient ischemic attack (TIA), gout, kidney stones, lung cancer, liver cancer, migraines, vertigo, Ménière's disease, neuropathy, diabetes, hypoglycemia, adrenal fatigue, shingles, Lyme disease, anxiety, Epstein-Barr virus (EBV)/mononucleosis, osteomyelitis, Hashimoto's thyroiditis, Graves' disease, thyroid cancer, low reproductive system battery, infertility, sleep apnea, pelvic inflammatory disease (PID), acne, bursitis, celiac disease, connective tissue damage, polycystic ovarian syndrome (PCOS), heavy metal toxicity, herpes simplex 1 (HSV-1), herpes simplex 2 (HSV-2), hiatal hernia, fibroids, anemia

SYMPTOMS

If you have any of the following symptoms, try bringing asparagus into your life:

Twitches, spasms, tingles and numbness, ringing or buzzing in the ears, slurred speech, body odor, fatigue, hypothyroid, hyperthyroid, pins and needles, neuralgia, weight gain, weight loss, premenstrual syndrome (PMS) symptoms, lack of motivation, listlessness, loss of libido, loss of energy, abdominal pain, menopause symptoms, urinary urgency, back pain, joint pain, neck pain, rib pain, adhesions, abdominal distension, canker sores, chronic loose stools, constipation, enlarged spleen, ovarian cysts, leg cramps, muscle spasms, muscle stiffness, inflammation

EMOTIONAL SUPPORT

Asparagus is a very helpful food if you struggle with shyness, self-consciousness, concern over what others think of you, fear of breaking out of your shell and exposing yourself, or dread of venturing out in public. If you truly need help in these areas (as opposed to if you're just a natural introvert who's comfortable with who you are, despite others' misguided opinions that you should act more like an extrovert), asparagus will come to your aid and give you the confidence to rise up and claim your place in the world.

SPIRITUAL LESSON

When we harvest asparagus, it's really just a sprout on its way to becoming a much larger plant. If we were to let asparagus fern out and go to seed, though, it would become woody and inedible. Over time, humans have learned to recognize when a spear of asparagus is at its peak for consumption. It's a lesson that transfers to our own lives. Sometimes people push circumstances too far, aiming for more and more growth, trying to see something through to the bitter end. We don't always have to let a full cycle play out. We can learn to recognize when a project, meeting, or conversation has reached its best moment, and to gracefully end it at that point, harnessing the power of that peak time for the best ultimate outcome.

TIPS

- Look for thicker, fatter asparagus spears, as these tend to be the most nutritious. (Though if all you can find are bunches of skinny asparagus, don't shy away from them—they still have value.)
- Try juicing a few stalks of raw asparagus along with your favorite other vegetable juice ingredients, such as celery and cucumber. Consuming asparagus in this form makes it especially effective.
- For an incredible spring organ detox, eat one bunch of asparagus per day for the entire month of April or May.

ASPARAGUS SOUP

Makes 2 to 4 servings

This creamy soup is perfect for those spring nights that still have a bit of chill in the air and yet give you hope of all the renewal the season has to offer. And when fresh asparagus is unavailable, it's the perfect comfort food to make with frozen asparagus instead. Either way, it's a hit that's sure to win fans from the moment they smell it cooking on the stove.

5 cups chopped asparagus

½ yellow onion, roughly chopped

2 garlic cloves

½ teaspoon poultry seasoning

¼ teaspoon sea salt

1 tablespoon olive oil

½ cup almonds

Black pepper to taste

Place the asparagus, yellow onion, and garlic in a saucepan. Add 2 cups of water; cover and bring to a simmer. Steam the asparagus for 5 to 7 minutes, until tender. Remove from heat. Drain off any excess water and transfer the mixture to a blender*. Add all the remaining ingredients and blend until smooth. Allow steam to escape the top of the blender as you go.

*You may also use an immersion blender, if desired. Leave the asparagus in the pan and add all the remaining ingredients before blending.

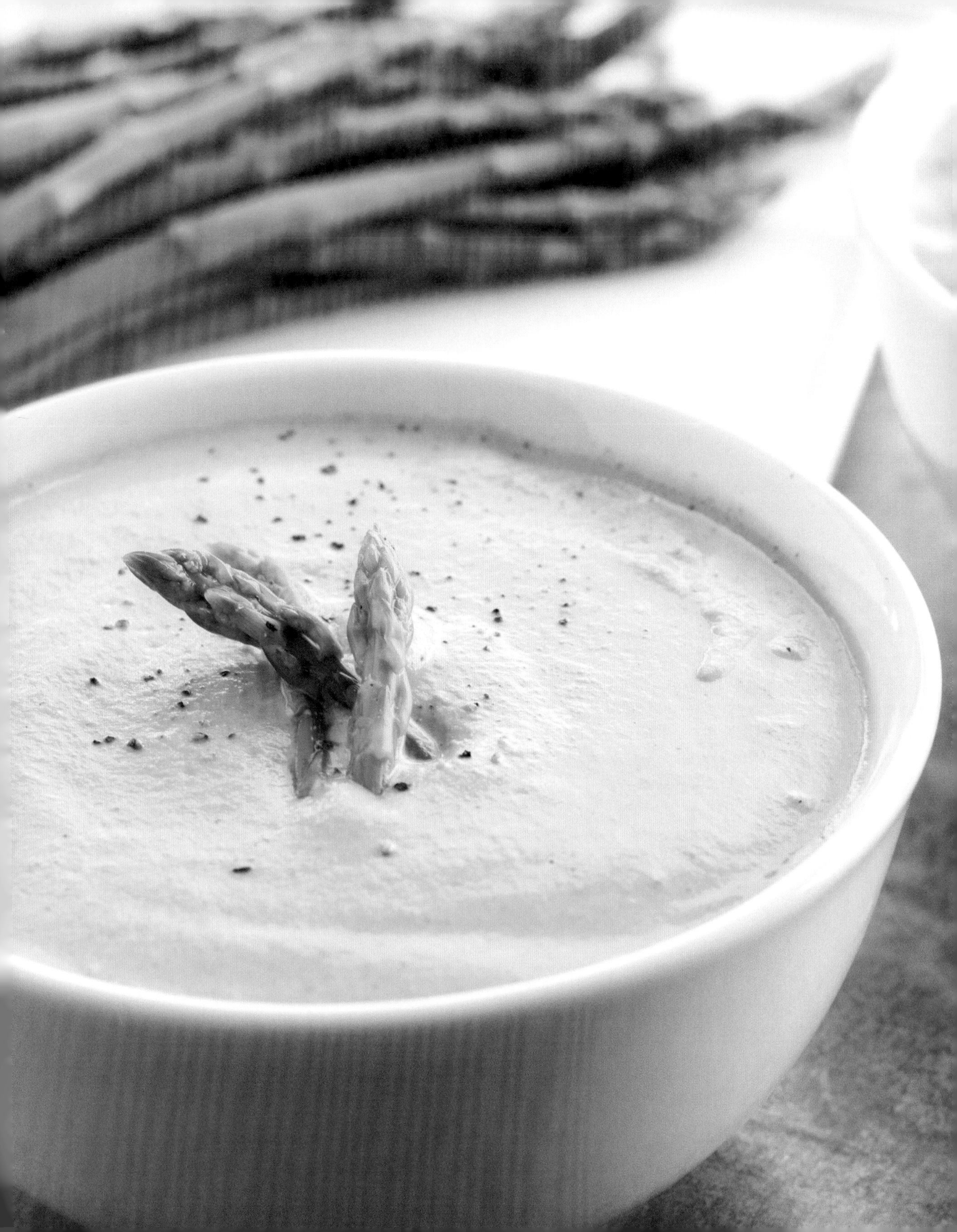

Celery

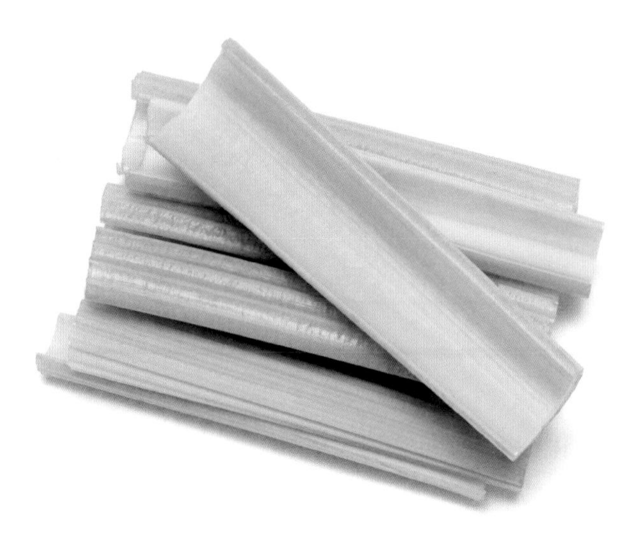

Celery is one of the most powerful anti-inflammatory foods, because it starves unproductive bacteria, yeast, mold, fungus, and viruses that are present in the body and flushes their toxins and debris out of the intestinal tract and liver. Pathogens like these are so often the underlying cause of inflammation—in their absence, your body is much better able to handle whatever life throws your way. At the same time, celery helps good bacteria thrive.

Consuming celery is the most powerful way to alkalize the gut. That's in part because celery (which is technically an herb, not a vegetable) is high in bioactive sodium. It also contains cofactor micro trace mineral salts as yet undiscovered in research. These are varieties of sodium and other trace minerals (more than 60 of them) that are present in celery and work symbiotically and systematically with each other and with celery's regular sodium to raise your body's pH and rid toxic acids from every crevice of your body, including your gut. This process is ideal to cleanse and repair intestinal linings.

At the same time, celery offers enzymes and coenzymes, and it raises hydrochloric acid in the stomach so that food digests with ease and doesn't putrefy. This helps prevent a multitude of gastrointestinal disorders. Adding celery juice to your diet is the best way to resolve ammonia permeability, an unrecognized condition in which ammonia gas seeps through the intestinal lining and causes health issues such as dental rot and brain fog. (You can read more on ammonia permeability and the misunderstood leaky gut syndrome in my first book.)

While celery may seem to some like a bland, boring food, it is anything but. In addition to the above, celery improves kidney function, helps restore the adrenals, and can even bring ease to one's mind and thought patterns, with its mineral salts feeding electrical impulse activity and supporting neuron function, which is key if you suffer with ADHD, brain fog, or memory loss. When it comes to celery, think electrolytes. It hydrates on a deep cellular level, lessening your chances of suffering from migraines. Celery is ideal to address each of the Unforgiving Four factors, plus it offers stress assistance and also repairs your DNA. I could go on and on about the benefits of celery juice for all manner of ills. It is one of the greatest healing tonics of all time.

CONDITIONS

If you have any of the following conditions, try bringing celery into your life:

Acne, attention-deficit/hyperactivity disorder (ADHD), autism, eczema, psoriasis, amyotrophic lateral sclerosis (ALS), leaky gut, infertility, Lyme disease, migraines, obsessive-compulsive disorder (OCD), pelvic inflammatory disease (PID), thyroid diseases and disorders, low reproductive system battery, diabetes, hypoglycemia, adrenal fatigue, anxiety, sepsis, urinary tract infections (UTIs), kidney stones, kidney disease, pancreatic cancer, pancreatitis, fatty liver, chronic fatigue syndrome (CFS), fibromyalgia, lupus, Sjögren's syndrome, Addison's disease, rosacea, lipoma, bladder cancer, interstitial cystitis, Crohn's disease, colitis, irritable bowel syndrome (IBS), thrush, hyperglycemia, hypertension, depression, apnea, thyroid cancer, bacterial vaginosis, edema, injuries, parasites, yeast infections, insomnia, mold exposure, bacterial infections, viral infections, ammonia permeability

SYMPTOMS

If you have any of the following symptoms, try bringing celery into your life:

Intestinal spasms; cysts; low hydrochloric acid; sluggish liver; low cortisol; high cortisol; brain fog; food allergies; acidosis; hypothyroid; hyperthyroid; blurry eyes; joint pain; headaches; bloating; gas; abdominal pressure; abdominal distension; chronic dehydration; eye dryness; frozen shoulder; acid reflux; inflamed gallbladder, stomach, small intestine, and/or colon; rashes; nausea; white film on tongue; *Candida* overgrowth; anxiousness; memory loss; high blood pressure; food sensitivities; swelling; inflammation; muscle spasms; leg cramps; fatigue; mineral deficiencies; brain inflammation; sleep disturbances

EMOTIONAL SUPPORT

We tend to hold a lot of fear in our guts. Nervousness causes those sensations we know as tummy flips or butterflies in the stomach, and anxiety can run deep through the nervous system, putting our guts in knots. Celery restores the entire digestive system. Use it for its calming effects when you are feeling frightened, panicky, shocked, fretful, nervous, threatened, unsure, afraid, or defensive.

SPIRITUAL LESSON

All too often, we make life more complicated than it needs to be—or else we oversimplify what's truly a complex issue. This push-and-pull happens in all areas of life, especially health. In one approach, people overthink health problems and throw all kinds of potential solutions at them. In the other approach, people take a health challenge that's actually a delicate interplay of many factors and try to make it seem like it's just a simple case of the body going haywire out of the blue.

For true healing to occur, we have to embrace a balance of the simple and the complex—and celery teaches us this. Drinking celery juice is the simplest of measures, so simple that people often write it off as too easy to make a difference in how they feel. They figure that adding several other ingredients to their green juice will add that many more nutrients. While green-juice blends can be very healing (see the recipe on the next page, for example), there is nothing that equals the simple power of pure celery juice. It is as healing, transformational, and life-changing as it gets—and that's due to its complex nutritional makeup, which needs to be left undisturbed to work its magic. It's an important reminder for other areas of life. Where else do we need to have an intricate understanding of a situation to conclude that the simplest approach is the best?

TIPS

- To press the reset button on your body, juice celery by itself. For the full effect, drink a full 16 ounces of fresh celery juice daily—and make sure it's on an empty stomach to raise hydrochloric acid levels most efficiently. For dramatic results, drink *two* 16-ounce glasses of fresh celery juice a day.
- If your goal is to cleanse your body of toxic heavy metals such as mercury, aluminum, lead, copper, cadmium, nickel, and arsenic, add a half cup of fresh cilantro when you're juicing your celery.
- An easy way to get more celery into your diet is to add two to four sticks of it when blending the smoothie of your choice.

EASY GREEN JUICE

Makes 1 to 2 servings

This green juice is clean and sweet, making it an easy way to get in an extra dose of greens. It's the perfect way to start off any morning, and you may be surprised that the kids in your life will love it, too.

1 head of celery, stalks separated

1 large apple, sliced

1 lemon

½ bunch parsley or cilantro

4 sprigs fresh mint

Run all the ingredients through a high-speed juicer. Pour into a tall glass and enjoy immediately.

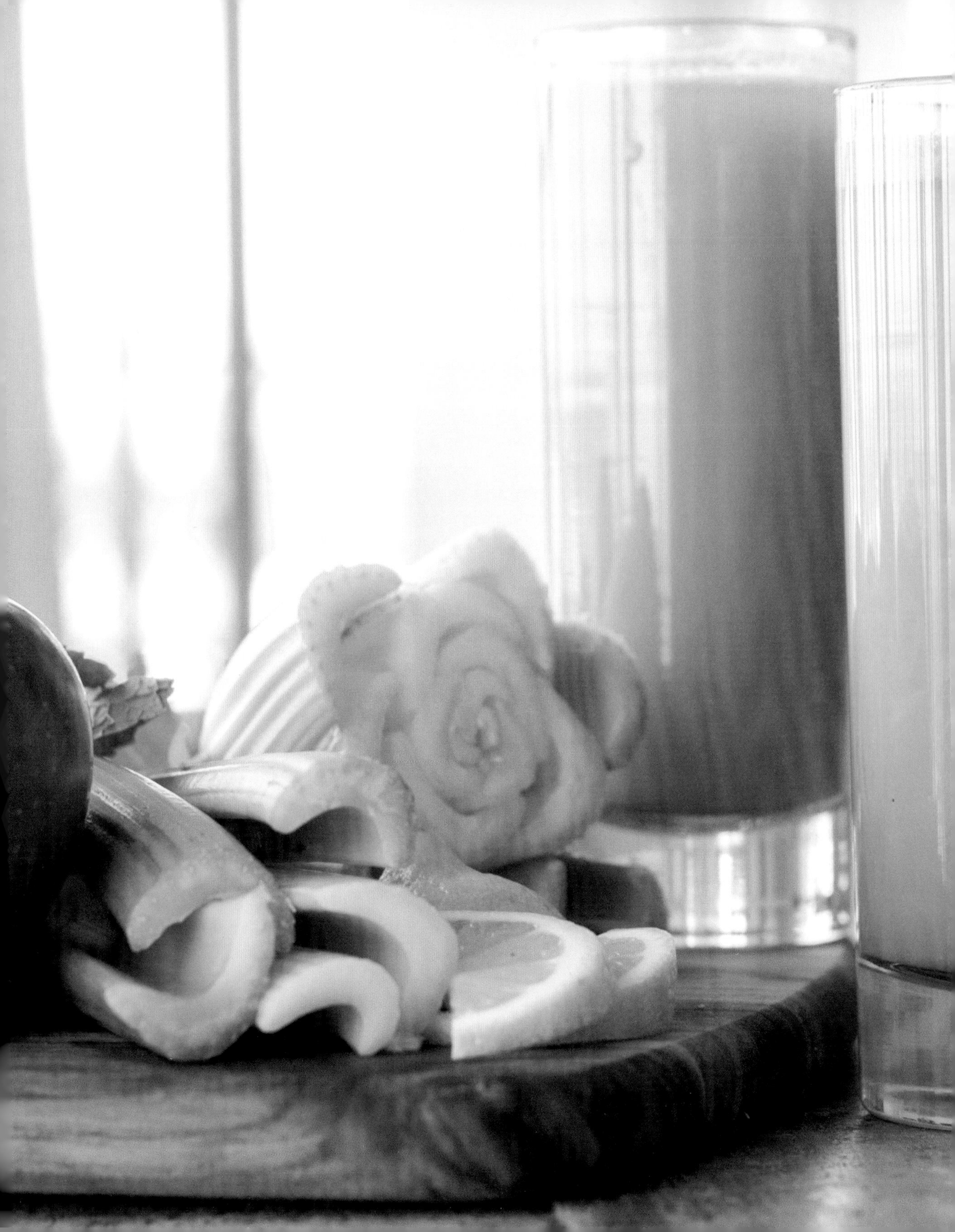

Cruciferous Vegetables

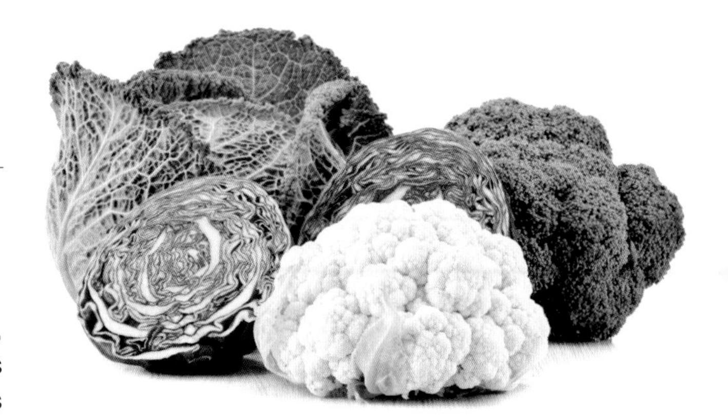

Foods such as cabbage, collard greens, broccoli, broccoli rabe, cauliflower, brussels sprouts, kale, arugula, and mustard greens belong to the cruciferous family. Cruciferous vegetables are like the most charismatic of people—those individuals who have sparkling personalities and who also bring out the best in their companions. That's because in addition to the amazing properties of crucifers you'll read about below, they also have the undiscovered miracle ability to ignite hidden cleansing and healing abilities in other foods when eaten in certain combinations. (See "Tips" for details.)

This group of foods has gotten negative attention lately due to misinformation. If you've heard that these foods are "goitrogenic" and therefore bad for the thyroid, rest assured—this couldn't be further from the truth. (For more on this, see the chapter "Harmful Health Fads and Trends.") Cruciferous vegetables are a thyroid's best friend—they pull out radiation from the thyroid that's gotten there from dental and medical exposure. They also protect against the viral explosion that's behind so much of thyroid disease.

Crucifers help stave off a variety of cancers, including breast cancer, reproductive cancers (such as ovarian, uterine, and cervical), brain cancer, intestinal cancers, and lung cancer. They're especially good for lung health; because of their sulfur-rich nature, every single vegetable in this family restores and stimulates the growth of lung tissue. Sulfur is one of the only minerals that branches out into other forms of itself—a chemical process that science has discovered at a surface level and has yet to tap into in its full meaning. Cruciferous vegetables contain two types of sulfur, one in macromineral form and the other as an accompanying micro-sulfur trace mineral. Together they permeate lung tissue to help stimulate growth, regeneration, and healing, and they also restore and recover lung scar tissue. Crucifers are also rich in vitamins such as B vitamins and A, C, E, and K.

Let's take a closer look at some of the individual crucifers:

- **Red cabbage:** The coloring agents that give this crucifer its red-purple hue are at the top of the heap when it comes to disease-fighting pigments. The sulfur in the cabbage carries the phytochemicals from these pigments into the liver with great ease, making red cabbage one of the most rejuvenating foods for the liver. In fact, red cabbage can help retard and reverse scar tissue in the liver.

- **Kale:** When connective tissue is under attack by a virus, inflamed, highly sensitive, and/or weak, it is one of the fastest paths to chronic illness. For the person dealing with connective tissue damage, aches and pains, or inflammation of the joints, kale is a secret weapon, providing a double whammy: while its anti-inflammatory compounds help destroy viruses, its bioavailable phytochemicals help stimulate cell growth and the production of healthy, new connective tissue.
- **Collard greens:** These possess nutrients in the stems that hold antibacterial properties. Steaming collard greens or adding them to a soup draws out their medicinal properties so that when you consume them, their nutrients travel through your body and act as an antibiotic. (If Grandma's chicken soup were made with collard greens, it truly would be an antibiotic.)
- **Cauliflower:** This crucifer contains the trace mineral boron, which is also known to help the endocrine system—and yet cauliflower gets more attention for the so-called goitrogens it contains. Cauliflower does the very opposite of what the hype says—it *helps* the thyroid and the rest of the endocrine system (including the hypothalamus and adrenal glands) to stave off the viruses that are truly behind issues such as thyroiditis. Cauliflower has a unique ability to be easily digested in its raw state, which is ideal, because eating it raw gives you the best chance at easily assimilating and using the full potential of what it has to offer.
- **Broccoli:** When you were a kid and your parents told you to eat your broccoli, they were right. Broccoli is an all-purpose multivitamin for the body, plus it contains bioavailable trace minerals and other nutrients that enhance all body systems, including the entire immune system. Nature made broccoli in this way, with a balance that can't be matched, to offer a little something for every organ, gland, bone, nerve, and more in the body.
- **Brussels sprouts and green cabbage:** Green cabbage is very nutritious, wonderful for supporting the joints and reversing osteoporosis. If you enjoy this vegetable, it's definitely worth eating. If you're looking for maximum nutrient density, though, go with brussels sprouts—they have 10 times the nutrition found in green cabbage. Brussels sprouts take the joint factor to the next level, plus they help lower bad cholesterol, increase good cholesterol, purify the liver and other dense sponge organs such as the spleen, and purify the blood.

CONDITIONS

If you have any of the following conditions, try bringing cruciferous vegetables into your life:

Hepatitis C, cirrhosis of the liver, connective tissue damage, Hashimoto's thyroiditis, Graves' disease, nutrient absorption issues, nodules on bones and glands, breast cancer, reproductive cancers (such as ovarian, uterine, and cervical), brain cancer, intestinal cancers, lung cancer, adrenal fatigue, macular degeneration, osteoporosis, high cholesterol, mold exposure, hypertension, depression, herpes simplex 1 (HSV-1), herpes simplex 2 (HSV-2), HHV-6, obsessive-compulsive disorder (OCD), low reproductive system battery, pelvic inflammatory disease (PID), diabetes, hypoglycemia, migraines, acne, anxiety, attention-deficit/hyperactivity disorder (ADHD), autism, eczema, psoriasis, Epstein-Barr virus (EBV)/mononucleosis, shingles, urinary tract infections (UTIs), chronic obstructive pulmonary disease (COPD)

SYMPTOMS

If you have any of the following symptoms, try bringing cruciferous vegetables into your life:

Weight gain, aches and pains, scar tissue in the liver, premenstrual syndrome (PMS) symptoms, food allergies, joint inflammation, joint pain, knee pain, scar tissue in the lungs, hypothyroid, sluggish liver, liver congestion, hyperthyroid, histamine reactions, hot flashes, hives, inflammation, menopause symptoms, leg cramps, loss of smell, nerve inflammation, shortness of breath, snoring, swollen lymph nodes, fatigue, tingles and numbness, ringing or buzzing in the ears, heart palpitations

EMOTIONAL SUPPORT

Cruciferous veggies are great at supporting anyone who is mired in confusion. If you know someone who seems baffled, bewildered, befuddled, or confounded, sit down with her or him over a salad of kale and red cabbage, some cauliflower soup, or a side dish of broccoli or brussels sprouts. Even if all you have time to do is drop off one of these ingredients at your friend's house, it will make a difference in her or his emotional state.

SPIRITUAL LESSON

Have you ever lovingly taken care of someone, looked out for her or his needs, provided nurturing, given everything you had and more, supported and believed in and protected that someone, only to be betrayed in the end? Have you ever felt stranded and alone, with the very person you once coddled now spreading false rumors about you?

If so, you've got a friend in the cruciferous family. These vegetables have recently been disgraced and shunned on the false premise that they harm the thyroid, when in fact, it's just the opposite. They've been supporting the thyroid all along. For decades to come, misinformation will cause people to turn against the food source that would most help them—until someday, the misguided theory of goitrogenic foods is finally proven wrong.

Kale, broccoli, cauliflower, and all their cousins teach us to make room for patience and thankfulness in our lives, for ourselves and others. If you've been the one whom others have turned on, sustain yourself with the knowledge that you are not alone, and that adversity does not diminish your truth. We must remember also to have respect for others who have devoted time, energy, love, and guidance to our lives, even if we didn't see their efforts, honor them, or if we quickly forgot what they did for us. Just as the cruciferous family has been looking out for us, keeping us safe by protecting us from illness, hold a candle in your life for those who have worked hard for you.

TIPS

- Cauliflower and seaweed together create a powerful detoxification tool to help expel chlorine, harmful fluoride, and radiation from the sensitive endocrine glands. One delicious way to enjoy this combination is to chop raw cauliflower in the food processor until fine, then to use it as rice in nori roll-ups.
- Apples and red cabbage eaten at the same time are especially effective at expelling bacteria, worms and other parasites, and viruses from the liver, spleen, and intestinal tract. For a filling and flavorful dish, combine apples, red cabbage, tahini, and garlic in the food processor and chop until shredded and well combined. Serve in wraps or over leafy greens.
- When eaten with asparagus, broccoli heightens the cancer-fighting compounds in asparagus. Broccoli also strengthens the kidney-cleansing phytochemicals in asparagus. An easy way to enjoy these vegetables together is to add them to the same steam pot.
- On their own, collard greens and pumpkin seeds are both rich in zinc. When eaten together, though, the zincs combine and become more bioavailable, for maximum absorption and use by the body. Try making a pumpkin-seed pâté, then spread it onto collard-green leaves, top with your favorite fillings, and roll up into burritos.

ASIAN KALE SALAD

Makes 2 servings

The best thing about this salad is that it just keeps getting better as it sits in the fridge and the flavors combine. Make an extra-large batch, and you'll have an awesome lunch waiting for you for up to two days afterward. The trick to kale salad is to roll up your sleeves and massage the kale until it is really tender. It will be well worth the effort when you take your first bite!

¼ cup raw tahini
¼ jalapeño, seeds removed
¼ cup lime juice
1 garlic clove
½ cup cilantro leaves
2 dates, pitted
2 cups peeled cubed zucchini
2 heads of curly kale, chopped
1 cup shredded red cabbage
3 scallions, chopped
Sesame seeds (optional)

For the dressing, blend the first 7 ingredients in a blender until smooth. Add water only if needed for a smoother consistency. Massage the mixture thoroughly into the kale leaves until the kale is well softened. Top with the red cabbage, scallions, and a sprinkle of sesame seeds, if desired.

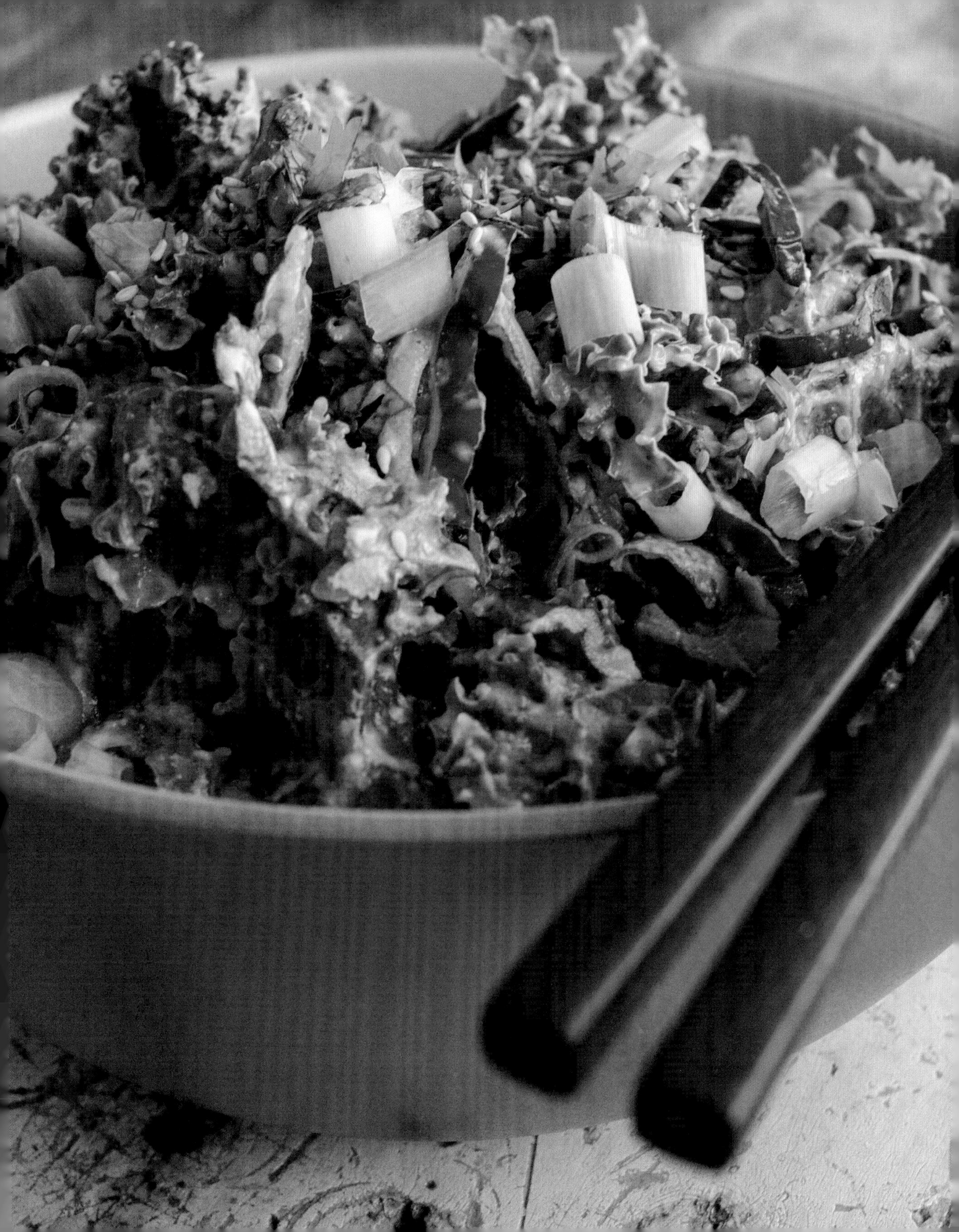

Cucumbers

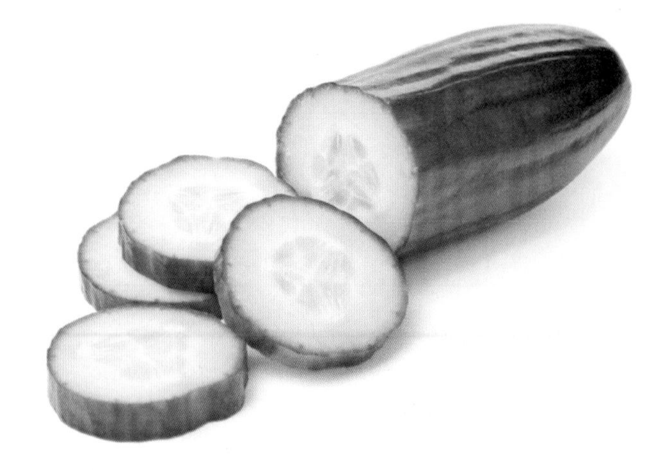

So many people go through life with chronic dehydration, with no idea of the negative effect it's having on their health. Cucumbers are the perfect antidote. They have a fountain-of-youth effect, hydrating us at the deepest cellular level possible. Plus, cucumbers' cooling effect makes them excellent at rejuvenation and especially effective at cooling a hot, stagnant liver. When eaten on a daily basis, cucumbers can reverse liver damage, dialing back 10 to 15 years of toxin exposure (including from heavy metals and pesticides such as DDT) and poor diet. It makes this vegetable (really, a fruit) a particular ally in reducing bloat.

Fresh cucumber juice is the best rejuvenation tonic in the world. It contains electrolyte compounds specifically geared toward nourishing and cooling down overused adrenal glands and kidneys that are struggling with their task of filtering out toxic debris and getting overheated from toxic uric acid. If you have kidney disease, are on dialysis, or you're missing a kidney, drinking cucumber juice every day can be extremely beneficial. Cucumbers' cooling effect on the glands and organs also makes them wonderful fever reducers for both children and adults. Juicing cucumbers unleashes their magical anti-fever compounds and agents that help calm a fever like water on a fire.

Cucumbers' traces of the amino acids glycine and glutamine, combined with their extreme and highly active content of enzymes and coenzymes, plus their abundance of more than 50 trace minerals, make them an excellent delivery system for neurotransmitter chemicals. This is great news if you're dealing with anxiety or other neurological conditions. Cucumbers provide other critical nutrition, too, such as chlorophyll in their skins that's bonded to B vitamins and vitamins A and C. And cucumbers support digestion; they contain undiscovered coenzymes that will one day be called *talafinns*. Alongside enzymes that have been discovered by medical research (such as erepsin), talafinns help the body's protein digestion process so you can get the most out of everything you eat.

CONDITIONS

If you have any of the following conditions, try bringing cucumbers into your life:

Kidney disease, kidney failure, missing kidney, adrenal fatigue, anxiety, Epstein-Barr virus (EBV)/mononucleosis, diabetes, hypoglycemia, migraines, amyotrophic lateral sclerosis (ALS), eczema, psoriasis, transient ischemic attack (TIA), mystery infertility, pelvic inflammatory disease (PID), low reproductive system battery, colds, influenza, cytomegalovirus (CMV), HHV-6, shingles, chronic fatigue syndrome (CFS), fibromyalgia, multiple sclerosis (MS), lupus, postural tachycardia syndrome (POTS), dysautonomia, sepsis, yeast infections, *E. coli* infection, *Streptococcus* infection, sunburn

SYMPTOMS

If you have any of the following symptoms, try bringing cucumbers into your life:

Fever, dandruff, bloating, gastric spasms, stagnant liver, dehydration, headaches, dry and/or itchy skin, hot flashes, weight gain, menopause symptoms, premenstrual syndrome (PMS) symptoms, anxiousness, neuralgia (including trigeminal neuralgia), food sensitivities, inflammation, blood toxicity, acidosis, back pain, all neurological symptoms (including tingles, numbness, spasms, twitches, nerve pain, and tightness of the chest), low hydrochloric acid

EMOTIONAL SUPPORT

There's a reason we use the expression "cool as a cucumber." If you or a loved one are dealing with an anger issue, bring cucumbers into the diet. Offer cucumber slices to anyone who you know can be easily infuriated, disgruntled, crabby, cranky, irritated, heated, or downright hostile.

SPIRITUAL LESSON

Because they're green and we eat them in salads, we often think of cucumbers as a vegetable. When we open one up, though, we remember that all those little seeds mean a cucumber is truly a fruit. It's a powerful reminder that outside appearances and the boxes other people put us into don't make up the full truth of who we are. Very often we, too, have a talent, quality, or gift that someone couldn't guess just by looking at us. Cucumbers teach us to look deep inside ourselves and each other for the miracles we all contain.

TIPS

- For results you can see, try to eat two cucumbers daily.
- Instead of juicing a multitude of vegetables and fruits at one time, try juicing cucumber on its own. Like celery juice, straight cucumber juice has unique healing qualities. If you drink 16 ounces of pure cucumber juice on a regular basis, it can have a life-changing effect.
- If you're trying to keep grains out of your diet, turn cucumbers into noodles with a spiralizer or julienne peeler. Cucumber noodles are more hydrating and tastier than the more popular zucchini noodles. Try English cucumbers for best noodle results.
- When using conventional cucumbers, make sure to peel off the skin before eating to avoid consuming the toxic wax coating.

CUCUMBER NOODLE BOWL

Makes 2 servings

This clean, cool noodle bowl will leave you feeling light and refreshed. The Asian-inspired flavors of lime and sesame are tossed with cucumber, carrot, and cashews in a beautiful mix of color and crunch. This nice, mild dish can easily be made spicier by adding extra red pepper flakes at the very end to find your perfect flavor. You'll end up with a bowl that is just as beautiful as it is delicious.

4 cucumbers
2 large carrots
2 teaspoons sesame oil
2 teaspoons sesame seeds
Lime juice (from about 2 limes)
Red pepper flakes (optional)
½ cup chopped cilantro
½ cup chopped basil
½ cup chopped cashews

Cut the cucumbers and carrots into thin strips using a julienne peeler, knife, or spiralizer. In a large bowl, toss the cucumber and carrot "noodles" with sesame oil, sesame seeds, lime juice, and red pepper flakes, if using. Just prior to serving, top the mixture with chopped cilantro, basil, and cashews. Enjoy!

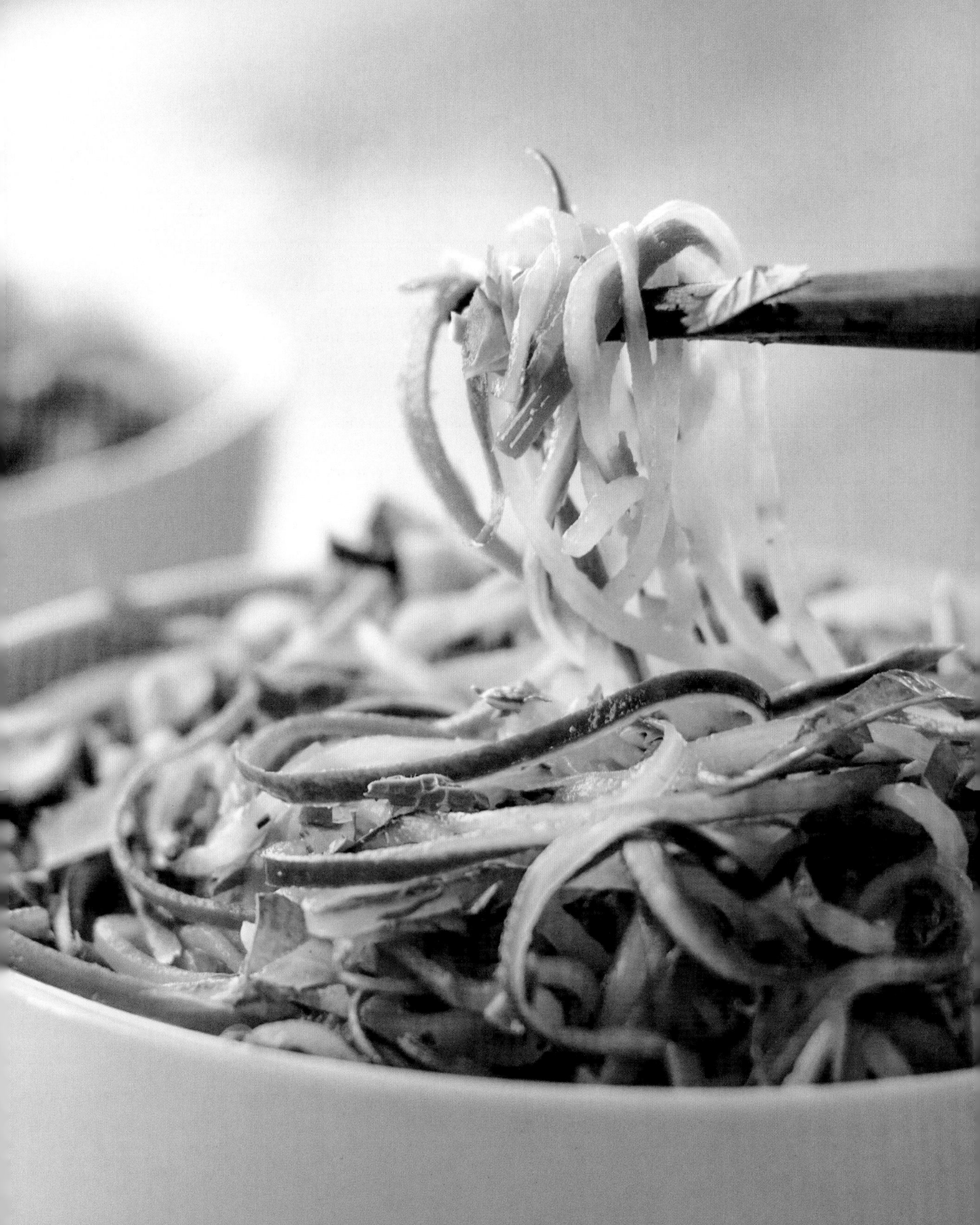

Leafy Greens

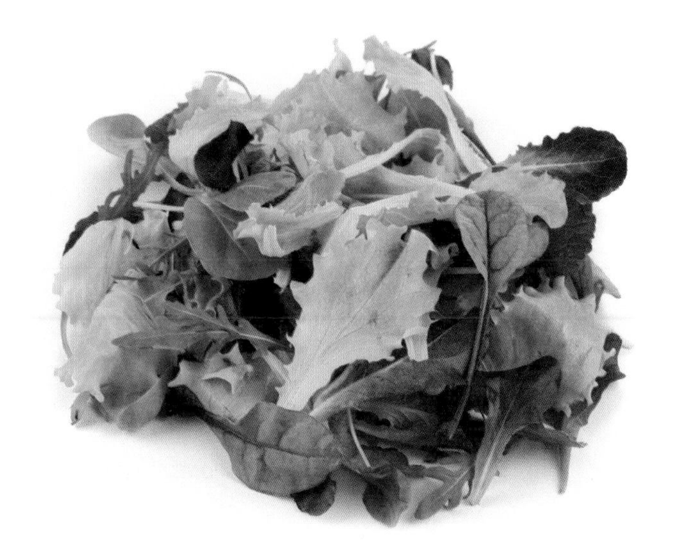

When we hear the advice, "Eat your veggies," we often think of classic dinnertime side dishes like carrots, broccoli, peas, and green beans. Leafy greens, on the other hand, are often written off as boring and lesser—the base of a salad in which all the other ingredients are much more interesting. Really, leafy greens such as lettuce, spinach, Swiss chard, mâche, and watercress deserve accolades for the power they hold to restore your health. (Numerous other leafy greens have made it into this book too: for kale, collard greens, mustard greens, and arugula, see "Cruciferous Vegetables"; for radish greens, see "Radishes"; and for dandelion greens, parsley, and cilantro, see their individual write-ups.) Far from blasé, salad greens are vegetable royalty.

One common misunderstanding is that eaten raw, these greens, labeled "roughage" are difficult to digest. On the contrary, leafy greens are practically predigested and therefore require very little work on the part of your digestive system. What does occur is that these leaves scrub and massage the linings of your stomach, small intestine, and colon, loosening old, trapped yeast, mold, and other types of fungus, along with debris and pockets of waste matter, so they can be carried out, making elimination very productive. Discomfort from eating raw salads is usually due to sensitive nerves or inflammation in the intestinal tract, or the simple sensation of fiber doing its job to "sweep out the chimney." If this describes you, add butter leaf lettuce, red leaf lettuce, and/or spinach to your daily diet in small amounts.

Over time, leafy greens are wonderful healers of intestinal disorders. They help create a more alkaline stomach composition by raising beneficial hydrochloric acid levels, which in turn kills off the unproductive bacteria that create the bad acids responsible for GERD and other forms of acid reflux. One of the specific types of bacteria that leafy greens reduce is *H. pylori*, which is often responsible for stomach ulcers.

Leafy greens create true alkalinity in the body systems, especially the lymphatic, which can become the most acidic system due to a barrage of chemicals, acids, plastics, pesticides, heavy metals, and pathogens constantly entering the lymphatic passages. Medical communities are unaware that alkalinity of the blood, organs, endocrine system, reproductive system, and central nervous system hinges completely on the lymphatic system being alkaline. Leafy greens help to expel, purge, and drain the lymphatic system of these toxins so that it can remain alkaline. This is where these greens really have a critical role in our healing process.

Leafy greens also hold precious and vital mineral salts, partially composed of a group of cofactors associated with sodium, such as trace bioavailable iodine, chromium, sulfur, magnesium, calcium, potassium, silica, manganese, and molybdenum, which are critical for neurotransmitter and neuron support, and are also the fundamental basis of building electrolytes. On top of which, leafy greens are high in enzymes, vitamin A, B vitamins such as folic acid, healing alkaloids (plant compounds that fight disease), micronutrients for restoring the endocrine system, and forms of chlorophyll and carotenes that are specific to these vegetables. This unique group of nutrients works together to feed all organs and body systems, making leafy greens a foundation of our health. Leafy greens are antiviral, antibacterial, and anti-mold—and great for staving off every one of the Unforgiving Four. While they don't have carbohydrates to sustain our energy, they cover the other side of the equation necessary to keep us alive, and to stave off disease and chronic illness.

If you worry about getting enough protein, fret no more. Leafy greens have the most bioavailable and assimilable proteins you can find, readily available for your body to take up. Leafy greens help reverse all protein-related diseases, such as gout, kidney disease, kidney stones and gallstones, gallbladder disease, hepatitis C, lymphedema, connective tissue damage, osteopenia, osteoporosis, osteoarthritis, and heart disease, which all arise from protein sources that are not breaking down or assimilating, and are instead causing deterioration of the body.

The next time you hear someone refer to a salad as "rabbit food," remember what you've just read. Leafy greens are anything but a joke.

CONDITIONS

If you have any of the following conditions, try bringing leafy greens into your life:

Gastroesophageal reflux disease (GERD), thyroid disease, celiac disease, diverticulitis, gallbladder disease, gallstones, gout, kidney disease, anemia, irritable bowel syndrome (IBS), kidney stones, peptic ulcers, heart disease, *H. pylori* infection, hepatitis C, osteoporosis, osteopenia, osteoarthritis, low reproductive system battery, lymphedema, dyspepsia, skin disorders (including eczema and psoriasis), nodules on bones and glands, mold exposure, endocrine disorders, adrenal fatigue, insomnia, acne, amyotrophic lateral sclerosis (ALS), anxiety, attention-deficit/hyperactivity disorder (ADHD), depression, infertility, Lyme disease, thyroid cancer, migraines, obsessive-compulsive disorder (OCD), herpes simplex 1 (HSV-1), herpes simplex 2 (HSV-2), pelvic inflammatory disease (PID), diabetes, hypoglycemia, Epstein-Barr virus (EBV)/mononucleosis, shingles

SYMPTOMS

If you have any of the following symptoms, try bringing leafy greens into your life:

Heartburn, acidosis, iron deficiency, constipation, mineral deficiencies, trace mineral deficiencies, swelling, fluid retention, inflamed liver, weakened kidneys, low hydrochloric acid, stomach upset, muscle cramps, food allergies, spasms, bone loss, receding gums, stagnant liver, joint pain, inflammation, weight gain, menopause symptoms, premenstrual syndrome (PMS) symptoms, hormonal imbalances, acid reflux, dry skin, scaly skin, calcifications, low platelet count, abdominal cramping, arrhythmia, heart palpitations, balance issues, blisters, body aches, brain fog, cavities, chest tightness, dandruff, dizziness, earwax buildup, enamel loss, jaw pain, knee pain

EMOTIONAL SUPPORT

When your body is filled with toxins on a physical level, it can lead to toxic buildup on an emotional level. So many people feel stuck, stagnant, confined, lost, or otherwise held back in life. Leafy greens are a way forward. Just as they flush out physical debris, they loosen stored-up toxic emotions and guide them out of your life. Adding more leafy greens to your diet can be an incredibly freeing experience, helping you to feel clean and clear again—your rightful state of being.

SPIRITUAL LESSON

How many times have you missed a window of opportunity? Time can slip by so fast, and before we know it, the birthday wishes we're sending a friend are belated, or we're getting to the beach when the tide is too high to enjoy it. Leafy greens teach us to seize the moment. Their short shelf life means that the earlier we eat them after they're picked, the better they are for our health. Getting in tune with this awakens us to the other fleeting moments of life—the other opportunities to nourish ourselves on every level if only we have the presence of mind to recognize what's in front of us.

TIPS

- Create a schedule for leafy greens, so that you feature a different green in your salad (or other meal) each day of the week. This can be a fun way to ensure that you're getting variation for maximum nutritional benefits.
- If you find raw greens too difficult to chew, try selecting one to juice along with cucumbers or celery.
- For another nutritious green drink, blend spinach with fresh-squeezed orange juice.
- Try growing your own greens. This will not only give you the chance to take advantage of their powerful natural probiotics (see the chapter "Adaptation" for more on these elevated biotics); it will also mean that they grow specifically for your benefit, as though your name becomes written into each leaf.
- When growing your own greens, try to pick some at an early phase of development. Eating them at this stage prepares your body to receive even more of the greens' benefits later on, when they become full-grown.
- Lettuce leaves make great alternatives to tortillas. Try filling them with your desired ingredients for taco- or burrito-style roll-ups.
- If you avoid avocado because you dislike the texture, try making guacamole with an ample amount of chopped mâche and a tablespoon of raw honey. This will alter the texture at the same time that it adds the greens' nutty flavor and the honey's sweetness to the dish, changing your avocado experience. Over time, eating this special guacamole will alter your avocado aversion, leading you to enjoy avocado on its own.

LEAFY GREEN SALAD WITH LEMON DRESSING

Makes 2 to 4 servings

This simple salad is full of flavor and perfect for lunch at work. Just keep the dressing separate until right before eating, and you can enjoy a delicious, vibrant lunch right at your desk. Make sure to look for raw pistachios if you can. They're tender and absolutely perfect alongside the sweetness of the strawberry and the brightness of the lemon.

½ cup lemon juice
¼ cup olive oil
2 tablespoons raw honey
8 cups leafy greens
2 cups sliced strawberries
½ cup unsalted raw pistachios

For the dressing, blend the lemon juice, olive oil, and honey until smooth. Toss the leafy greens with the dressing in a large bowl until the greens are evenly coated. Divide the salad into individual bowls. Top with the strawberries and pistachios.

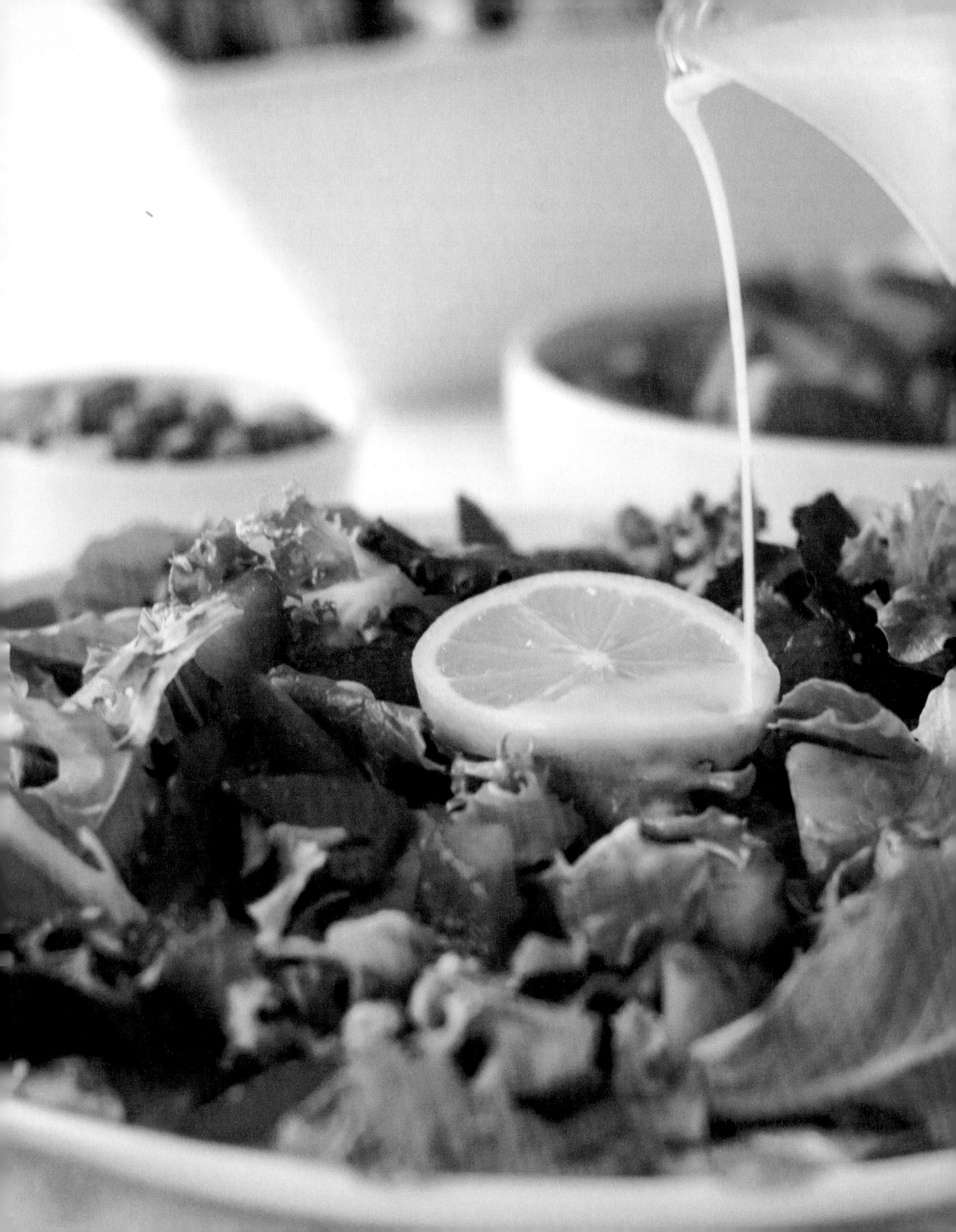

Onions

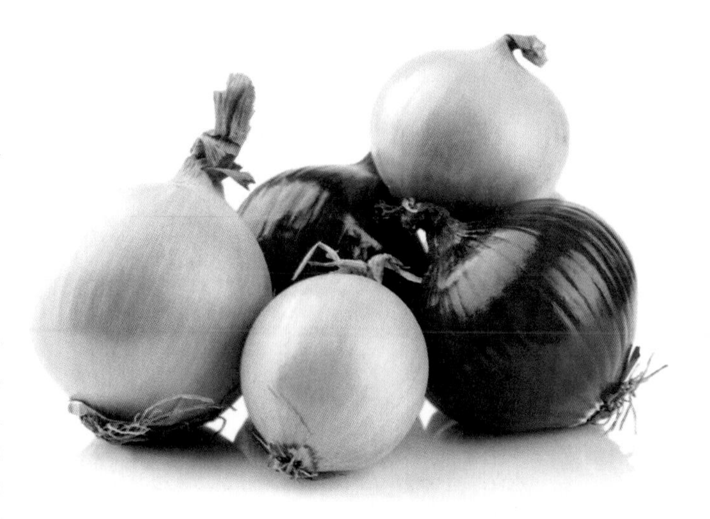

Leeks, chives, ramps, scallions, red onions, yellow onions, white onions, shallots, and any other type of allium you enjoy are nature's antibiotics. Unfortunately, people don't often eat a high volume of onions—maybe just a wedge in soup once a month, or a slice once a week on top of salad. To truly benefit from onions' antibacterial qualities, we have to make them more central to our lives.

Some people complain of digestive distress when they eat onions. Contrary to popular belief, though, onions are not irritants. Rather, they're highly medicinal. An upset stomach from onions is an indication that someone has an elevated level of unproductive bacteria in the digestive tract. The onions are working to eliminate that bacteria, and the resulting die-off can translate to temporary discomfort.

One particular condition that many people deal with these days is SIBO, which is largely a mystery to the medical field. What's usually responsible for this small intestinal bacterial overgrowth are *Streptococcus* A and B, various strains of *E. coli*, *C. difficile*, *H. pylori*, *Staphylococcus*, and/or different varieties of fungus (excluding *Candida*, the natural fungus that we need to survive). Onions are one of the most accomplished foods on the planet for keeping down bacterial overgrowth in the body, making them a star for anyone who deals with SIBO. This quality also enhances the body's production of B_{12}. If you avoid onions because of a sensitive digestive tract, try adding them back into your diet in very small amounts at first. Over time, their cleansing effect will enable you to tolerate larger servings of them.

We'd all do well to make friends with onions. The sulfur they contain (including the phytochemical allicin, other organosulfides, and sulfur compounds that haven't yet been uncovered in research) is part of what makes onions nature's antibiotic. It's also responsible for ridding the body of radiation exposure, casting out viruses, and drawing out DDT and other pesticides, herbicides, and toxic heavy metals. The sulfur in onions makes them wonderful for alleviating joint pain, degeneration, discomfort, and for repairing tendons and connective tissue. If you have an iron deficiency, onions are also very helpful, because their sulfur content slows iron loss.

High in the trace minerals zinc, manganese, iodine, and selenium, onions help rejuvenate the skin and protect the lungs. If you'd like your skin to look younger, it's a great idea to eat onions daily. Same goes if you used to be a smoker, and you'd like to repair some of that damage to your lungs. Onions are very helpful for addressing colds and flus that cause bronchitis, and for bacteria-caused pneumonia. They're also the ultimate anti-inflammatories for the bowels, helping to heal ulcers, eliminate mucus from the stool, and soothe the intestinal tract.

In old folklore, garlic was used to keep ghosts and ghouls away. Onions should share a similar reputation—for keeping pathogenic ghouls away. Making them part of your diet will give you a powerful immune boost and safeguard against the pathogenic world. The next time you go out to buy cough syrup or decongestant, pick up a few different types of onions at the same time—though they may not be in the same aisle, onions truly are medicine.

CONDITIONS

If you have any of the following conditions, try bringing onions into your life:

Gastroesophageal reflux disease (GERD); asthma; chronic obstructive pulmonary disease (COPD); emphysema; breast cancer; bone cancer; diverticulitis; ear infections; influenza; conjunctivitis; sties; hypertension; leukemia; migraines; prostate cancer; ringworm; rosacea; staph infections; small intestinal bacterial overgrowth (SIBO); halitosis; Lyme disease; liver disease; fatty liver; herpes simplex 1 (HSV-1); herpes simplex 2 (HSV-2); HHV-6; HHV-7; the undiscovered HHV-10, HHV-11, and HHV-12; urinary tract infections (UTIs); colds; Epstein-Barr virus (EBV); yeast infections; transient ischemic attack (TIA)

SYMPTOMS

If you have any of the following symptoms, try bringing onions into your life:

Bad breath, heartburn, canker sores, iron deficiency, joint inflammation, tendon inflammation (particularly Achilles inflammation), eye issues, cold hands and feet, scars, snoring, joint pain, joint discomfort, shortness of breath, all neurological symptoms (including tingles, numbness, poor circulation, spasms, twitches, nerve pain, and tightness of the chest), restless leg syndrome, gastritis, body stiffness, body aches and pains, dizziness, dry skin, enlarged spleen, hot flashes, inflammation, jaw pain, knee pain, tremors, weakness, mineral deficiencies

EMOTIONAL SUPPORT

When you're dealing with chronic frustration, anger, and aggravation—whether toward other people, events, or yourself—it's critical to bring onions into your routine. Onions purge anger from the body, helping to loosen up resentment, fury, vexation, and disappointment so you can be free to live your life.

SPIRITUAL LESSON

Onions are wrongly blamed for bad breath. In fact, the opposite is true—onions help alleviate bad breath. What's really responsible for halitosis is unproductive bacteria in the gut that rises up to the mouth. Because onions are antibacterial, they help combat this problem, so that your breath becomes sweeter-smelling over time. Right after you eat an onion, there may be a lingering scent—this is just the onion's natural sulfur, and a sign that it's doing its job. While we focus on different toothpastes, mouthwashes, and breath mints as the answer for halitosis and scorn the onion as the enemy, it's really our savior.

Have you ever seen this phenomenon take place in your life, where someone who worked hard to alleviate a problem mistakenly got the blame for creating the issue? It happens so often, from a supervisor at work whom employees disrespect even though that supervisor is saving their jobs, to a parent who gets flak from a child for pointing out a mistake on homework, when learning the right answer will be a key to the child's success that semester. The next time you're in a situation where you're quick to point a finger, keep in mind the plight of the onion, and take a moment to analyze every angle.

TIPS

- Avoid the tip you'll hear out there to rinse or soak onions to make them less pungent. This technique lowers onions' potency, because it dilutes the medicinal properties that kill off bacteria and boost your immune system to keep you healthy.
- Whenever you eat a food that you know isn't a healthy choice, incorporate some onions to counteract the detrimental effects. (This doesn't mean you should order a plate of onion rings. Dipped in bad batter and fried in bad oil, onion rings are not advisable. Rather, if you're eating a hot dog, pile some chopped raw onion on top.)
- When you're eating out at restaurants and are concerned about picking up flu viruses, norovirus, or food poisoning, order something with onions. For example, if you order a salad, get it with onion to kill off any contaminants.
- When picking out onions at the market, make sure each onion is firm and doesn't cave in when you squeeze it. Try to avoid onions that are sprouting new green tips. (This is different from buying a fresh-picked onion with its greens still attached—those onion greens are very beneficial.)
- Experiment with different varieties of onions in different dishes. Try chives in guacamole, scallions in hummus, red onions in salads and stir-fries, leeks in soups, or try steamed yellow or white onions.
- If you're dealing with sinus congestion, cold, or flu, try placing chopped onion in a bowl of warm to hot water, draping a towel over your head and the bowl, and inhaling. This is a great technique for breaking up mucus and loosening congestion.
- If you get chilly easily, have difficulty warming up, always have to wear a sweater, and/or struggle with cold hands and feet, try to incorporate onions into your daily routine to increase circulation.

ONIONS STUFFED WITH MASHED POTATOES AND MUSHROOMS

Makes 4 to 6 servings

These beautiful baked onions look like a restaurant-quality dish and are surprisingly easy to make. They look stunning on any dinner table and worthy of any party occasion. If you don't enjoy mushrooms, feel free to get creative and substitute the sautéed vegetable of your choice.

- 8 large onions
- 8 cups diced potatoes
- 2 teaspoons olive oil
- ½ teaspoon fresh rosemary leaves
- 8 cups chopped mushrooms
- 2 garlic cloves, minced
- 1 teaspoon sea salt
- 1 teaspoon poultry seasoning
- 2 tablespoons pine nuts

Preheat the oven to 350°F. Prep the onions by cutting off the top quarter of each. On the opposite end of each onion, cut off the root so that the onion can rest on a flat surface. Do not peel. Place the onions in a large baking dish and add an inch of water. Bake until the onions are cooked through, checking periodically, 45 to 60 minutes. (Onions are done when they are soft and fragrant.) Remove from the oven and allow to cool. Peel the onions, then carefully remove the inner layers using a fork until only 2 layers remain, forming a cup. Reserve the insides of the onions for later use.

Fill a large sauté pan with an inch of water and bring to a boil. Place the potatoes in the pan, cover, and steam for 15 to 20 minutes, or until tender, stirring occasionally and adding more water if needed to prevent sticking. Place the potatoes in a food processor with 1 teaspoon of olive oil and ½ teaspoon of rosemary leaves. Process until the potatoes are smooth. Set aside.

For the mushroom filling, sauté the mushrooms and garlic in 1 teaspoon of olive oil until the mushrooms are tender and juicy, adding water as needed to prevent sticking. Transfer all but 1 cup of the sautéed mushrooms to a food processor with 1 teaspoon sea salt, 1 teaspoon poultry seasoning, and 2 cups of the reserved onion. Process until the mixture is roughly combined.

Fill the onion cups with alternating layers of mushroom filling and mashed potatoes. Top with sautéed mushrooms and pine nuts. Serve and enjoy!

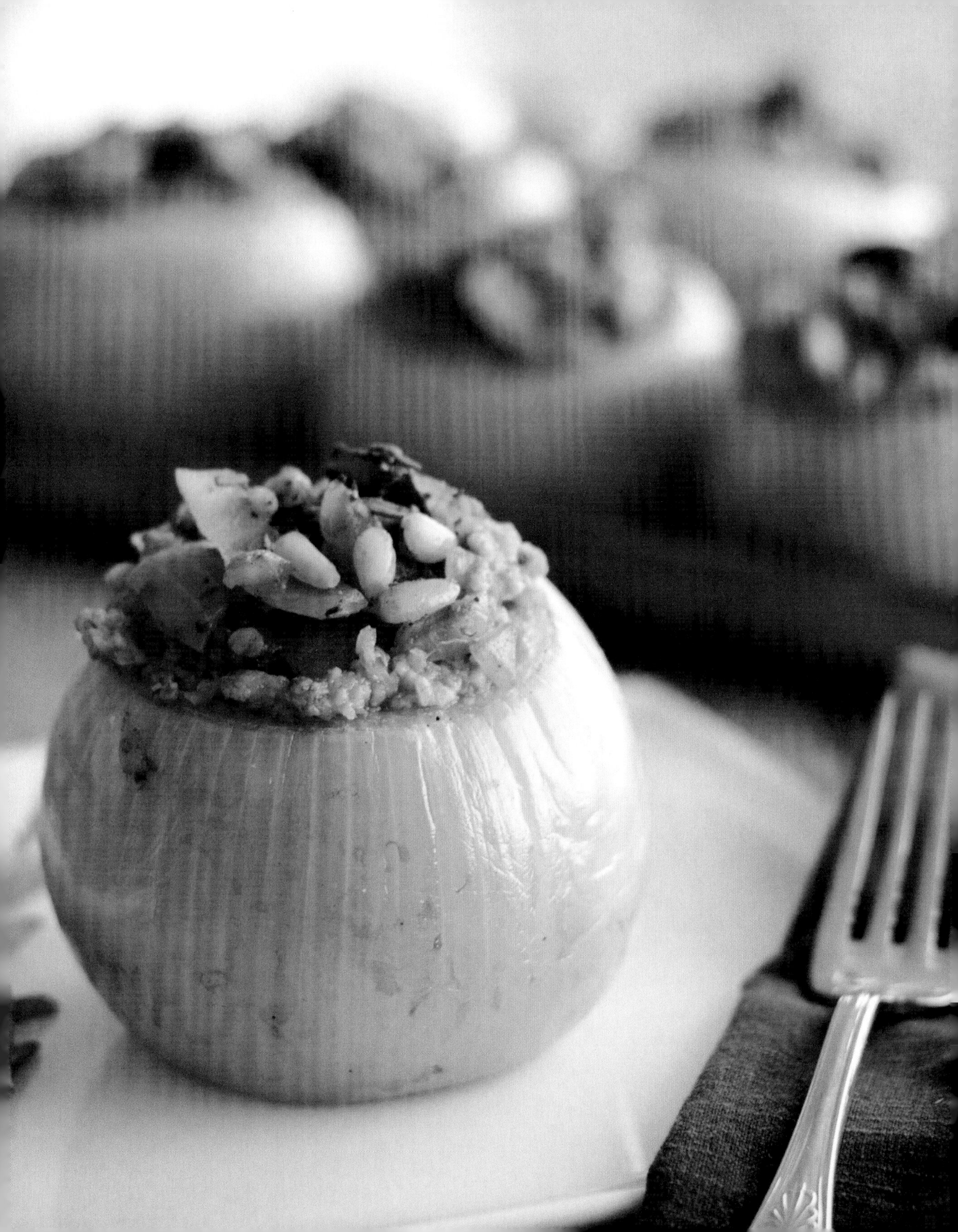

Potatoes

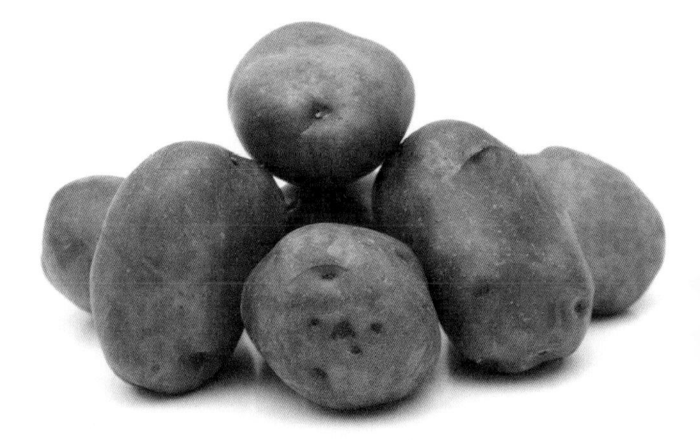

Was there ever a time, maybe in your childhood, when you got in trouble for someone else's mischief—when you were judged as guilty by association? Then you understand the plight of the potato. Potatoes have gotten a bad rap for far too long. As victims of the war on foods mistakenly categorized as "disease-producing," potatoes have been blamed for ills they never caused. Potatoes are wrongly accused of contributing to obesity, diabetes, cancer, *Candida* overgrowth, and many other conditions, while in truth these miraculous tubers can *reverse* these illnesses. That's right! Potatoes are actually good for people with diabetes, because they help stabilize blood sugar.

One common misconception is that potatoes are poisonous because they're nightshades. Potatoes, tomatoes, eggplants, and other edible nightshades *do not* aggravate conditions such as arthritis; you can put aside the worry that potatoes are inflammatory. (For more on this, see the chapter "Harmful Health Fads and Trends.") Truth is, the toxic oil that potatoes are fried in, the cheese sauce ladled on top, and the butter, milk, and cream mashed in are what have the world convinced that potatoes are bad for us. The frying process and the high-fat/high-sugar content of dairy products are the real instigators of insulin resistance and A1C levels that reach the diabetic zone. This combination of fat plus lactose also feeds every type of cancer. Potatoes don't cause health issues; the other ingredients served with them do.

We should also be careful not to lump potatoes in with the fear of grains and processed foods. If you're avoiding "white" foods such as white rice, white flour, white sugar, and dairy products (such as milk, cheese, yogurt, and cream), don't cut out potatoes! After all, a potato in its whole, natural state isn't white—it's covered in nutrient-rich red, brown, gold, blue, or purple skin. This skin of the potato is one of the best nutrition sources on the planet—it's a miracle of amino acids, proteins, and phytochemicals. Only once you cut into a potato might you see a white interior—which doesn't mean it's lacking in value. After all, we don't think of apples, onions, or radishes as white and therefore useless, even though when you cut into them, they're devoid of color. And a cultivated blueberry is colorless inside (whereas wild blueberries are saturated with color inside and out); this doesn't mean it shows up on white food lists. Instead, we picture these foods in their whole forms, which is exactly how we need to start thinking of potatoes.

The entire potato, inside and out, is valuable and beneficial for your health: potato plants draw some of the highest concentration of macro and trace minerals from the earth. Potatoes are also high in potassium and rich in vitamin B_6, as well as a fantastic source of amino acids, especially lysine in its bioactive form. Lysine is a powerful weapon against cancers, liver disease, inflammation, and the viruses such as Epstein-Barr and shingles that are behind rheumatoid arthritis, joint pain, autoimmune disease, and more.

Potatoes will be your allies if you're looking to fight any chronic illness—to fend off liver disease, strengthen your kidneys, soothe your nerves and digestive tract, and reverse Crohn's, colitis, IBS, or peptic ulcers. In addition to being antiviral, they're antifungal and antibacterial, with nutritional cofactors and coenzymes plus bioactive compounds to keep you healthy and assist you with stress. Further, potatoes are brain food that helps keep you grounded and centered.

As a kid, did you ever do that science project where you stick some toothpicks in a potato, balance it in a cup of water, and watch it sprout on the windowsill? How many other foods can transform and thrive like that, coming to life before your eyes? That's the power of a potato—a power that's not to be underestimated—and we witness it firsthand as children. How does it happen that when we're adults, we're taught that it's a weak, empty, ridiculous food, as though we're supposed to forget the miracle we witnessed way back when? What we should really be saying about potatoes is, "Where would we be without you?" They are that vital to our existence.

Maybe you've steered clear of the potato misinformation all these years. If that's the case, your body thanks you for it—and now you have even more reason to appreciate potatoes. On the other hand, if you've been led to believe that potatoes are nothing but starch that will add to your waistline, it's time to see this root vegetable in a whole new light. If you're bold enough to overcome the conditioning of popular food culture to appreciate the potato in its unadulterated form, you will give yourself one of the greatest gifts on this earth.

CONDITIONS

If you have any of the following conditions, try bringing potatoes into your life:

Heart disease; colon cancer; breast cancer; pancreatic cancer; prostate cancer; liver disease; liver cancer; kidney disease; kidney cancer; hypoglycemia; diabetes; obesity; arthritis (including rheumatoid); peptic ulcers; hemorrhoids; irritable bowel syndrome (IBS); Crohn's disease; celiac disease; colitis; small intestinal bacterial overgrowth (SIBO); all other intestinal conditions; insomnia; depression; Graves' disease; Hashimoto's thyroiditis; low reproductive system battery; herpes; endometriosis; mystery infertility; shingles; anxiety; Addison's disease; all autoimmune diseases and disorders; chronic obstructive pulmonary disease (COPD); ear infections; eye infections; inflamed uterus, ovaries, and/or fallopian tubes

SYMPTOMS

If you have any of the following symptoms, try bringing potatoes into your life:

Inflammation; fungus; fatigue; brain fog; difficulty sleeping; dizziness; ringing or buzzing in the ears; diabetic neuropathy; tingles and numbness; malaise; listlessness; hearing loss; hypothyroid; canker sores; restless leg syndrome; food allergies; anxiousness; skin discolorations; frozen shoulder; *Candida* overgrowth; Bell's palsy; hyperthyroid; loss of libido; spasms; twitches; cold sores; central nervous system sensitivities; inflamed gallbladder, stomach, small intestine, and/or colon

EMOTIONAL SUPPORT

Potatoes offer us foundation and strength when we're feeling blurred, dizzy, foggy, troubled, or adrift in our lives. If your ego is consuming you, potatoes can tap into the humble confidence within, overriding the toxic emotions that keep you from succeeding in the areas of life that truly matter. Potatoes reorient us, help us to feel pleased and gratified by our experiences, and guide us to make choices not based on ego but out of true grounding and stability.

SPIRITUAL LESSON

Have you ever felt like you had so much to offer, only you remained unseen by those around you? The potato is the ultimate underdog—full of potential, yet perpetually overlooked and trampled on (sometimes literally). Potatoes remind us of all our hidden gifts, our life purposes and talents that get trapped inside, held back, stifled by the earthly traffic known as everyday life.

Potatoes' humble strength is due in part to how they grow: in clusters, surrounded by other potatoes, like a large extended family. If you come from a small family or had a difficult upbringing, potatoes will energetically pass along the grounding and sense of belonging that comes from being raised with a wide familial support network. If you come from a large, adoring family, potatoes will help you continue your connections. Potatoes come in numbers for a reason: so that, like an army of loved ones, they can fight for you.

When you feel like you're living by an arbitrary belief system that dictates what you're supposed to do and who you're supposed to be, connect with the wisdom and grounding of the potato. Remind yourself that so much of who you are is beneath the surface, that you are supported and witnessed, and that you deserve to unearth your true nature and share it with the world.

TIPS

- Potatoes are one instance where it's definitely best to seek out organic if possible.
- When preparing potatoes to eat, the best way to maximize the healing benefits and keep the nutrients intact is to steam them. If you normally eat your potatoes with butter, cheese, sour cream, or the like, try avocado as a dairy replacement, either cubed or mashed on top. Salsa and tahini are other tasty additions.
- After you've steamed a batch of potatoes, set some aside to cool. Later, pull them out of the fridge, slice or cube them, and add them to a spinach or kale salad. The enzymes from the potatoes will enhance the healing alkaloids in the leafy greens, maximizing the medicinal power of the meal.
- If you're dealing with a cold sore, try putting a slice of raw potato on it for relief.
- Potatoes can absorb and help diminish the negative effects of wireless Internet signals, cell phone signals and emissions, and other electromagnetic fields (EMF). They can even soak up and neutralize the negative emotional energy we sometimes pick up during the day and bring home with us. To tap into this feature of potatoes, select one to keep out in a bowl on the kitchen counter or elsewhere in your home. Discard the potato every five to seven days (don't eat it) and replace it with a fresh one.
- Whenever you're celebrating, make potatoes part of the meal. Whether it's a wedding, engagement, birthday, graduation, promotion, holiday, or other festive occasion, including potatoes will support and enhance the joyful emotions and help sustain them for days afterward.

CHILI-LOADED BAKED POTATOES WITH CASHEW "SOUR CREAM"

Makes 6 to 8 servings

This chili is the perfect hearty, warming meal for colder months, though it's great eaten any time of year. While it requires some chopping and a little time, the end result is a nice big batch of chili that will feed a hungry crowd or keep well for meals all week long. Feel free to add more red pepper for some extra spice.

6 potatoes

1 pound black beans or kidney beans, soaked overnight*

1 tablespoon coconut oil

4 cups diced onion

4 garlic cloves, minced

2 cups diced carrots

2 cups diced celery

2 cups diced mushrooms

2 cups diced red bell pepper

2 teaspoons each cumin, poultry seasoning, garlic powder, and chili powder

1 teaspoon sea salt

teaspoon red pepper flakes (optional)

2 tablespoons tomato paste

2 cups diced tomatoes

1 avocado, diced

1 jalapeño, minced

¼ cup minced cilantro

FOR CASHEW "SOUR CREAM":

1 cup raw cashews

½ lemon, juiced

½ date, peeled, pitted

1 garlic clove

½ cup water

Preheat the oven to 425°F. Pierce the potatoes in several places with a fork. Bake for 45 to 60 minutes, until tender.

Drain the beans, place in a 4-quart pot, and cover with an inch of water. Bring to a full boil, then reduce heat to a simmer. Cook the beans for 1 hour, or until tender, adding more water as needed to keep the beans covered with liquid. Drain and set aside.

For the chili, heat 1 tablespoon coconut oil in a large pot; add the onions and garlic. Sauté over high heat until the onions are translucent and fragrant, adding water as needed to prevent sticking. Add the carrots, celery, mushrooms, bell pepper, spices, sea salt, and red pepper flakes, if using. Continue to cook, stirring occasionally, until vegetables begin to soften, about 15 minutes. Add beans, tomato paste, and tomatoes, stirring until well combined. Cover and continue to simmer on medium heat for 15 minutes. Reduce heat to low.

For the "sour cream," blend all the ingredients until smooth, adding ½ cup water slowly (just enough to keep things moving).

Halve the baked potatoes. Serve topped with chili, cashew "sour cream," avocado, jalapeño, and cilantro.

*You may use 6 cups of salt-free canned beans, if desired.

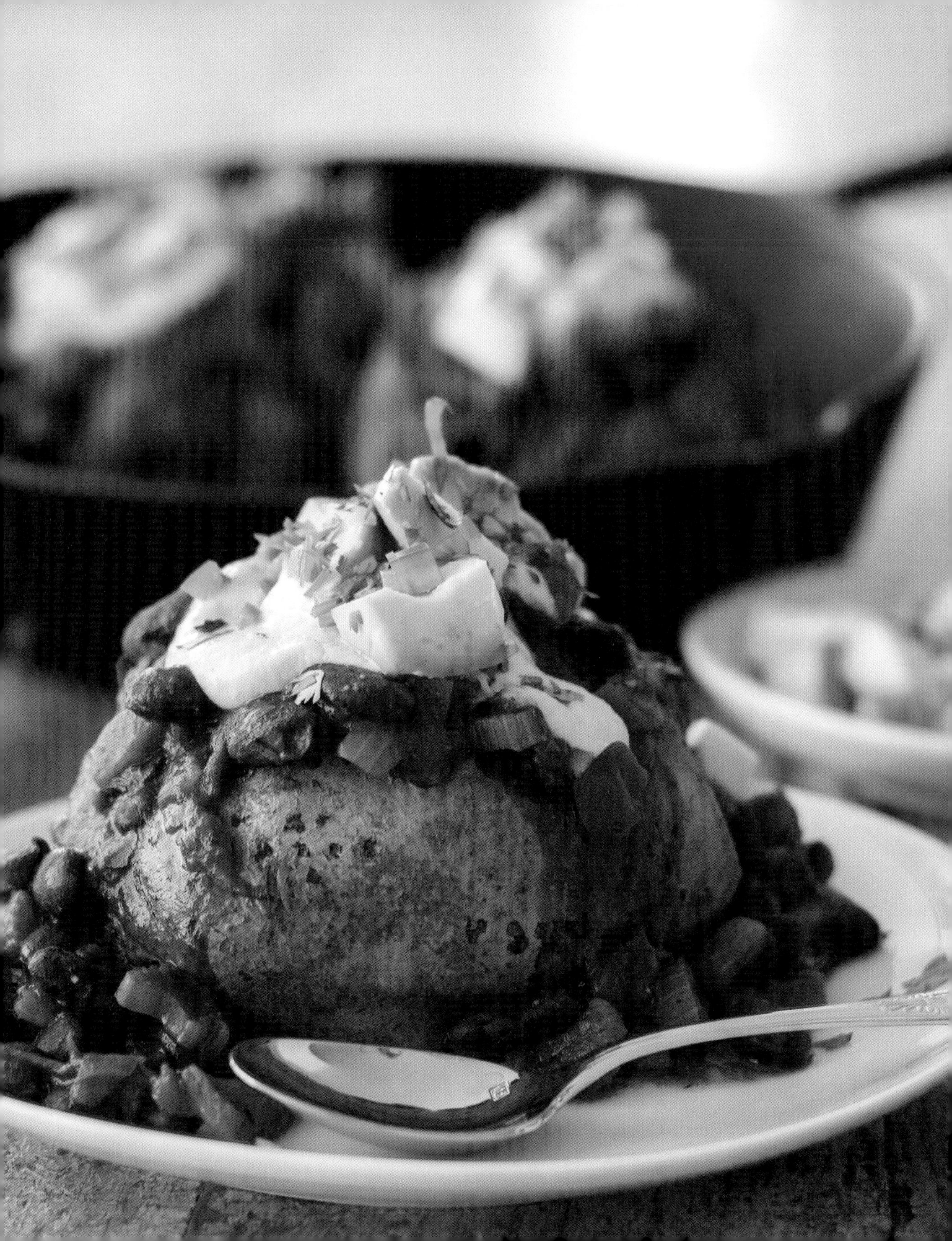

Radishes

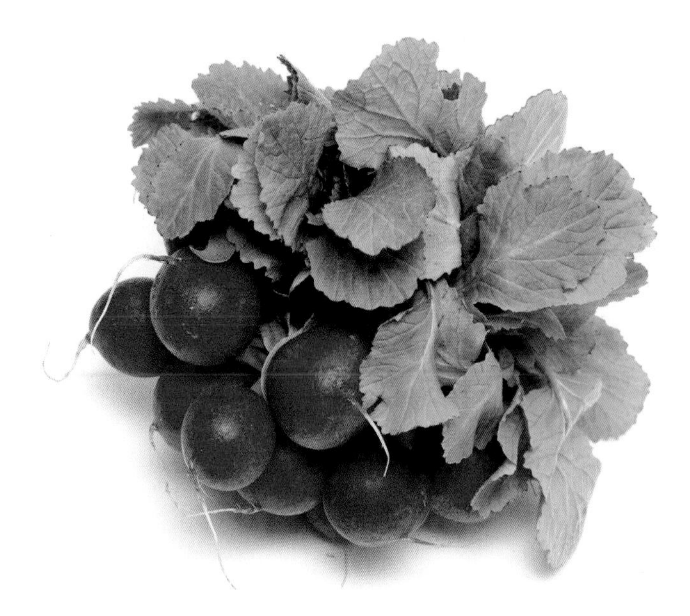

Radishes are a standout cruciferous vegetable that deserves its own time in the limelight. If the term "food as medicine" applies to anything, it applies to radishes. And what makes radishes unique from other crucifers is that they have two components, defined by different characteristics.

To begin with, there is the root of the radish plant—what we think of as the radish itself. Overall, radishes are an immune-system replenisher. When consumed, the sulfur in radishes repels any type of pathogen and acts as a wormicide to kill off intestinal worms and other parasites. The organosulfides in radishes also keep arteries and veins clean, creating a protective barrier in blood vessels so plaque doesn't adhere to their linings. Radishes are incredible heart food, excellent for helping to prevent heart disease and other cardiovascular issues in part by increasing good cholesterol and lowering bad cholesterol. Meanwhile, the skin of the radish repels virtually every type of cancer, which makes these little root vegetables a go-to food for helping to prevent the disease. And we can't forget that radishes are very restorative for the kidney, liver, pancreas, and spleen.

Then there are the radish greens—one of the most healing foods possible, and they're thrown away. These leaves of the radish are the second most powerful prebiotic there is (next to wild blueberries). Radish greens hold a plethora of nutrients such as vitamins, minerals, antioxidants, phytochemicals, and cancer-fighting alkaloids, plus the greens possess antibacterial and antiviral properties. They repair the colon and other parts of the intestinal tract that have lost the ability to absorb nutrients. Radish greens' nutrition absorbs into the most dysfunctional digestive tracts, assimilating better than any other food, thanks to their high enzymatic profile; the greens contain various enzymes that are not yet documented by scientific study and that allow for the uptake of nutrients.

For what they offer, radish greens are really a wild food, even when cultivated in your garden bed or a farmer's field. Radish greens help remove all of the Unforgiving Four from the body. In particular, they cleanse heavy metals to an extreme degree, removing mercury, lead, arsenic, and aluminum from your system—they hold almost as much power as cilantro in this department. Radish greens help stave off every neurological condition, including MS, ALS, and neurological Lyme. By far, radish greens are the most powerful leafy green for someone's health.

CONDITIONS

If you have any of the following conditions, try bringing radishes into your life:

Brain tumors, brain cancer, gastroesophageal reflux disease (GERD), arthritis, breast cancer, asthma, bronchitis, pneumonia, fibromyalgia, epilepsy, herpes simplex 1 (HSV-1), herpes simplex 2 (HSV-2), hypertension, kidney disease, Parkinson's disease, severe acute respiratory syndrome (SARS), skin cancers, thyroid disease, thyroid cancer, intestinal worms and other parasites, nutrient absorption issues, multiple sclerosis (MS), amyotrophic lateral sclerosis (ALS), Lyme disease, pneumonia, bronchitis, insomnia, pelvic inflammatory disease (PID), rheumatoid arthritis (RA)

SYMPTOMS

If you have any of the following symptoms, try bringing radishes into your life:

Fatigue, dizziness, brain fog, burning sensations in or on the body, moving pain, joint pain, sleep disturbances, nutrient deficiencies, heartburn, high blood pressure, food sensitivities, inflammation, sensations of humming or vibration in the body, ringing or buzzing in the ears, nervousness, rashes, balance issues, chest tightness, congestion, cough, dark under-eye circles, difficulty breathing, ear pain, frozen shoulder, gum pain, hearing loss, high cortisol, loss of energy, melancholy, neck pain

EMOTIONAL SUPPORT

When *fail* is the key word in how you're feeling—whether you feel like a failure yourself, or that someone is failing you, or that your body has failed you by developing an illness—radishes are a miracle for lifting you out of the doldrums. Because eating them shows you results so rapidly, radishes get you out of the rut of despair.

SPIRITUAL LESSON

When you grow radishes, you want to harvest them when the greens and the radishes themselves are young and tender. This is when they're at their peak, offering the most advanced nutrition you can get just about anywhere. Picking radishes at the right moment, before their skin becomes tough, their flesh fibrous, and their greens overgrown, means you have to be in tune with the plants, ready to pluck them out of the ground when your instincts say "go." It doesn't have to all be in one shot, though. You can practice succession planting—that is, sowing new seeds every week—so that you have a continuous supply of new chances to get the harvest timing right.

In this way, radishes teach us the value of choosing the right moment for important conversations and decisions. You don't want to put something off too long and find out that an opportunity to reap a situation's benefits has passed. At the same time, radishes teach us to persevere. As long as we're planting new seeds along the way, there's always another chance to seize the moment.

TIPS

- Look for black radishes at the farmers' market (or buy the seed and grow your own). Black radishes are the most powerful radish variety. They take everything we've just looked at about the value of radishes and radish greens to the next level.
- If you grow your own radishes, try to pick them when they're not quite full-grown. This is when they have the best chance of advancing your health rapidly. Try to eat at least three radishes a day.
- Radishes, celery, and onions make an incredibly healing broth (one that's especially good for those struggling with pneumonia or bronchitis) when combined.
- You can eat radish greens raw or cooked. Treat them like any leafy green. One great way to enjoy them is to chop them up and sprinkle on a salad.

RADISH SALAD

Makes 2 servings

This simple salad packs a health punch with the earthy radish and the light cucumber tossed in herbs, olive oil, and lemon juice. Finish it off with a sprinkle of sea salt and what results is a gorgeous dish worthy of any brunch or lunch gathering. Make sure to use the freshest, most beautiful radishes available to make this dish sing—and don't forget to save the radish greens for use in juice, soup, and other dishes!

2 cups sliced radishes
2 cups sliced cucumbers
2 tablespoons minced tarragon
4 tablespoons minced dill
2 tablespoons olive oil
¼ lemon, juiced
⅛ teaspoon sea salt

Place the radish and cucumber slices in a medium bowl and toss with all the remaining ingredients. Allow the salad to chill in the refrigerator for 15 minutes before eating.

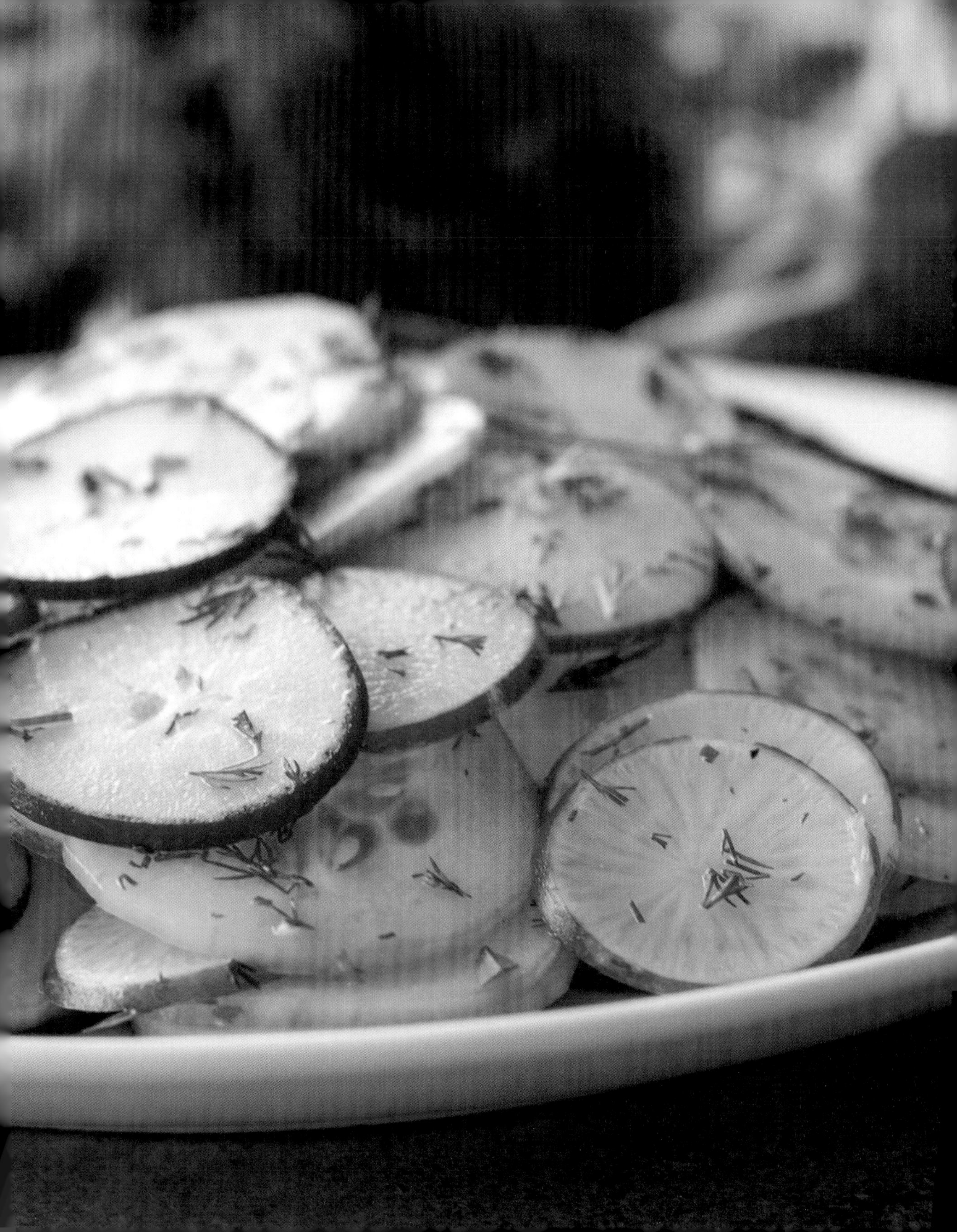

Sprouts & Microgreens

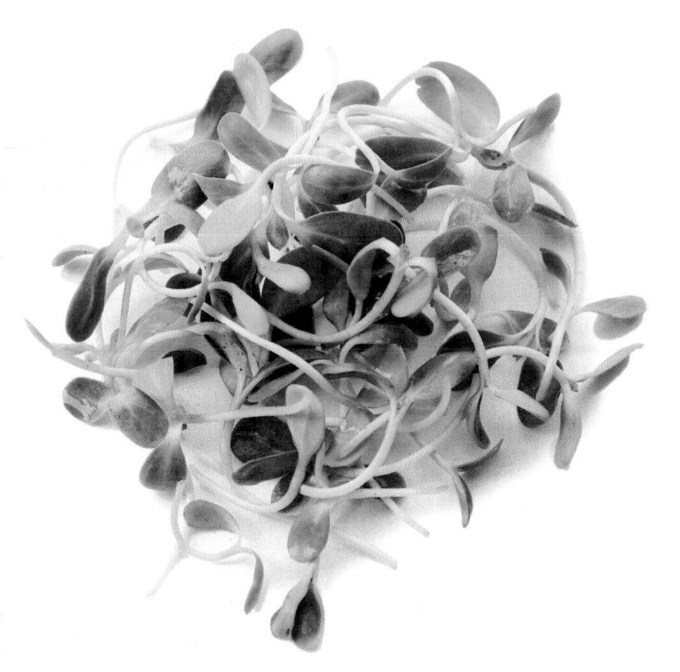

Just like the vegetables they would become if they grew to full size, sprouts and microgreens are packed with nutrients like vitamin A, B vitamins, minerals, trace minerals, disease-reversing compounds, and other phytochemicals. When we eat greens in this early phase of life, though, the digestion process is a fraction of what it would otherwise be to assimilate their powers. The most important role that sprouts and microgreens play is to bring back vitality to people who are always exhausting themselves for others. When you put your heart and soul into everything you do, whether at home or work, sprouts have the unique ability to support you.

Sprouts and microgreens are wonderful reproductive foods. They are one of the ultimate tools for renewing an exhausted reproductive system and revitalizing a new mom who hasn't been getting much sleep while caring for her baby. Sprouts and microgreens are phytoestrogenic and critical for rebalancing and restoring hormones such as progesterone, estrogen, and testosterone, and for regenerating hormone production of the adrenal glands, thyroid, and the rest of the endocrine system after a woman has given birth.

High in mineral salts that are involved with neurotransmitter chemical production, sprouts and microgreens also support the brain with amino acids and enzymes, pull toxic heavy metals from the brain, and help rejuvenate and strengthen neurons—which ultimately helps the body in reversing Alzheimer's, dementia, brain fog, and memory loss. Sprouts and microgreens are wonderful for skin repair, and they're also high in more than 60 trace minerals, including iron, iodine, selenium, zinc, copper, manganese, sulfur, magnesium, chromium, and molybdenum. As antiproliferatives, sprouts and microgreens stave off infection and unwanted cell growth (such as cancer). Further, they are the best possible source of the elevated biotics critical to your body's production of vitamin B_{12}. And in this early stage of growth, sprouts and microgreens hold thousands of phytochemicals to supercharge your body.

Choosing sprouts is like choosing friends; they all have different personalities. Do you have that friend who you know is a great person, and yet is a little edgy—you can only handle him in small doses? That describes the broccoli sprout. Strong in flavor with a bit of bite, broccoli sprouts are wonderful to strengthen digestion by raising hydrochloric acid levels.

And do you have a friend whom you sometimes hold back from sharing everything with, because you know that her fiery, explosive disposition will mean she'll leap to your defense before you're even finished speaking? That's the radish sprout, which is remarkable for its ability to purge the liver (an organ that's fiery in its own right in so many of us).

What about the friend who's very gentle and laid-back, who listens to everything you say and offers words of comfort? This describes the red clover sprout, which is very soothing as it gently cleanses our lymph and blood, removing toxins and purifying our bodies.

Then there's the friend who's very emotional and cries very easily, whether happy or sad tears. The fenugreek sprout is all heart and soul, perfect for supporting our emotions and the endocrine system, both of which are tied up in the heart, soul, and brain. Fenugreek sprouts are especially helpful for balancing the adrenals' cortisol production and regulating thyroid hormone production.

And we can't forget about that friend with the muscle, the person you call to show up with a pickup truck and help move you out of your house. This is the lentil sprout. Very dense energetically, high in fortifying protein that your body can assimilate with ease, lentil sprouts also give you a carbohydrate base to help propel you through whatever needs to get done. Lentil sprouts love to pass their brute strength on to you. Eating them is like getting the fortification of a Thanksgiving dinner—and yet having tremendous energy afterward, rather than wanting to fall asleep on the couch.

On and on the list goes. Also keep your eye out for mung bean sprouts, sunflower greens, pea shoots, and micro-kale, among other advocates. Just like the people who support you in life, all the different sprouts and microgreen varieties have special qualities that you'll discover as you get to know them.

CONDITIONS

If you have any of the following conditions, try bringing sprouts and microgreens into your life:

Human papilloma virus (HPV), fibroids, all types of cancer, polycystic ovarian syndrome (PCOS), low reproductive system battery, depression (including postpartum), jaundice, anxiety, anemia, infertility, miscarriage, Alzheimer's disease, dementia, Epstein-Barr virus (EBV)/mononucleosis, Hashimoto's thyroiditis, diabetes, hypoglycemia, adrenal fatigue, Graves' disease, eczema, psoriasis, food allergies, attention-deficit/hyperactivity disorder (ADHD), autism, nutrient absorption issues, insomnia, herpes simplex 1 (HSV-1), herpes simplex 2 (HSV-2), HHV-6, HHV-7, thyroid disease, celiac disease, Lyme disease, strep throat

SYMPTOMS

If you have any of the following symptoms, try bringing sprouts and microgreens into your life:

Abnormal Pap smear results, fatigue, lack of energy, weight gain, tooth decay, enamel loss, gum recession, hot flashes, night sweats, blurry eyes, bruising, pelvic pain, iron deficiency, memory loss, brain fog, sleep disturbances, acid reflux, all neurological symptoms (including tingles, numbness, spasms, twitches, nerve pain, and tightness of the chest), blood sugar imbalances, belching, bone loss, brittle nails, cravings, fluid retention, gastritis, leg cramps, listlessness, stagnant liver, mucus in the stool, muscle spasms, sweets cravings, sore throat, hyperthyroid, hypothyroid

EMOTIONAL SUPPORT

When you're feeling a sense of loss, whether grieving for a career, friendship, or an object you've lost, sprouts and microgreens are exceptionally helpful. These tiny messengers of hope help you get out of a mindset of mourning and plant the seeds for new life and new opportunities.

SPIRITUAL LESSON

Sprouts and microgreens are highly adaptogenic. They don't demand the perfect environment. Even though in other circumstances these seeds would be given ample soil, space, sunlight, rain, and fresh air to take root and rise up to their fullest, when they're cultivated in countertop gardens, they manage to grow crowded together in a jar or tray with just enough light and water to survive. All it takes is a little routine (sprouts need regular rinsing, and microgreens need regular misting), for these shoots to adapt to their circumstances. And they do so happily—if sprouts and microgreens had faces, you'd see a smile on each one.

This cheerful adaptability transfers to us when we eat them. As long as we have the absolute necessities and give ourselves a bit of routine to normalize life, then even in the most difficult situations, we can take strength from our little friends and find a way to thrive.

TIPS

- For noticeable benefits, eat two cups of sprouts per day.
- When growing your own sprouts, think of them like little pets: they feed off of companionship, and they pick up on the energy of their environment and whatever is said around them. Always try to approach your sprouts with happiness. Talk to them, offer encouragement, and run your fingers over their tops as you pass by. As I wrote about in the chapter "Food for the Soul," growing your own food means that that food picks up on your individual needs and adjusts its nutrition so it will feed you in the best way possible. Sprouts and microgreens are especially adept at aligning with your specific health requirements, because they're so adaptogenic.
- Don't cook your sprouts if you want maximum benefit. Sprouts and microgreens are an amazing source of elevated biotics, those microorganisms so critical to gut health and production of vitamin B_{12}. Elevated biotics only remain intact when sprouts and microgreens are eaten raw. (And when those elevated biotics are on sprouts and microgreens you've grown yourself, they're geared to benefit your own flora.)
- Spraying liquid sea minerals mixed with water on your home-grown sprouts and microgreens daily mineralizes them as they develop, supercharging them for your health.
- Sprouts and microgreens such as radish, broccoli, fenugreek, kale, and sunflower should be eaten at lunchtime, because they support your energy levels during the day. Bean and lentil sprouts should be eaten at dinnertime, because they help calm and relax your nervous system in the evening.
- A juice made from cucumber, pea shoots, and sunflower greens can over time amplify a person's ability to see at night.

SPROUT-FILLED COLLARD WRAPS WITH MANGO-TOMATO DIPPING SAUCE

Makes 1 to 2 servings

These fresh, colorful collard wraps are a great way to fill your day with veggies. It's a fun lunch option to set out a tray of sliced veggies and let people build their own. Plus, you can make a variety of dipping sauces using some of the other recipes in the book—try the cilantro pesto (page 190), the garlic tahini salad dressing (page 194), or the nori rolls' avocado dip (page 228).

- 6 large collard leaves
- 1 bell pepper, any color
- 1 avocado
- ¼ red cabbage
- 2 medjool dates, pitted
- 2 cups sprouts
- 2 cups microgreens
- 1 cup diced mango
- 1 cup diced tomato
- 1 quarter-size slice ginger
- ¼ inch slice of jalapeño (optional)

Rinse the collard leaves and trim off their stems. Set aside for later use in a soup or smoothie. Slice the bell pepper, avocado, and cabbage into thin strips. Finely chop and mash the dates to form a paste. With the stem side facing you, start at the right side of the collard leaf and fill with the sliced veggies, sprouts, and microgreens. Roll toward the left like a burrito, folding the top of the leaf in as you go. Use the date paste along the left edge of the collard green to seal. Repeat with the remaining collard leaves, filling, and paste.

For the dipping sauce, blend the mango, tomato, ginger, and jalapeño, if using, until smooth.

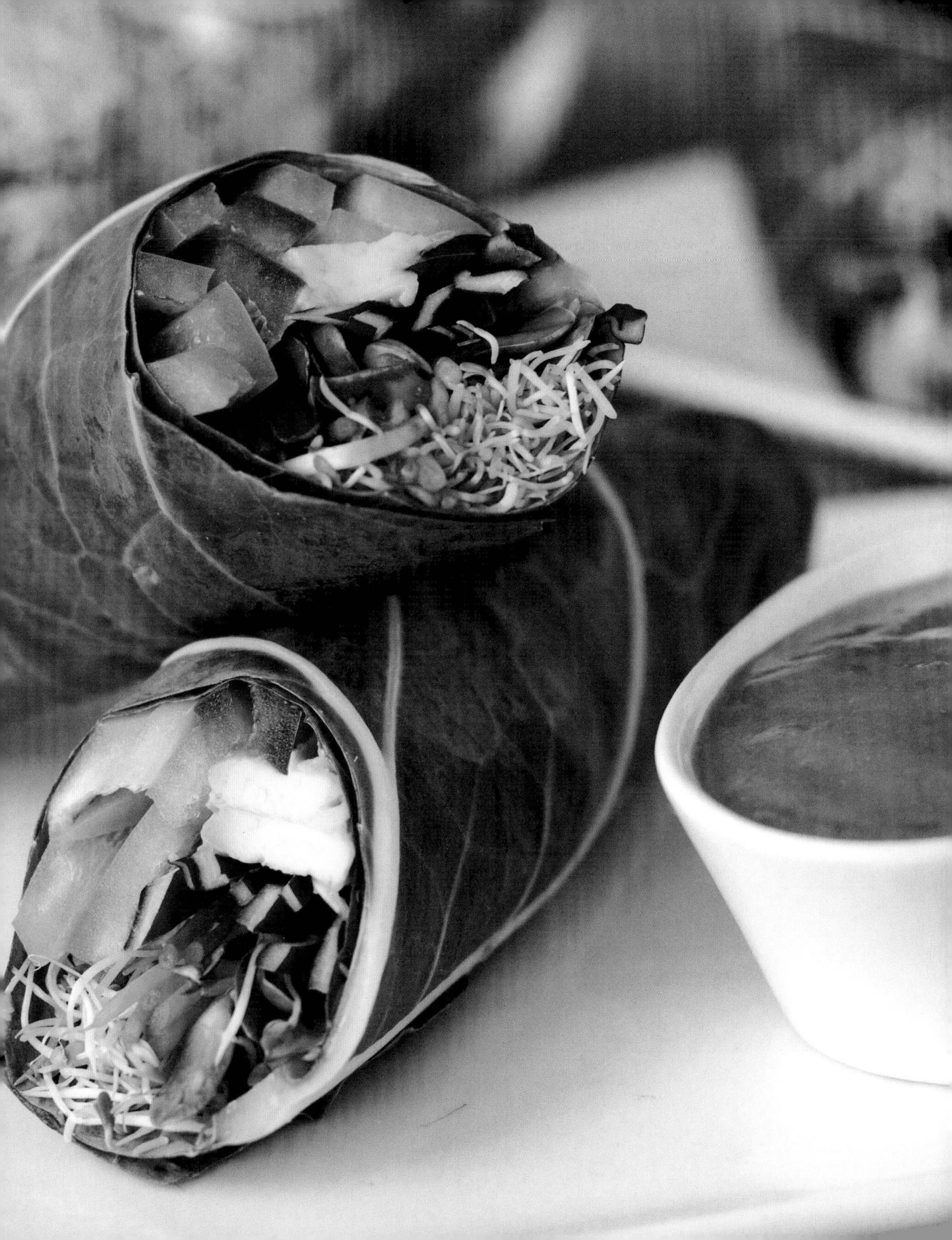

Sweet Potatoes

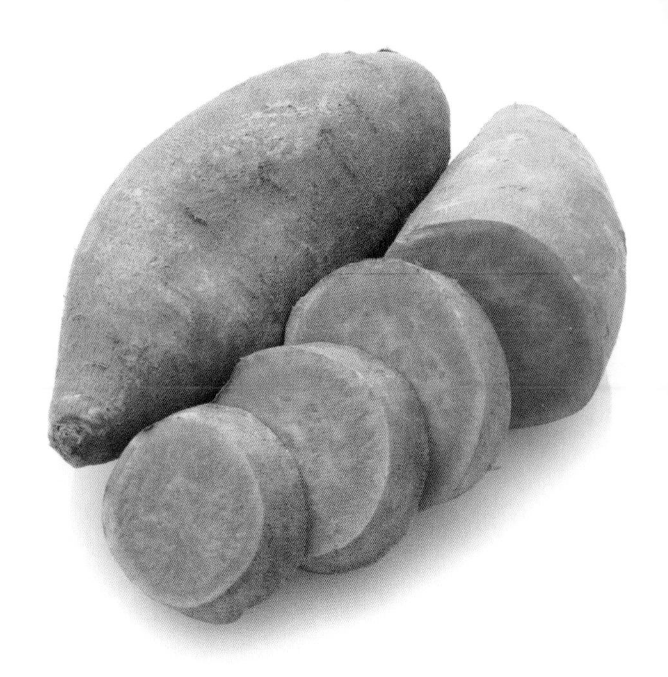

While the regular potato has been mistakenly villainized, the brighter, flashier sweet potato has gotten some of the acclaim it deserves. As with any of the life-changing foods in this book, though, it deserves more credit than it gets—sweet potatoes and yams are better for us than anyone realizes.

To start with, sweet potatoes promote productive bacteria in the stomach, small intestine, and colon, while at the same time, they starve out unproductive bacteria and fungi such as mold that are camping out there. By keeping these microbes at bay, sweet potatoes are standouts at enhancing the body's production of B_{12}. Also, sweet potatoes help prevent a condition called megacolon—that is, an expansion of the colon due to proliferation of *C. difficile*, *Streptococcus*, *Staphylococcus*, *E. coli*, *H. pylori*, *Chlamydia*, and/or other bacteria. Plus, this superfood helps alleviate narrowing of the intestinal tract due to the chronic inflammation that's so commonly diagnosed as Crohn's or colitis.

Abundant in vitamins, minerals, and other nutrients, orange-fleshed sweet potatoes are especially praised for being packed with carotenoids such as beta-carotene and lycopene, and rightfully so. These phytochemicals are extremely powerful. If you are fair and eat a sweet potato daily, before long you'll see your skin take on a glow, as if it's been sun-kissed. The lycopene, combined with sweet potatoes' abundant amino acids, is a recipe for drawing radiation from the body. On top of which, the anti-cancerous phytochemicals in sweet potatoes help protect you against skin cancers, breast cancer, reproductive cancers, stomach cancer, intestinal cancers, esophageal cancer, and rectal cancer.

Sweet potatoes are also phytoestrogenic and perform the vital function of ridding the body of unusable, destructive, cancer-causing estrogen that interferes with the body's hormone function. These estrogens come from plastics, pharmaceuticals, food, and environmental toxins, as well as from the body producing an overabundance of the hormone (due to a diet high in estrogen-producing foods). Because it's more than the body can use, this estrogen becomes inactive and builds up in the organs, negatively affecting the endocrine system. By purging this excess estrogen, sweet potatoes make room for healthier estrogens to take their place. Sweet potatoes are also important for regulating hair growth; they stimulate it where needed and prohibit hair when it tries to grow in the wrong places, as in the condition hirsutism.

If you struggle with insomnia or another sleeping disorder, sweet potatoes are very useful. They provide a critical form of glucose that stimulates the development of neurotransmitters such as glycine, dopamine, GABA, and serotonin, all of which aid in the ability to sleep soundly. Whether you like orange, yellow, white, pink, or purple sweet potatoes, eat up. Each type holds medicinal qualities that will power you through life.

CONDITIONS

If you have any of the following conditions, try bringing sweet potatoes into your life:

Megacolon, hirsutism, colitis, Crohn's disease, skin cancers, breast cancer, ovarian cancer, cervical cancer, stomach cancer, intestinal cancers, esophageal cancer, colorectal cancer, sleep disorders, chronic fatigue syndrome (CFS), heart disease, kidney disease, attention-deficit/hyperactivity disorder (ADHD), insomnia, alopecia, sunburn, Asperger's syndrome, depression, irritable bowel syndrome (IBS), psoriatic arthritis, epilepsy, hiatal hernia, adrenal fatigue, neuropathy, posttraumatic stress disorder (PTSD), anxiety, depression, eczema, psoriasis, shingles, urinary tract infections (UTIs), chlamydia, polycystic ovarian syndrome (PCOS), endometriosis, scleroderma, lichen sclerosus, celiac disease, social anxiety disorder

SYMPTOMS

If you have any of the following symptoms, try bringing sweet potatoes into your life:

Dandruff, temporomandibular joint (TMJ) issues, diarrhea, anxiousness, intestinal tract discomfort, inflamed colon, colon spasms, heartburn, scar tissue, muscle cramps, muscle spasms, food sensitivities, heart palpitations, hot flashes, abdominal cramping, accelerated aging, brain lesions, colon spasms, depersonalization, digestive disturbances, abnormal Pap smear results, eye dryness, swelling, age spots, weight gain, scaly skin, intestinal polyps

EMOTIONAL SUPPORT

When you need some coddling, there's nothing more comforting than a baked sweet potato. Unlike greasy, fried, or sugar-filled and processed "comfort" foods that leave you feeling bloated, lethargic, and more depressed, a sweet potato has properties that actually give you the sensation that the world around you has shut down. This is an important function that makes you feel safe and soothed, like you're getting a hug even if no one's there to give you one, so that you can draw up the strength to deal with hard times.

SPIRITUAL LESSON

Have you ever baked a sweet potato and seen the natural sugars that bubble up and drip down the sides? A sweet potato in and of itself is as rich as anything you could ask for—and yet that doesn't seem to be enough for us. Popular sweet potato recipes call for butter, cream, brown sugar, or marshmallows. Even though sweet potatoes are sweeter than sweet and already perfect, we adulterate them, obscure their natural qualities, and overindulge.

Where in your life are you unnecessarily piling on the extra toppings? Sweet potatoes teach us to evaluate other circumstances where we've been handed a pure and complete gift, and out of fear or a lack of appreciation, we've felt like that wasn't enough.

TIPS

- To reap sweet potatoes' maximum benefits, try to eat one per day.
- If you crave a creamy accompaniment to your sweet potato, scoop out some fresh avocado and mash it in as though it were butter.
- After you've cooked a batch of sweet potatoes (steaming and baking are the healthiest preparations), set some aside to save for later in the fridge. Chopping them up and serving over salad helps your body absorb and assimilate more nutrients from leafy greens. And a few bites of sweet potato when you're having trouble sleeping in the middle of the night will help you get some rest.
- Try rubbing a piece of raw sweet potato on a scar. It has medicinal qualities that stimulate healing and tone the skin to help reduce scar tissue.
- People often use cucumber slices to get rid of bags under the eyes. For variety, try cold slices of cooked sweet potato instead. This will infuse the under-eye tissue with beta-carotene, bringing back vitality to your appearance.
- When you're dealing with sunburn, try eating sweet potato to recover faster.
- If you have a lot of internal scar tissue from past surgeries, try a routine of eating two sweet potatoes daily for one week, then one sweet potato daily for three weeks. Repeat every month until your condition improves.
- When you're scheduled to see a movie you know will be scary or action-packed, eat a sweet potato beforehand. It will support your adrenals as you experience the excitement, fear, and adventure on-screen.

SWEET POTATOES STUFFED WITH BRAISED CABBAGE

Makes 2 to 4 servings

A great dish for weekly dinners, the components of this dish can be made ahead of time and assembled just prior to serving. Bake sweet potatoes and cook the cabbage in advance and store them in the fridge for up to four days for a quick, easy dinner that takes minutes to prepare. For best results, make the sauce right before serving and ladle it piping hot over the stuffed sweet potatoes.

4 sweet potatoes
4 cloves of garlic, minced
1 onion, diced
1 tablespoon coconut oil
1 red cabbage, shredded
½ teaspoon sea salt
½ lemon

FOR SAUCE:

1 tablespoon olive oil
1 tablespoon raw honey
1 tablespoon lemon juice
1 tablespoon grated fresh ginger

FOR GARNISH:

4 tablespoons minced parsley

Preheat the oven to 400°F. Bake sweet potatoes on a baking sheet for 45 to 60 minutes, or until easily pierced with a fork.

In a large pan, sauté garlic and onions in 1 tablespoon of coconut oil over medium-high heat for 5 to 10 minutes, stirring occasionally, until the onions are translucent and soft. Add the cabbage and sea salt, along with ½ cup of water. Cover and cook over medium heat for 30 to 40 minutes until the cabbage is tender, continuing to stir occasionally and adding a splash of water as needed to moisten.

Split open sweet potatoes and mash each side slightly with a fork. Stuff as much braised cabbage into the openings as possible.

Make the sauce just before serving the sweet potatoes. (For 4 servings, double the ingredients for the sauce.) Add all the ingredients to a small pan. Heat the mixture over medium-high heat until it bubbles slightly. Continue stirring for 1 to 2 minutes until the sauce is well combined and slightly thickened. Pour over the sweet potatoes, garnish with parsley, and enjoy!

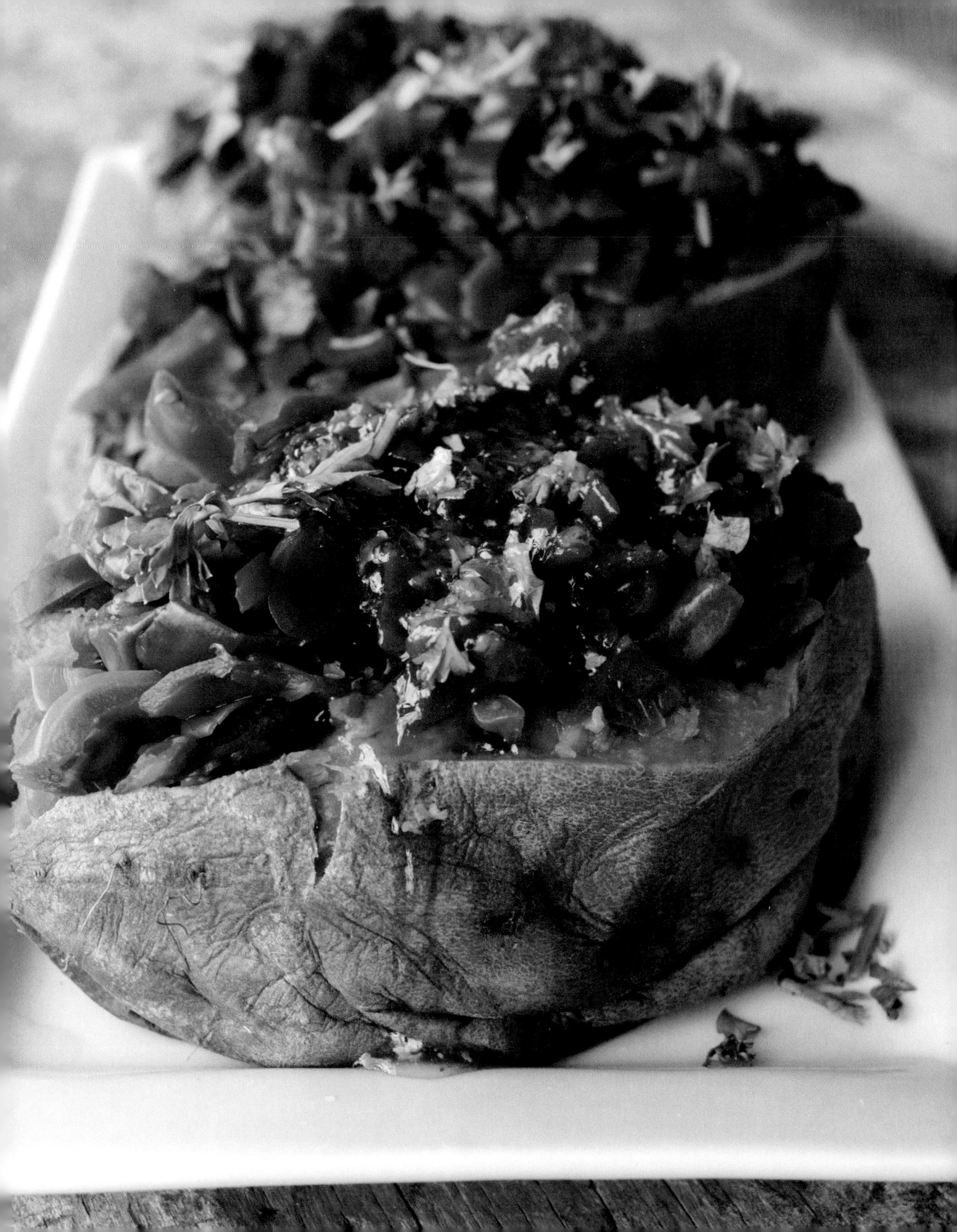

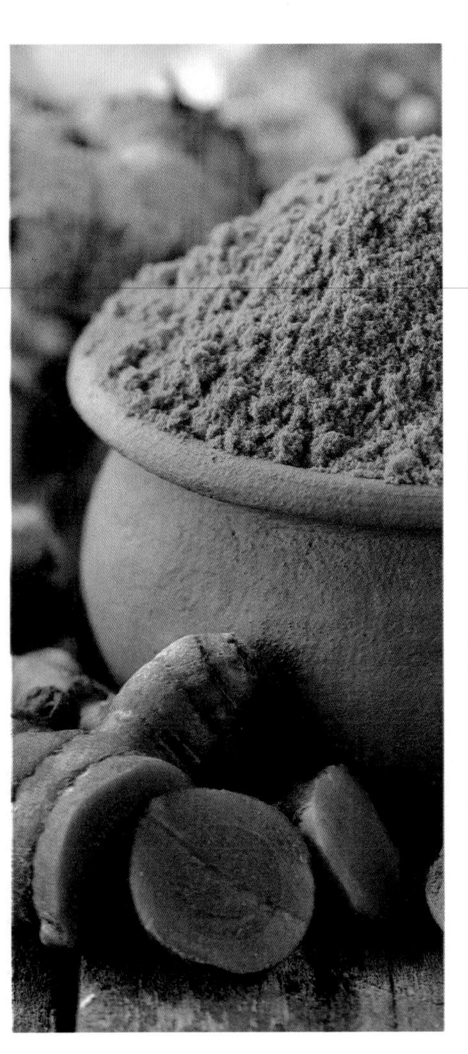
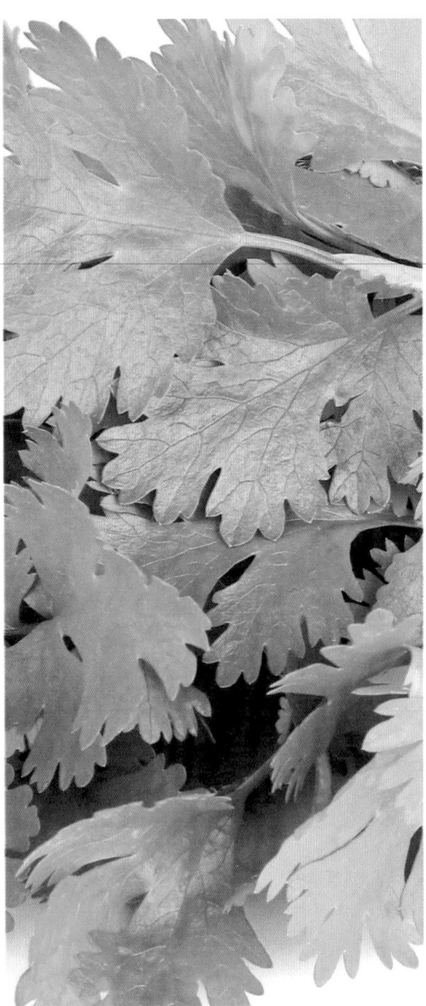
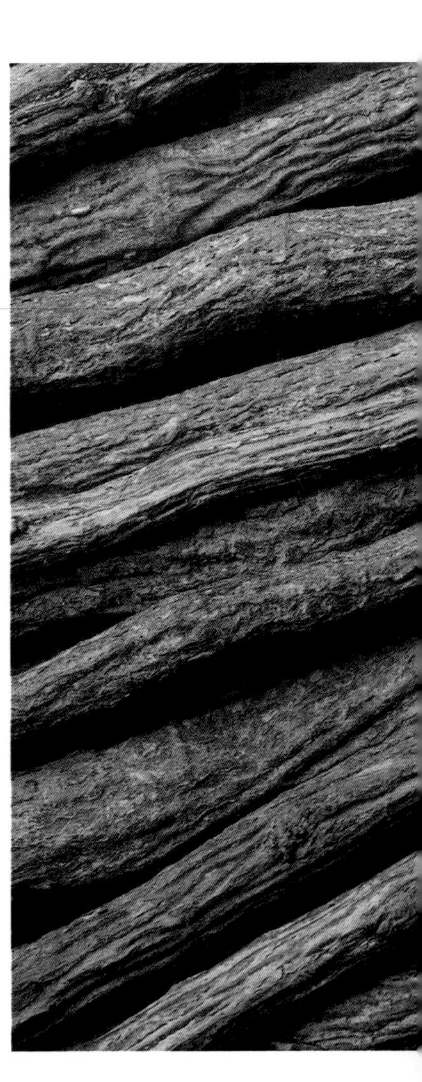

HERBS AND SPICES

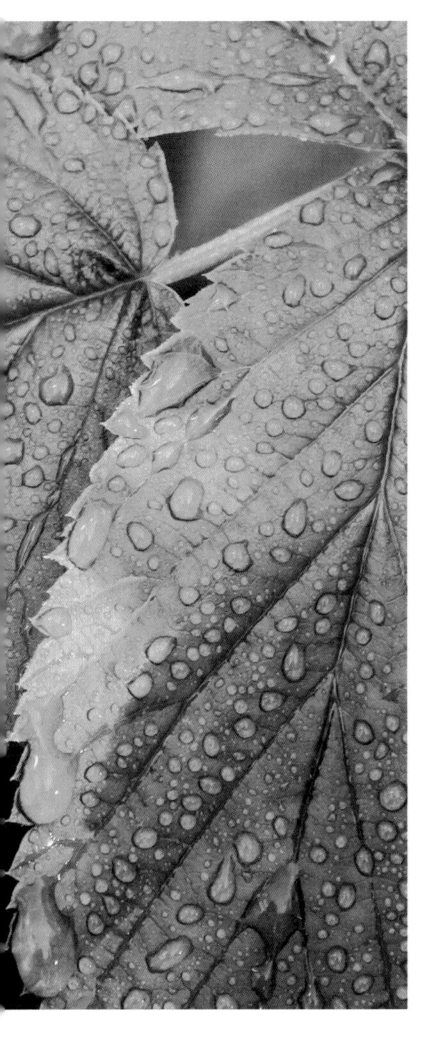
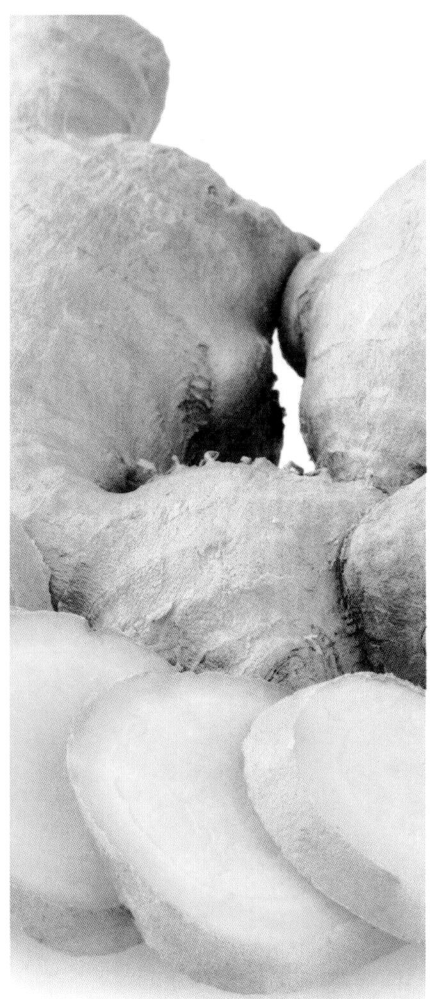
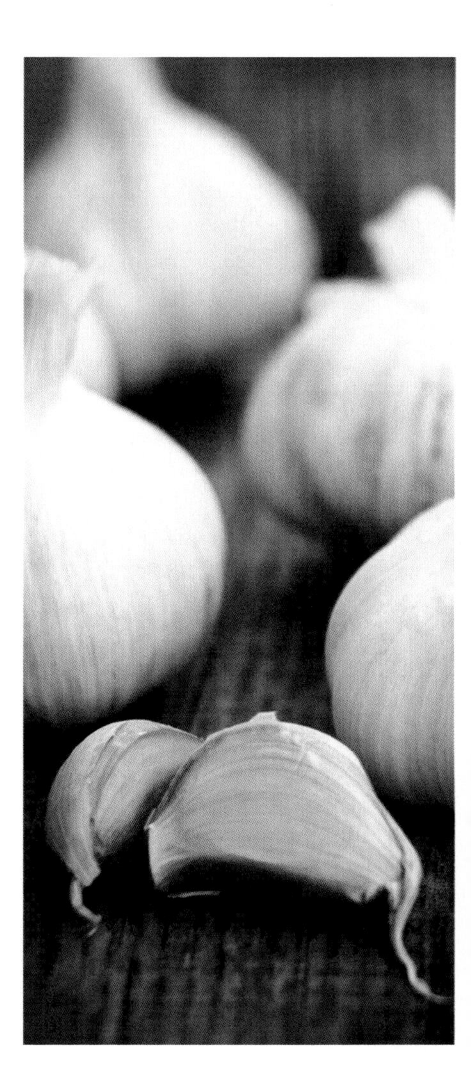

Aromatic Herbs

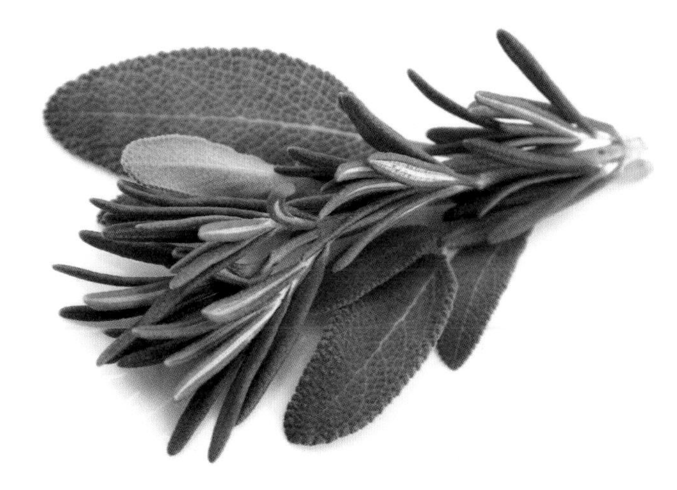

Oregano, Rosemary, Sage & Thyme

The aromatic herbs oregano, rosemary, sage, and thyme possess complementary qualities. Each has a different specialization, and when you consume them all on a regular basis (whether in diet, supplementation, or a combination), their disease-fighting phytochemical compounds and extremely high levels of a broad spectrum of minerals provide a well-rounded, powerful defense against the pathogenic world. (Parsley is another aromatic herb covered in this book, and it gets its own feature, because it's more of an individual.)

Aromatic herbs get much of their power from being very close to wild, even when cultivated. They need very little care to establish themselves and thrive; when they're neglected, they're still able to miraculously get what they need to provide you with the high levels of nutrients you need. It is unknown to scientific communities that aromatic herbs release an antifungal compound from their roots that earthworms love. The roots of aromatics become a gathering place for earthworms, as the worms ingest this antifungal to keep themselves healthy. In return, the earthworms aerate the soil around the roots and leave behind a rich fertilizer that can't be matched. This symbiosis is what gives aromatic herbs their unique healing properties. (If you grow these herbs in pots, or if you don't have earthworms in your garden, make sure you use a mineral solution and enough organic fertilizer.)

Here's a closer look at each of these standout aromatics:

- **Oregano**: Amazing for killing off unproductive bacteria such as *H. pylori*, *Streptococcus*, and *E. coli*, which minimizes the possibility of SIBO, peptic ulcers, strep throat, ear infections, and sinusitis. Oregano oil is an incredible antibacterial, especially for killing off the *E. coli* that causes diverticulitis and diverticulosis. It's also effective against ringworm.
- **Rosemary**: Another antibacterial, rosemary specializes in fighting antibiotic-resistant bacteria, such as those that take hold in hospitals. Bringing this herb into your diet is a game changer if you're dealing with the sorts of bacteria (such as *C. difficile* and multi-drug-resistant *Staphylococcus aureus*, or MRSA) that can result in conditions such as megacolon, severe infection, and can even lead to death.
- **Sage**: This herb's nature is geared toward fighting fungus. Consuming sage is wonderful for healing fungal infections such as athlete's foot and jock itch from the inside out, as well as tackling mutant strains of fungus in the intestinal tract. If you've been exposed

to toxic mold, turn to sage to help detoxify. Also, sage helps remove toxic heavy metals from the intestinal tract.

- **Thyme**: This antiviral's main job is to destroy viruses such as the flu, enteroviruses, norovirus, and the whole gamut of herpetic viruses that are responsible for autoimmune disease and Lyme disease. (For more on Lyme, see the extensive chapter on the subject in my first book.) Thyme's ability to cross the blood-brain barrier makes it a secret weapon against viruses that have started to attack the brain or spinal cord, resulting in neurological conditions.

CONDITIONS

If you have any of the following conditions, try bringing aromatic herbs into your life:

H. pylori infection; *Streptococcus* infection; *E. coli* infection; small intestinal bacterial overgrowth (SIBO); peptic ulcers; strep throat; ear infections; sinusitis; diverticulitis; diverticulosis; ringworm; megacolon; *C. difficile* infection; MRSA; influenza; enteroviruses; norovirus; Epstein-Barr (EBV)/mononucleosis; cytomegalovirus (CMV); Lyme disease; all Lyme disease cofactors (including *Borrelia*, *Bartonella*, *Babesia*, and mycoplasma); respiratory infections; gum infections; tinnitus; vertigo; cholera; sciatica; fibromyalgia; chronic fatigue syndrome (CFS); lupus; psoriatic arthritis; multiple sclerosis (MS); shingles; rheumatoid arthritis (RA); edema; migraines; herpes simplex 1 (HSV-1); herpes simplex 2 (HSV-2); HHV-6; HHV-7; HHV-8; HHV-9; the undiscovered HHV-10, HHV-11, and HHV-12; shingles; pelvic inflammatory disease (PID); B cell disease; bacterial infections; eye infections; ammonia permeability

SYMPTOMS

If you have any of the following symptoms, try bringing aromatic herbs into your life:

Stomachaches, food allergies, abdominal pain, dizziness, fatigue, discharge (e.g., vaginal or from the eyes), flatulence, nausea, cough, anxiousness, itching, blisters, rashes, headaches, anal itching, mold exposure, all neurological symptoms (including tingles, numbness, spasms, twitches, nerve pain, and tightness of the chest), appendix inflammation, blisters, bladder pain, balance issues, clogged ears, congestion, ear pain, excess mucus, fever, jaw pain, neuralgia

EMOTIONAL SUPPORT

In the stressful times we live in, it's understandable when emotional reactions are heightened. When heightened emotional response becomes chronic, though, and you can't get yourself out of a cycle of overreacting, turn to oregano, rosemary, sage, and thyme. These herbs help break the cycle of feeling consistently overstimulated, so that you can take what comes on more of an even keel.

SPIRITUAL LESSON

These aromatic herbs have been around in one form or another, one species or another, since the beginning of humankind. All this time, they've been right there beside us, adapting along with the changing world so that we can adapt, too. Oregano, rosemary, sage, and thyme are important teachers this way—they remind us of who we are and who we can become. What else in your life, whether a longtime hobby or long-term relationship, can you always count on to cut out the distractions and connect you back with your most essential self?

TIPS

- Remind yourself to use these aromatic herbs in your daily cooking. Experiment with how many of your mainstay dishes can benefit from a sprinkle of oregano, rosemary, sage, and thyme.
- Try incorporating the essential oils of these herbs into your daily life for cleansing of mind, body, and soul. For example, add essential oil of rosemary to a bath to ignite the water's purification process.

HERB-BATTERED ROOT VEGETABLE FRIES

Makes 3 to 4 servings

These may be the best veggie fries you'll ever eat. The trick is to boil the root vegetables and then shake them vigorously before baking. The herbs and garlic generously coat the outside and the smudged edges will turn crispy in the oven. If you're pressed for time, you can omit the extra steps and send them straight to the oven, though those few extra minutes will yield truly amazing results. Make a big enough batch to share—these won't last long!

3 pounds assorted root vegetables (such as potatoes, sweet potatoes, parsnips, carrots, and celery root)

2 tablespoons coconut oil

1 teaspoon sea salt

2 tablespoons finely minced garlic

1 tablespoon each finely minced sage, oregano, rosemary, and thyme

Preheat the oven to 400°F. Peel and slice the root vegetables into "fries." Transfer the vegetable fries to a large pot, cover with water, and bring to a boil. Boil the fries for 5 to 7 minutes, until just cooked through but not soft. (Watch carefully so as not to overcook.) Drain the water. Add the coconut oil, sea salt, garlic, and herbs to the fries and stir briefly. Cover the pot and shake vigorously until the fries are well mixed with their edges slightly mashed.

Line a baking tray with parchment paper. Arrange the fries on the tray so none are overlapping. Place in the oven and bake for 20 to 25 minutes, flipping once halfway through. Remove when the edges turn golden and crispy.

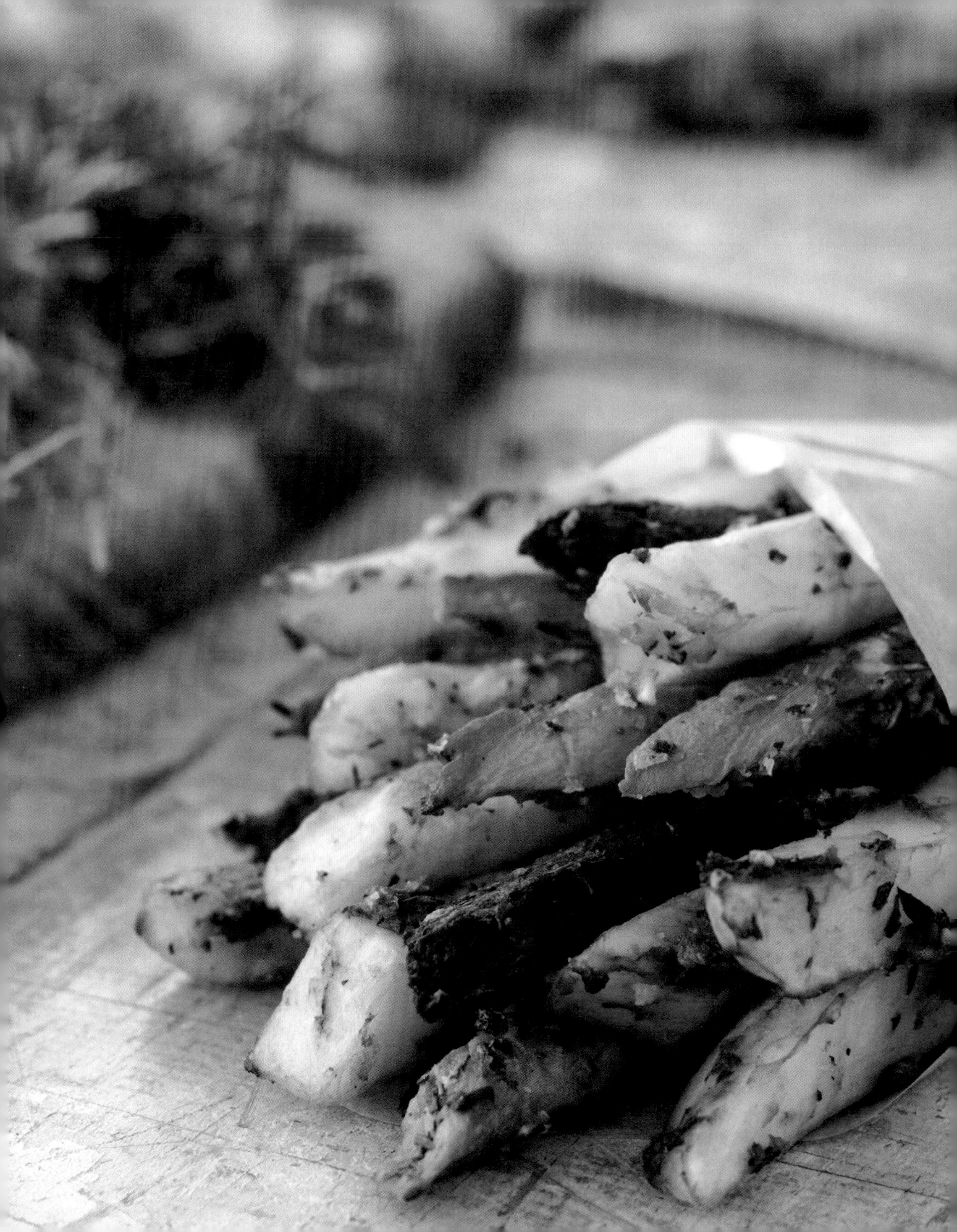

Cat's Claw

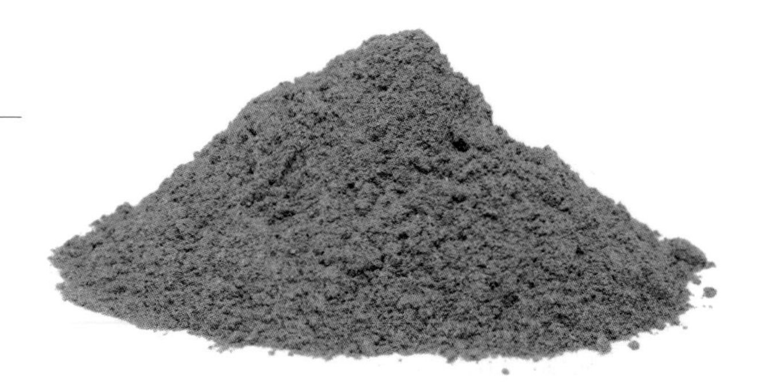

While inflammation has been pinpointed as a part of persistent illness, what has yet to be discovered by medical research is the real story about why this inflammation is present in the first place. So often the viral explosion in our modern world is to blame. Various strains and varieties of the Epstein-Barr virus, shingles, HHV-6, and other herpetic viruses, along with bacteria and parasites, are behind a great many people's suffering. To get rid of this widespread inflammation and the other debilitating symptoms of chronic illness, we have to get rid of the pathogens. Enter cat's claw, the herb also known by the Spanish name *uña de gato*. Cat's claw is one of the most powerful resources for reversing the epidemic of chronic and mystery illness in the 21st century.

Cat's claw can aid in alleviating almost any symptom, from neurological to digestive. While cat's claw has gotten some attention for its healing properties, it is as yet unknown to science that the herb contains bioactive pharma-compounds that supersede synthetic pharmaceuticals. All too often, antibiotics are employed against certain illnesses such as Lyme disease. The world would be a different place if cat's claw took the place of antibiotics; the rate of illness would reduce, and recovery would quicken, regardless of the diagnosis for a given illness. Of course, pharmaceutical antibiotics have their place and purpose. Cat's claw is unique, though, in that pathogens such as bacteria cannot become resistant to it, as they sometimes can to antibiotics.

Parasites such as *Babesia* and bacteria such as *Bartonella* cannot withstand the wrath of cat's claw. The herb eliminates these and other bugs without the so-called Herxheimer die-off reaction so common with antibiotics, because the bioactive pharma-compounds in the herb regulate the destruction of pathogens so that it's at a level the individual person can tolerate. Cat's claw is also incredible at fighting viruses. Eventually medical research will discover a group of antiviral adaptogens, and scientists will realize that cat's claw is at the top of that list. The herb is the ultimate secret weapon for battling PANDAS (pediatric autoimmune neuropsychiatric disorders associated with streptococcal infections), ALS, strep throat, MS, mystery aches and pains, and more.

Cat's claw is also remarkable for its ability to rid the body of the infamous strep, which is frequently misdiagnosed as yeast or *Candida*. Millions of women go on antibiotics and antifungals that only end up making problems worse, because the *Streptococcus* bacteria that causes urinary tract infections is so often antibiotic-resistant. Cat's claw lowers strep without issue, making it the ultimate UTI-alleviating herb and a fundamental tool of our time.

Note that if you're pregnant or trying to conceive, keep cat's claw out of your medicinal regimen.

CONDITIONS

If you have any of the following conditions, try bringing cat's claw into your life:

Every type of cancer; Lyme disease; all Lyme disease cofactors (including *Borrelia*, *Bartonella*, *Babesia*, and mycoplasma); small intestinal bacterial overgrowth (SIBO); amyotrophic lateral sclerosis (ALS); laryngitis; PANDAS; strep throat; multiple sclerosis (MS); dyskinesia; rheumatoid arthritis (RA); urinary tract infections (UTIs); kidney infections; lymphoma (including non-Hodgkin's); *Chlamydia pneumoniae*; yeast infections; migraines; irritable bowel syndrome (IBS); ulcers; Epstein-Barr virus (EBV)/mononucleosis; shingles; HHV-6; HHV-7; HHV-8; HHV-9; the undiscovered HHV-10, HHV-11, and HHV-12; nodules; herpes simplex 1 (HSV-1); herpes simplex 2 (HSV-2); acne; pelvic inflammatory disease (PID); vitiligo; sleep disorders; transient ischemic attack (TIA); plantar fasciitis; psoriatic arthritis; Morton's neuroma

SYMPTOMS

If you have any of the following symptoms, try bringing cat's claw into your life:

Inflammation, aches and pains, ringing or buzzing in the ears, *Candida* overgrowth, temporomandibular joint (TMJ) issues, gastritis, tingles and numbness, neurological heart palpitations, headaches, brain fog, parasitical and bacterial infection, twitches, Bell's palsy, frozen shoulder, spasms, tics, weakness of the limbs, burning sensations in or on the body, digestive disturbances, pins and needles, tremors, swallowing issues, slurred speech, nervousness, seizures, rashes, restless leg syndrome, dizziness, balance issues, moving body pain, muscle cramping, muscle tightness, muscle weakness, neck pain, joint pain, jaw pain, inflammation

EMOTIONAL SUPPORT

When someone is quick to judge or play the blame game, the first step is for that person to be aware that she or he is doing it. The next step is to take cat's claw. The herb is extremely helpful for reducing a sense of urgency, so that rather than automatically reacting to a situation, you can take some time to think, process, and address what has arisen with a level head.

SPIRITUAL LESSON

People are constantly on the search for the Holy Grail of health. As every new trend hits, we hope that this is the answer, the protection we've been waiting for, the discovery that will change our lives. Meanwhile, a miracle medicinal—cat's claw—sits on the shelf of the health food store, and we pass it by. Or we add it to our herbal tool kit and forget to use it. It comes from the tropical jungle, so you'd think its exotic origin would pique more interest. Yet it's within reach now, attainable, and so we figure it's too accessible to be the real thing. If we gave cat's claw a real chance, we would see that it really is a magical healer.

Throughout life, we overlook similar saving graces. Cat's claw teaches us to reevaluate them. Have you ever underestimated a person, resource, object, or opportunity, and then realized in hindsight that you'd passed up the gift of a lifetime? What's out there right now that could help if you let it? Cat's claw teaches us that sometimes what we seek is within reach. We just need to have the presence of mind to recognize those everyday miracles that have made their way to us, so we can seize them.

TIPS

- When choosing a cat's claw tincture, make sure it's not in an alcohol base. Alcohol cancels out the beneficial effects of the herb.
- Take a bottle of cat's claw tincture with you as part of your emergency kit when you're traveling. Over the course of your trip, when you can remember, take small doses of the tincture. It's a wonderful tool to protect your immunity and guard against malaria and bacterial infections.
- Regardless of what health issue you use cat's claw to address, take the tea or tincture in the evening, when its healing properties work most efficiently.

CAT'S CLAW TEA

Makes 4 cups

There's nothing like drinking a cup of this cat's claw tea as you watch the moon rise to activate your body's healing potential. It's an especially useful practice when you've done yoga or Pilates earlier in the day.

2 teaspoons cat's claw
½ lemon, sliced
Raw honey (optional)

Boil 4 cups of water. For each serving of tea, use 1 teaspoon of cat's claw per cup of hot water.* Steep for 5 minutes or more. Serve with lemon slices and raw honey, if desired.

*If a stronger, more medicinal tea is desired, use 2 teaspoons or up to 1 tablespoon of cat's claw per cup of hot water.

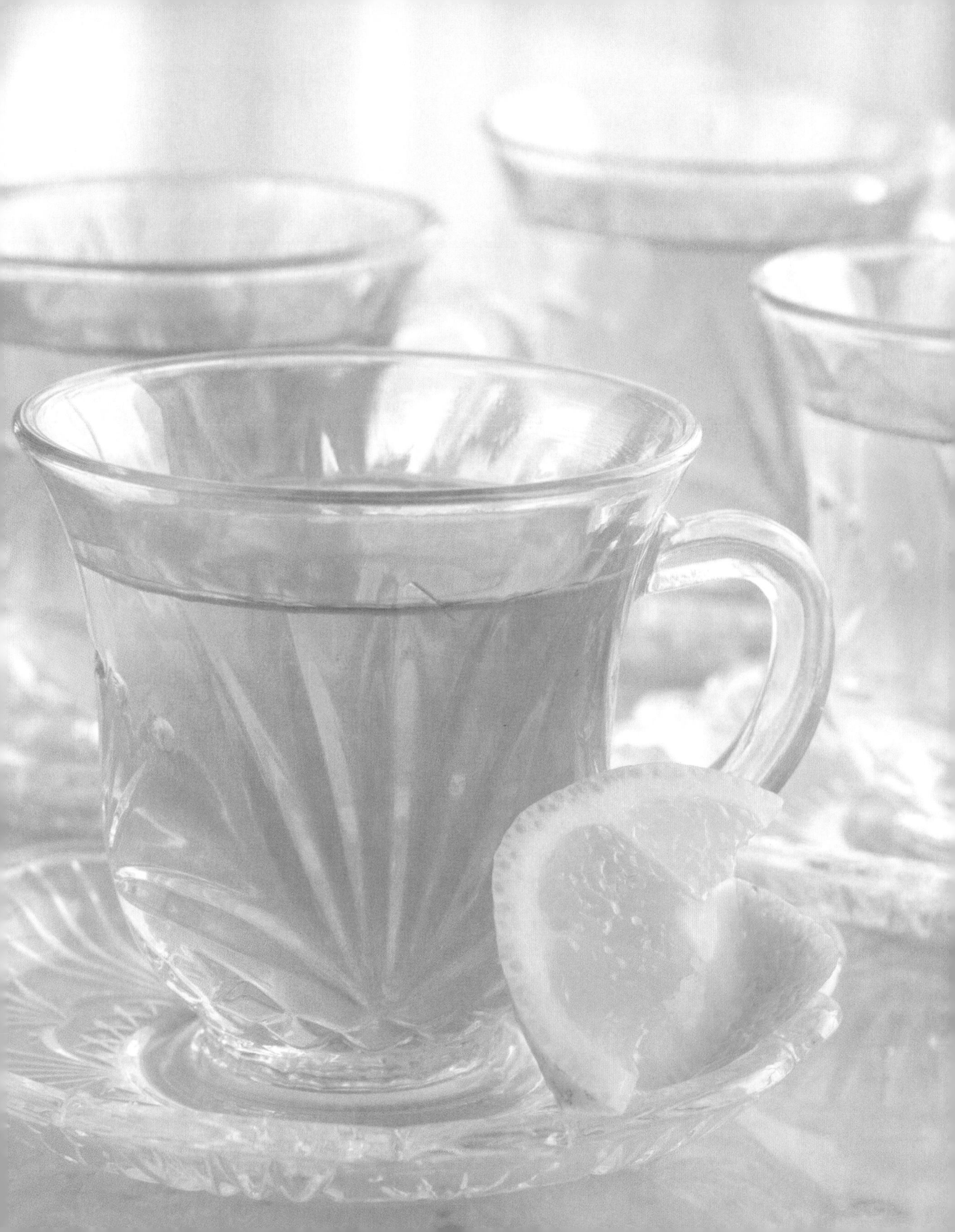

Cilantro

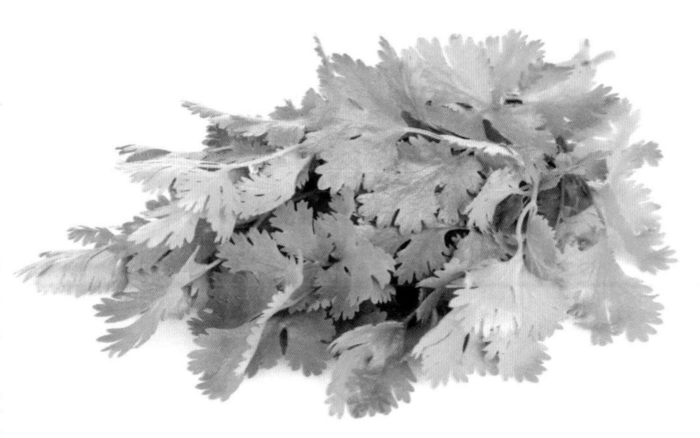

Cilantro, also called coriander and Chinese parsley, is the go-to herb for heavy metal detoxification. Cilantro's magic in detoxifying the brain lies in the living water in its stems and leaves. This is a critical aspect of how it can travel past the blood-brain barrier; in this living water are mineral salts comprised of minerals such as sodium, potassium, and chloride, which are bound to potent phytochemicals. When they enter the body, these precious salts join natural highways of other mineral salts that travel through the bloodstream, lymph fluid, and spinal fluid. As they come upon the amino acids glycine and glutamine in their travels, the mineral salts bind onto them, forming the ultimate neurotransmitters. The brain is a magnet for mineral salts, and when it draws up these precious mineral salt compounds from cilantro, a surprise package is attached: phytochemicals that deliberately remove toxic heavy metals from the brain, freeing up neurons from toxic heavy metal oxidized residue, so that they can function at their best.

While many people love the rich, savory flavor of cilantro, others get a bad taste in their mouths whenever they eat it. Try not to get caught up in the trend that theorizes that a dislike of cilantro has to do with genes. This genetic concept hasn't been studied widely enough—if it were, researchers would find that there is not a gene that determines whether or not a person has an aversion to cilantro. There are no genes that tell us not to eat a certain food.

What's really going on with cilantro aversion? When a person perceives an abrupt, harsh flavor from the herb, it means that she or he has a higher oxidative rate of heavy metals in her or his system. This doesn't mean the person possesses a higher level of toxic heavy metals. Rather, the heavy metals (in this case, usually a combination of aluminum, nickel, and/or copper, at whatever level) in her or his body are corroding rapidly. Corrosion means that there's toxic runoff, which makes its way into a person's lymphatic system and saliva. The moment cilantro makes contact with the mouth, its phytochemicals start to bind onto any oxidative runoff they encounter—if there's a lot of this debris in a person's saliva, it can result in a harsh sensation when eating cilantro. In other words, if someone dislikes cilantro, there's a good chance she or he really needs it.

Cilantro is also very valuable for extracting heavy metals and other toxins from other body systems and organs, particularly the liver. In fact, it's an amazing liver detoxifier in its own right. It's one of the best adrenal support herbs, too, and wonderful for balancing blood glucose levels and staving off weight gain, brain fog, and memory issues. And just when you thought cilantro had enough flare and flash, it's also antiviral—cilantro helps keep down levels of the Epstein-Barr virus, shingles, HHV-6, cytomegalovirus (CMV), and other herpetic viruses in all their various forms, as well as HIV.

It's also antibacterial; it helps to fight off virtually every form of bacteria and flush its waste from your body. Whether you like the taste of cilantro or not, parasites definitely don't like the taste of it; cilantro is an incredible worm deterrent especially. For any chronic or mystery illness, whether diagnosed, misdiagnosed, or undiagnosed, cilantro is a must-have.

CONDITIONS

If you have any of the following conditions, try bringing cilantro into your life:

Alzheimer's disease, dementia, depression, anxiety, obsessive-compulsive disorder (OCD), attention-deficit/hyperactivity disorder (ADHD), autism, posttraumatic stress disorder (PTSD), Epstein-Barr virus (EBV)/mononucleosis, shingles, HHV-6, cytomegalovirus (CMV), Parkinson's disease, Addison's disease, Cushing's syndrome, postural tachycardia syndrome (POTS), Raynaud's syndrome, chronic fatigue syndrome (CFS), fibromyalgia, multiple sclerosis (MS), migraines, vertigo, Ménière's disease, thyroid disease, ulcerative colitis, amyotrophic lateral sclerosis (ALS), autism, eczema, psoriasis, urinary tract infections (UTIs), insomnia, all autoimmune diseases and disorders, fibroids, injuries

SYMPTOMS

If you have any of the following symptoms, try bringing cilantro into your life:

Memory loss, brain fog, confusion, spasms, twitches, numbness, tingles, muscle cramps, foot drop, anxiousness, food allergies, sciatica, back pain, neck pain, jaw pain, headaches, dizziness, liver congestion, weight gain, trigeminal neuralgia, myelin nerve damage, mineral deficiencies, food sensitivities, heavy metal toxicity, blood toxicity, nervousness, constipation, inflamed liver, inflammation, hot flashes, sleep disturbances, joint pain, neuralgia, pins and needles, ringing or buzzing in the ears

EMOTIONAL SUPPORT

When you find yourself getting easily flustered, a little dizzy when faced with life's choices, perplexed about your life's purpose or about how someone in your life is behaving, turn to cilantro. This potent herb brings clarity, so that you can find your path and head in the right direction without getting distracted by other options or others' behavior.

SPIRITUAL LESSON

Cilantro teaches us that life is an ongoing cycle of extraction. It doesn't stop at pulling heavy metals out of our bodies—we're also meant to help our friends and family through life by listening to them without judgment as they work through difficult times. What pain can you help a loved one purge? What negative self-talk can you coach a friend to leave behind? Sometimes we hold on to beliefs or memories that no longer serve us, and we need some extra support to let them go. Just as cilantro is featured in cuisines from diverse cultures, emotional detox is a universal need. The next time you eat cilantro, think about who in your life could use a sympathetic ear. Try reaching out to that person, and—without overriding with your own opinion—let your loved one speak freely.

TIPS

- To remove toxic heavy metals from your body, cilantro needs to be in its fresh form.
- Frequently, cilantro is used as just a garnish. Try to acclimate yourself to using more than a sprig at a time. If you want results, it's best to incorporate it into your meals multiple times a day. You can juice some along with fresh vegetables, put a handful in a smoothie, add it to a chopped salad, soup, salsa, guacamole. The more cilantro you use, the more benefits it will bring.

CILANTRO PESTO

Makes 1 to 2 servings

Pesto gets a twist in this cilantro-inspired recipe. Use this pesto as a salad dressing, a veggie dip, or as a thick sauce over your favorite vegetables—it can do anything. It's a great way to get cilantro's healing benefits into your day.

2 cups packed cilantro
¼ cup walnuts
½ lemon, juiced
2 garlic cloves
2 tablespoons olive oil
⅛ teaspoon sea salt

Place all the ingredients in a food processor and process until well combined. Scoop the pesto into a small bowl and enjoy as a dip, salad dressing, or sauce.

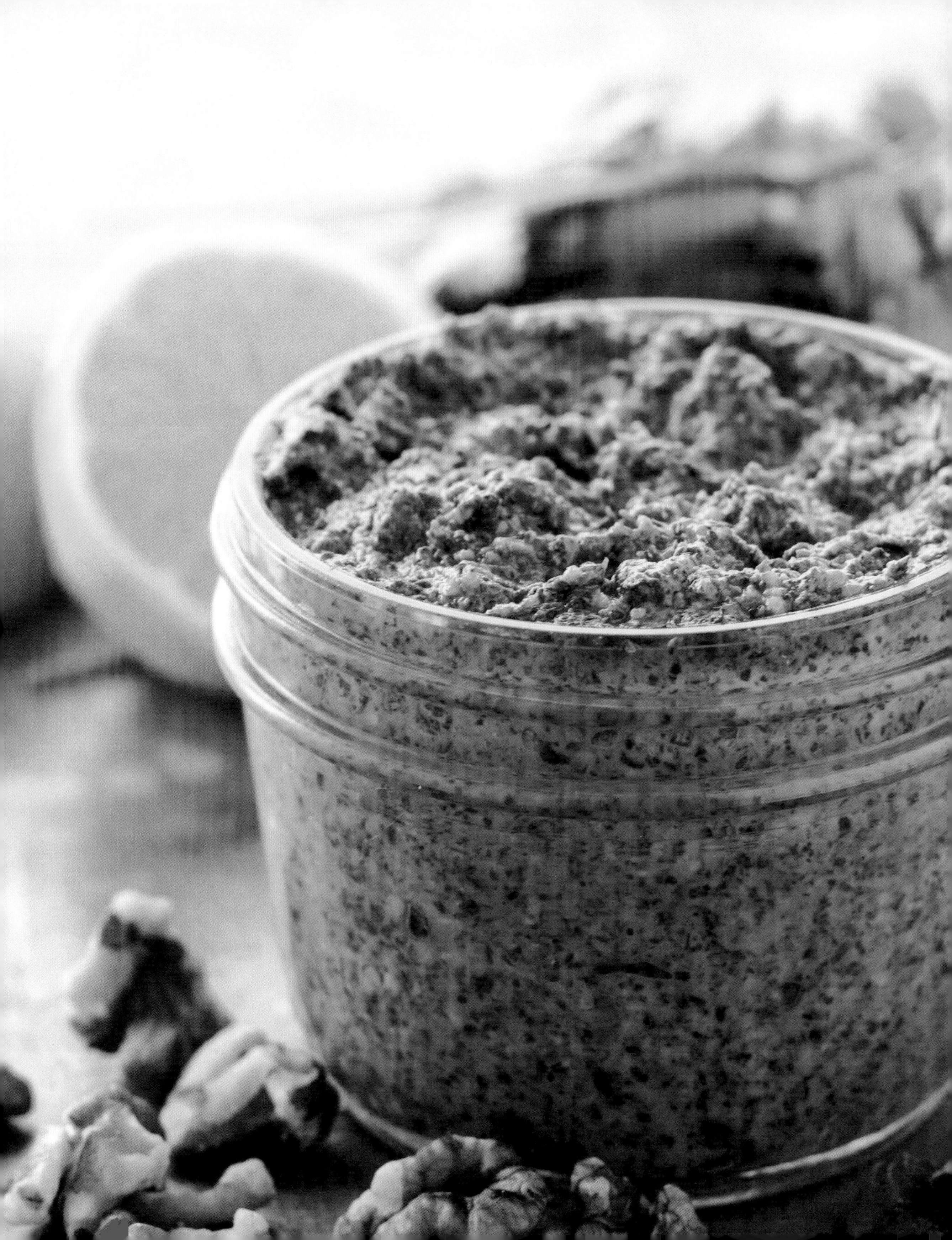

Garlic

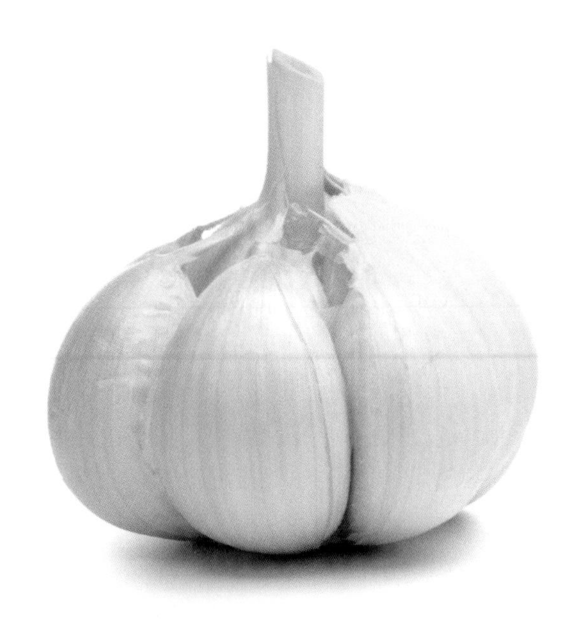

Whether you love garlic or take pains to avoid it, one thing's for certain: garlic deserves to be heralded as medicine for our world today. Used to enhance vitality since ancient times, garlic is more important for our well-being now than ever before. To give garlic its proper due would take a book on its own. Suffice it to say that like its relative the onion, garlic is multifaceted, playing many different roles in protecting a person's health, and has substantial reach in what it can do for someone. Garlic is antiviral, antibacterial, antifungal (including anti-mold), anti-parasitic, and rich in the phytochemical allicin, a sulfur compound that prevents disease.

Contrary to some mistaken theories, garlic does not kill productive bacteria in the intestinal tract. It only kills unproductive bacteria, which runs on a positive frequency. Don't confuse this with the term *gram-positive*, which doesn't actually refer to electrical charge. Both gram-positive and gram-negative bacteria that are harmful to humans run on a positive frequency. On the other hand, productive, beneficial bacteria (regardless of whether they're gram-negative or gram-positive) run on a negative frequency, the same frequency that humans run on. Not to be mistaken for negative, unfavorable energy, this negative charge is a good thing; it's our source of grounding. Unproductive bacteria, worms and other parasites, fungi, and viruses all run on a positive charge. When they take hold in our systems, they drain our batteries, and we lose our grounding. Then along comes garlic, which has anti-pathogenic properties that are positively charged. This like fights like, and garlic rids us of the pathogens that were harming us. Because beneficial bacteria in our guts and other microorganisms that benefit us are negatively charged and grounded, garlic doesn't wipe them out.

While there is a certain abrasive aspect to garlic, it is abrasiveness that's to your benefit. Rest assured that garlic does not disrupt anything that shouldn't be disrupted—it does not hurt you. On the contrary, it's perfect to fight colds, flus, strep throat, pneumonia-causing bacteria, and viral-related cancers. It also extracts toxic heavy metals in the colon and gives you a powerful immune boost.

CONDITIONS

If you have any of the following conditions, try bringing garlic into your life:

Strep throat, vaginal strep, strep-induced acne, other conditions related to *Streptococcus*

A and B, yeast infections, urinary tract infections (UTIs) such as bladder infections and kidney infections, staph infections, edema, sties, low reproductive system battery, ear infections, sinus infections, chronic sinusitis, immune system deficiencies, *H. pylori* infection, common colds, influenza, bacterial pneumonia, breast cancer, laryngitis, intestinal cancers, stomach cancer, esophageal cancer, prostate cancer, lymphoma (including non-Hodgkin's), Epstein-Barr virus (EBV)/mononucleosis, thyroid disease, adrenal fatigue, migraines, sleep apnea, Lyme disease, psoriatic arthritis, eczema, psoriasis, herpes simplex 1 (HSV-1), herpes simplex 2 (HSV-2), HHV-6, infertility, pelvic inflammatory disease (PID), ulcerative colitis, chronic bronchitis, small intestinal bacterial overgrowth (SIBO), thyroid nodules, thyroid cancer

SYMPTOMS

If you have any of the following symptoms, try bringing garlic into your life:

Swelling of the lymphatic system, inflammation, Bell's palsy, earache, postnasal drip, headaches, digestive distress, canker sores, enlarged spleen, all neurological symptoms (including tingles, numbness, spasms, twitches, nerve pain, and tightness of the chest), appendix inflammation, trouble breathing, back pain, bad breath, cough, chest pain, congestion, chest tightness, eye floaters, excess mucus, fever, fatigue, liver stagnation, headaches, neck pain, sinus pain, *Candida* overgrowth

EMOTIONAL SUPPORT

When you're at a fragile point and you feel vulnerable and exposed in your workplace, at home, or in a new relationship, turn to garlic. It's the food to bring into your life when you need protection and shelter.

SPIRITUAL LESSON

Before it can be harvested, garlic needs plenty of time to rest. It thrives on that time of nesting and quiet, covered over by the soil in the garden bed, when it can absorb nutrients and build up its own immune system against the pathogens that go after plant life, such as mold and other fungi, worms, and bugs; it strengthens during the growing season so it can pass on that strength to us. Take a cue from garlic, and stake out your own nesting period each year. In order to build up our physical reserves and spiritual immune systems, we all need a periodic time out from pollutions, pathogens, stress, and those people in our lives who drain our energy. Renewed, we can be better prepared for our own growing seasons.

TIPS

- Take a look at a bulb of garlic. It is perfectly packaged in little self-sealed doses—that is, cloves. This is God and Mother Nature's way of providing you with easy-to-take medicine to keep you healthy. Treat a bulb of garlic as if it were a bundle of premeasured medicinal supplements, and try to get into a rhythm where you consume one clove per day. Don't worry that the cloves are different sizes—smaller cloves have higher concentrations of nutrients, so each "dose" is comparable.
- Although roasting or otherwise cooking garlic is delicious and valuable, garlic is most effective when consumed raw. Try mixing raw garlic into your favorite dips, salad dressings, chilled soups, and other dishes.
- If you feel like you're coming down with something like a sore throat, cold, or flu, mince one raw clove of garlic and mash it into half an avocado, banana, or some cooked potato. Repeat this three times daily until you feel better.

GARLIC TAHINI SALAD DRESSING

Makes 1 to 2 servings

It's easy to make a big batch of this salad dressing and keep it in your fridge all week long. The classic Mediterranean flavors of olive oil and tahini blend wonderfully with garlic and the subtle sweetness from the dates. Enjoy this dressing atop any greens of your choice or use it as a dip for your favorite veggies.

¼ cup raw tahini
1 tablespoon olive oil
2 garlic cloves
2 medium dates (or 1 large date), pitted
½ cup water

Place all the ingredients in a blender and blend until smooth. Pour over your favorite salad greens and enjoy.

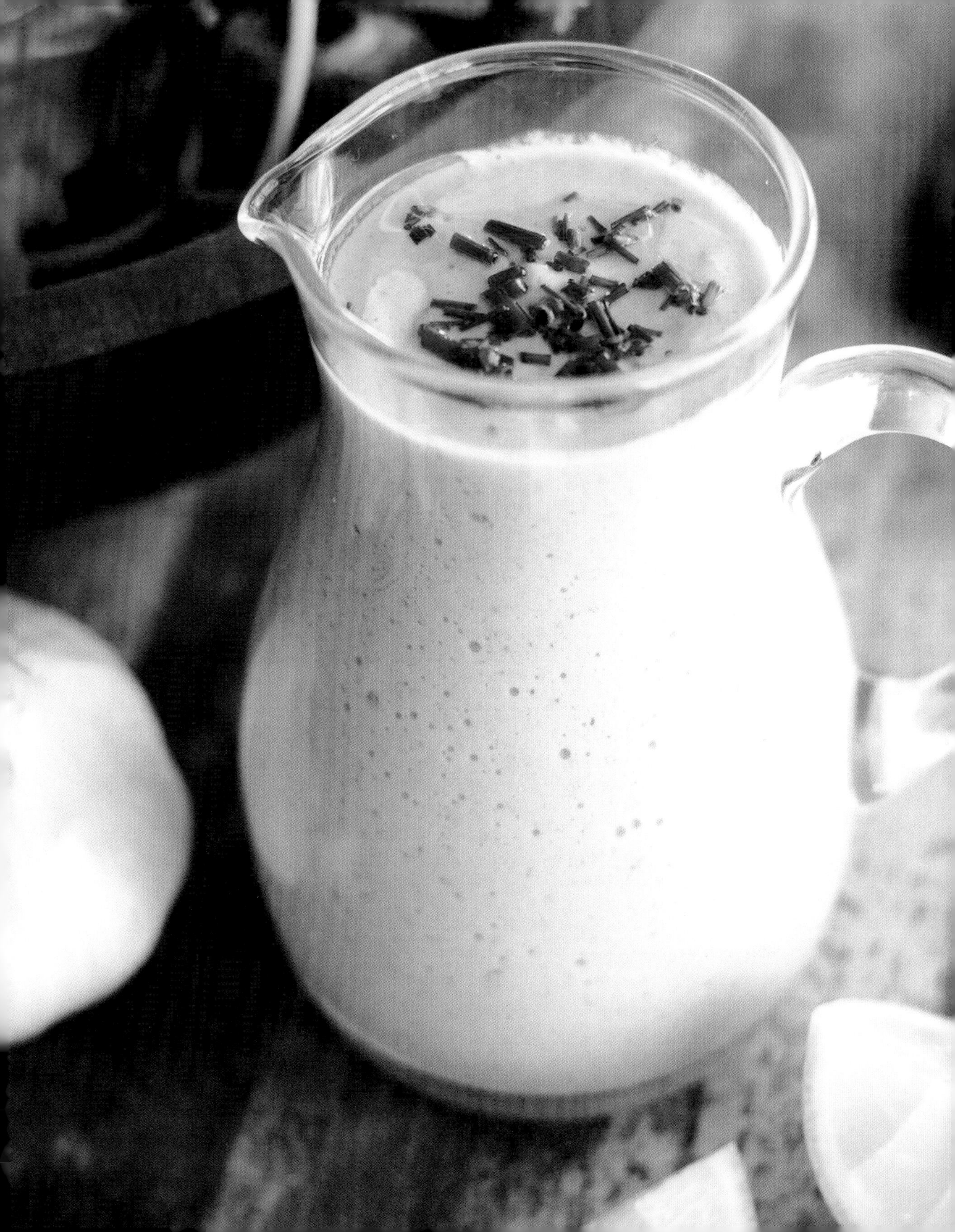

Ginger

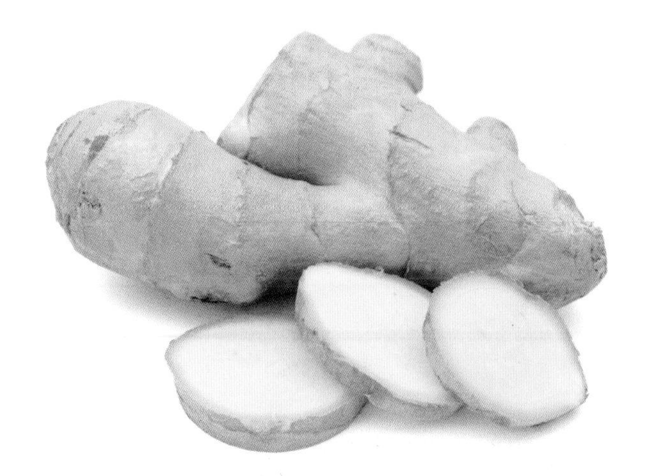

In this world, we live by reaction. We start the day with certain goals, and before we know it we get a phone call about a minor emergency, or an appliance breaks, or a client calls with an urgent request. Suddenly we're in crisis mode—and we may not be able to leave this state for the rest of the day, because the moment one issue is resolved, a new one takes its place. All day long, every day, we're dying out fires, large and small. This reactivity is what we need to survive the Quickening. At the same time, never winding down can set us up to be hyperreactive—like when there's traffic when you're already late to pick up your child from soccer practice, and without even thinking, you honk the horn at the car in front of you for stopping at a yellow light.

Ginger is one of the most important tools for giving ourselves respite from a reactive state. When you've been going a mile a minute from morning until night and you finally start to check out mentally and emotionally, the physical body often stays reactive, in a heightened, spasmodic state. This is how stress-related illnesses such as adrenal fatigue, acid reflux, sleep apnea, spastic bladder, insomnia, digestive issues such as spastic colon and gastritis, and chronic muscle pain can get kicked up. Ginger is the ultimate antispasmodic. A cup of ginger tea can calm an upset stomach and relax any other areas of tension for up to 12 hours. Rather than acting as a nerve tonic, it acts as a tonic for the organs and muscles, telling the body that it can let go, that everything is under control.

If your throat muscles are tight from speaking or yelling too much, or from having to hold in something you wish you could say, ginger is an amazing relaxant for the area. It also helps relieve tension headaches and flush excess lactic acid from muscle tissue into the bloodstream and out of the body—because it's not just strenuous exercise that causes the release of lactic acid; stress does, too. If you sit at a desk all day with stress pumping lactic acid through your muscles, it needs a way out, since you're not moving around to keep it flowing on its normal path.

Ginger's antispasmodic properties come from its more than 60 trace minerals, well over 30 amino acids (many of them undiscovered), and more than 500 enzymes and coenzymes all working together to calm reactivity. And as an antiviral, antibacterial, and anti-parasitic, ginger deserves all the accolades it gets for promoting a healthy immune system. Ginger is also ideal for stress assistance, DNA reconstruction, enhancement of your body's production of B_{12}, and so much more. It will be 100 years before research uncovers how much ginger truly holds.

CONDITIONS

If you have any of the following conditions, try bringing ginger into your life:

Pancreatitis, gallstones, adrenal fatigue, spastic colon, sleep apnea, spastic bladder, insomnia, laryngitis, common colds, influenza, hiatal hernia, Epstein-Barr virus (EBV)/mononucleosis, migraines, small intestinal bacterial overgrowth (SIBO), thyroid disease, pelvic inflammatory disease (PID), HHV-6, eczema, psoriasis, anxiety, amyotrophic lateral sclerosis (ALS), plantar fasciitis, Raynaud's syndrome, radiation exposure, all types of cancer (especially thyroid cancer and pancreatic cancer), celiac disease, chronic sinusitis, ear infections, fungal infections, hiatal hernia, human papilloma virus (HPV), insomnia, lymphedema, lupus, rheumatoid arthritis (RA), psoriatic arthritis, shingles

SYMPTOMS

If you have any of the following symptoms, try bringing ginger into your life:

Muscle spasms, muscle cramps, ganglia cysts, muscle tightness, muscle pain, temporomandibular joint (TMJ) issues, anxiousness, gastritis, bloating, stomach cramps, stomach pain, canker sores, acid reflux, upset stomach, headaches, gallbladder spasms, pelvic pain, back pain, dizziness, lightheadedness, sinus pain, congestion (particularly of the chest and/or sinuses), cough, urinary frequency, incontinence, urinary retention, weight gain, food allergies, abnormal Pap smear results, mineral deficiencies, food sensitivities, belching, diarrhea, brain fog, chronic nausea, colon spasms, cough, congestion, digestive disturbances, high cholesterol, sleeping disturbances, fatigue

EMOTIONAL SUPPORT

Ginger is ideal for those who feel forced to hold back what they have to say. When you are silenced, there are circumstances where the right course of action is to speak up anyway, and circumstances where you get the sense that saying your piece, however valid, would make the situation worse. Ginger is for the latter. Because holding in your true sentiments can make you feel locked up and stifled—and even put you into muscle spasm—it's very important to release all that tension, and ginger performs the job beautifully.

SPIRITUAL LESSON

Ginger teaches us that we don't always have to have an insight, breakthrough, or solution in order to let go of what's not helping us. We don't have to process everything or stress ourselves out reliving it. We don't have to react. There are enough other situations that require our reactions; there's no sense in taking on extra. Just like we can turn to ginger to work the kinks out of our muscles and the knots out of our stomachs, we can let it work that antispasmodic magic on our souls, cleansing us of wounds and damage without us having to do anything other than let it.

TIPS

- Ginger can be reused throughout the day. It's fine to keep using the same ginger for multiple servings of tea.
- Drinking ginger tea during a full moon increases the medicinal effects of the ginger by 50 percent.
- Consume ginger shortly before or during a time period when you have to make a serious life decision.
- Just before you take a therapeutic bath, drink ginger water or ginger tea to enhance the bath's healing power.

GINGER LIMEADE

Makes 2 to 4 servings

This ginger limeade is so refreshing. It will be especially helpful to anyone trying to transition off of caffeinated energy drinks. The subtle heat of fresh ginger juice makes this drink one you will come back to time and time again.

¼ cup honey

4 cups water, divided

1 tablespoon ginger juice (from about one 3-inch piece of ginger)

1 cup lime juice (from about 10 limes)

¼ cup fresh mint leaves

Heat ¼ cup of honey and 1 cup of water in a small pan until the honey dissolves completely. Set aside to cool.

Juice the ginger and limes into a large pitcher. Mix in the remaining 3 cups of water. Stir in the cooled honey water and the fresh mint leaves. Refrigerate until chilled.

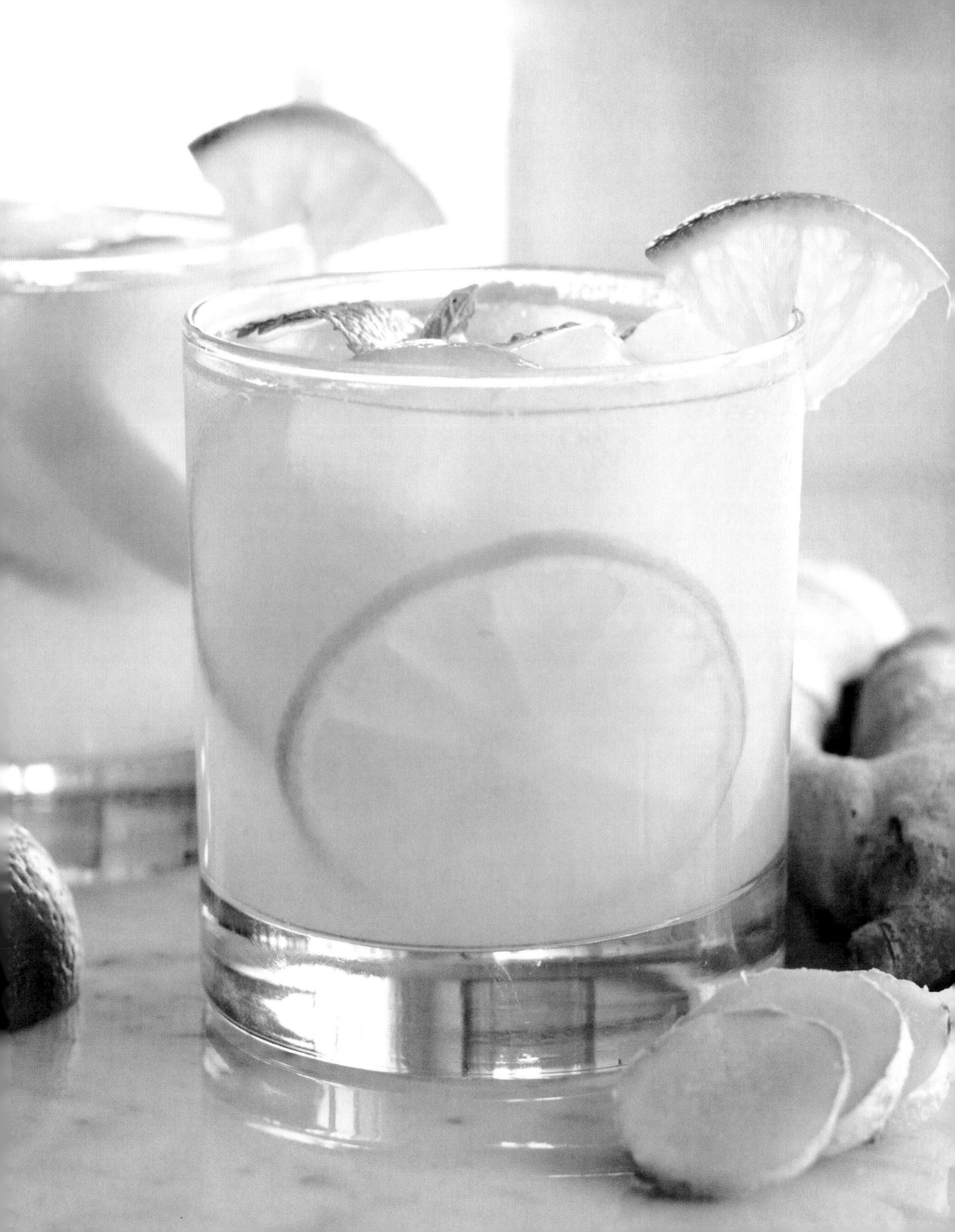

Lemon Balm

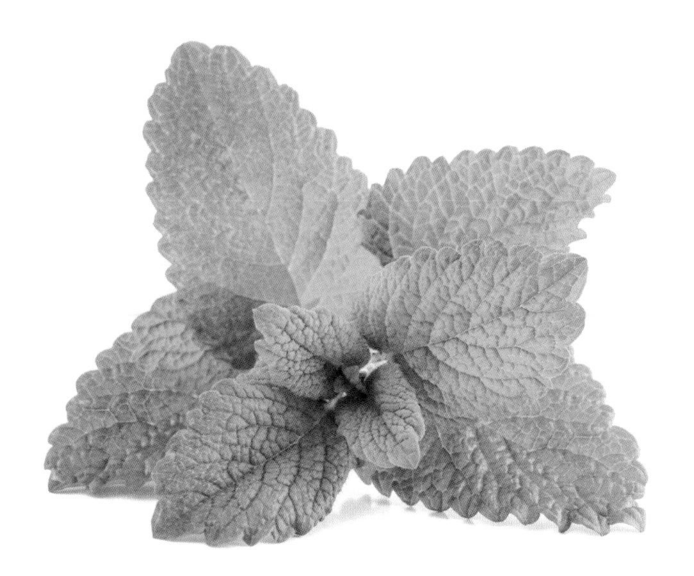

Lemon balm, also known as Melissa because of its botanical name *Melissa officinalis*, is an essential herb for calming the nerves—in particular, those involved with digestion. Many people suffer from various sensitivities in the gut, with complicated and confusing misdiagnoses involved. What's often behind these problems are nerve endings that have become hypersensitive around the digestive organs. Nerves play a role in much of the digestive distress we experience in this day and age. For instance, inflamed phrenic nerves (which control the diaphragm and therefore influence the stomach) and vagus nerves (which run through the diaphragm and govern the stomach and digestion) are sometimes behind digestive sensitivities, as are nerves that connect the spine and digestive tract.

If someone's stomach or intestines are irritated for no identifiable reason, it's usually due to sensitive nerves. One common occurrence is that a food (even something very easy to digest) rubs against the lining of the intestinal tract, which causes someone with sensitive nerves to feel discomfort. Nerve sensitivities can also trigger symptoms such as nausea, loss of appetite, and a sudden urgency to eliminate when nervous. Lemon balm is a gift from God and Mother Nature to deal with our frazzling world; it's wonderful for addressing all of these situations with its soothing properties, which come from bioactive phytochemicals such as undiscovered alkaloids that calm the nerve receptors at the digestive tract so that the nerves become less sensitized and inflammation reduces. This makes lemon balm a valuable herb for stress assistance.

And lemon balm doesn't stop there. It is a heal-all, with a high contribution factor to almost every part of the body. Extremely high in trace minerals such as boron, manganese, copper, chromium, molybdenum, selenium, and iron, lemon balm also has large amounts of the macromineral silica. Plus it's a B_{12}-conserving herb—which means that it monitors your stores of this vitamin and keeps your body from using it all up. Anti-parasitic, antiviral, and antibacterial throughout the body, lemon balm fights the Epstein-Barr virus, shingles, and other herpetic viruses such as HHV-6. It's an amazing herb for tonsillitis, which is inflammation caused by strep bacteria. Plus, lemon balm detoxifies the liver, spleen, and kidneys, and helps reduce bladder inflammation, which makes it a star for alleviating interstitial cystitis and urinary tract infections (UTIs).

CONDITIONS

If you have any of the following conditions, try bringing lemon balm into your life:

Nutrient absorption issues, laryngitis, interstitial cystitis, yeast infections, urinary tract infections (UTIs) such as bladder infections and kidney infections, tonsillitis, hypertension, Epstein-Barr virus (EBV)/mononucleosis, shingles, HHV-6, transient ischemic attack (TIA), staph infections, *H. pylori* infection, small intestinal bacterial overgrowth (SIBO), ear infections and other ear problems, hiatal hernia, neuropathy, ringworm, anxiety, depression, thyroid disease, adrenal fatigue, migraines, attention-deficit/hyperactivity disorder (ADHD), strep throat, autism, nodules on bones and glands, Lyme disease, amyotrophic lateral sclerosis (ALS), herpes simplex 1 (HSV-1), herpes simplex 2 (HSV-2), tonsillitis, rosacea, osteopenia, polycystic ovarian syndrome (PCOS), Ménière's disease

SYMPTOMS

If you have any of the following symptoms, try bringing lemon balm into your life:

Loss of appetite, trouble sleeping, anxiousness, nervous stomach, sensitive stomach, heart palpitations, hot flashes, night sweats, frozen shoulder, stomachaches, gastritis, abdominal pain, bloating, gas, nervousness, fatigue, diarrhea, urinary urgency, urinary frequency, weight gain, weakness of the limbs, weak digestion, trace mineral deficiencies, tooth pain, fever, seizures, nosebleeds, inflammation, histamine reactions, brain inflammation

EMOTIONAL SUPPORT

Stress and insecurities often cause us to feel fearful about what's around the bend. We find ourselves lying in bed at night, wondering what will happen to us and our families. If you're worried about what the future holds for yourself and others, lemon balm can take the worry away and replace it with a sense of peace.

SPIRITUAL LESSON

Lemon balm is practically an all-purpose plant, and it teaches us that we are just as well-rounded. We're not each here for just one reason. Within one lifetime, we have many different lives. We don't have to live with singular focus; we have many chances to explore different gifts and serve diverse purposes—some of which we'll discover along the way and some of which we'll live out without ever knowing how we're effecting change.

TIPS

- Make a sun tea with fresh lemon balm by steeping it in a pitcher of water for a few hours in bright, direct sunlight. The sun extracts and upgrades lemon balm's therapeutic properties, enhancing its nutrient profile to help you heal.
- Try using lemon balm leaves in small amounts as a culinary herb. Grow it in a pot on your windowsill so you always have some nearby to mince and add to salads for flavor and good medicine.
- Having lemon balm before bed will help calm your nerves and give you a better night's sleep.

LEMON BALM TEA

Makes 2 to 4 cups

This lemon balm tea is soothing and mild. The lemon doesn't overpower the herbs' subtle beauty, though if you want a stronger kick of lemon, go ahead and add more juice or zest to take the flavor to another level.

2 tablespoons lemon balm

1 teaspoon lemon zest

½ teaspoon minced fresh thyme leaves

1 teaspoon lemon juice

Mix the lemon balm, lemon zest, and thyme together in a small bowl. Boil 4 cups of water. For each serving of tea, use 1 teaspoon of the blend per 1 cup of hot water. Steep for 5 minutes or more. Just prior to serving, add ½ teaspoon of lemon juice to each cup.

*If a stronger, more medicinal tea is desired, use 2 teaspoons or up to 1 tablespoon of the tea blend per serving.

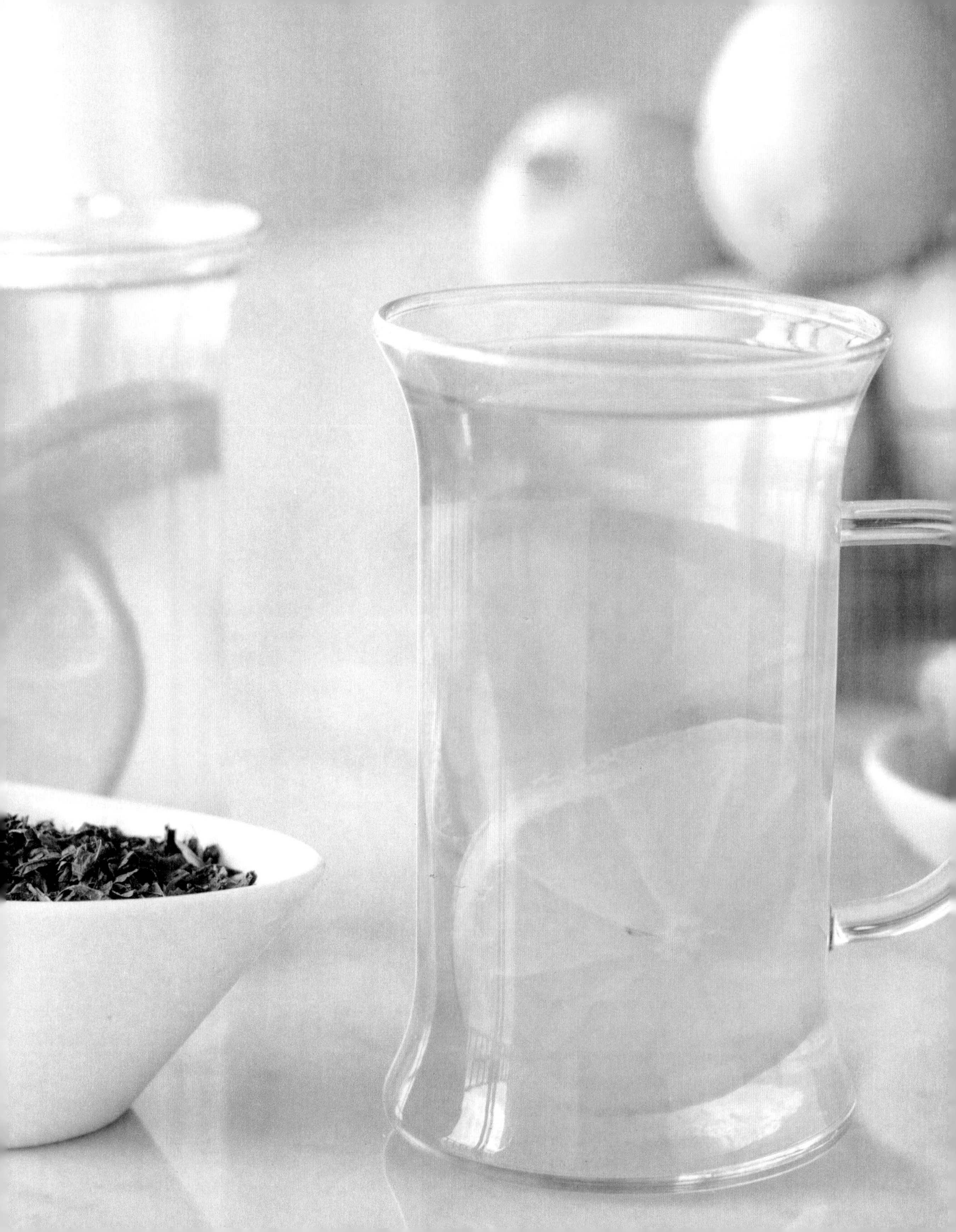

Licorice Root

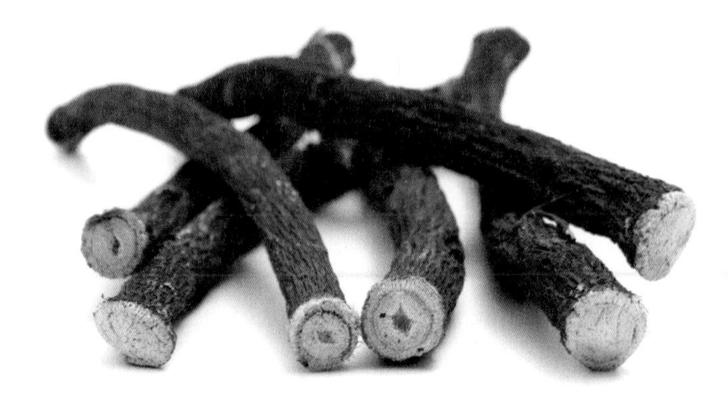

Licorice root is a savior. It is the most important herb of today's world, the camel to carry you through the desert of chronic illness. Why is licorice so critical? Because it is the ultimate weapon against the viral explosion. As you read about in the "Save Yourself" chapter, herpetic viruses (including Epstein-Barr, HHV-6, cytomegalovirus, and shingles) are so often behind mystery illnesses such as fibromyalgia, chronic fatigue syndrome, Lyme disease, Ménière's disease, and adrenal fatigue, as well as symptoms such as vertigo, dizziness, body aches and pains, and nerve pains in the jaw, neck, shoulder—not to mention those conditions such as rheumatoid arthritis and Hashimoto's thyroiditis that are labeled "autoimmune." (If you'd like full explanations of any of these illnesses, my first book covers them in detail.)

The body does not attack itself; strains and mutations of these herpes viruses do—which is why we need a potent antiviral on our side. That essential antiviral is licorice root. Its phytochemicals and antiviral properties stop a virus from procreating and at the same time push the virus out of the body, making your system as inhospitable as possible for viruses that want to take up residence there. In the autoimmune confusion of the 21st century, licorice root is one of the most powerful tools at our disposal.

Licorice root is also incredible for people with low blood pressure, and it helps soothe the liver by lowering liver heat. Not to mention that licorice is the most important adrenal restorative we have today. Popular herbs such as rhodiola, holy basil, ginseng, and even ashwagandha don't do a fraction of what licorice does for the endocrine glands. These other herbs are useful because they support the adrenals where they are, so if you have underactive adrenals, the herbs keep them from dropping even lower. Licorice root, on the other hand, acts like a battery charger for the adrenals: it brings them out of a fatigued state and increases their capacity to function to your advantage.

Note that there are conflicting views out there about licorice, including many misconceptions. Try not to get drawn into the negatives—you will be cheated out of healing.

CONDITIONS

If you have any of the following conditions, try bringing licorice root into your life:

Fibromyalgia, chronic fatigue syndrome (CFS), Lyme disease, Ménière's disease, adrenal fatigue, neuropathy, Graves' disease, interstitial cystitis, diverticulitis, diverticulosis, all autoimmune diseases and disorders (especially Hashimoto's thyroiditis, lupus, and rheumatoid arthritis), osteomyelitis, migraines, digestive disorders, strep throat, vertigo, Epstein-Barr virus (EBV)/mononucleosis, shingles, depression, insomnia, laryngitis, acne, adrenal fatigue, urinary tract infections (UTIs), sciatica, migraines, gastroesophageal reflux disease (GERD)

SYMPTOMS

If you have any of the following symptoms, try bringing licorice root into your life:

Dizziness, body aches and pains, anxiousness, nerve pain, jaw pain, neck pain, shoulder pain, brain fog, tingles and numbness, constipation, stomach pain, headaches, fatigue, nausea, hyperthyroid, appendix inflammation, hypothyroid, gastritis, food allergies, Bell's palsy, cold hands and feet, menopause symptoms, canker sores, acid reflux, ringing or buzzing in the ears, frozen shoulder, brain inflammation, temporomandibular joint (TMJ) issues, premenstrual syndrome (PMS) symptoms, low hydrochloric acid, vaginal burning, vaginal pain, ulcers (including peptic), tics, spasms, swallowing issues, heart palpitations, stagnant liver, pelvic pain, loss of libido, inflamed spleen

EMOTIONAL SUPPORT

Licorice root is wonderful for anyone who processes emotions through the gut instead of the head. If you feel like the simplest of misunderstandings give you a stress stomachache, or if you hold tension in your gut, deal with emotional agita, or get butterflies in the tummy, licorice helps prevent and relieve your suffering.

SPIRITUAL LESSON

When used correctly, licorice can bring back the health of people who have been struggling with illness for much of their lives. If you've ever been sick, you know that healing is a divine wonder. While those who haven't suffered may see others' healing as just getting back to normal, you know just what a miracle "normal" is—and anything that plays a role in restoring someone's well-being is a miracle in itself. Licorice teaches us that small miracles like these are all around us, though we'll only recognize them if we don't have on our blinders. What else in your life seems commonplace, and yet is a marvel of the universe?

TIPS

- If you're trying to get off of caffeine, try licorice root tea instead. First thing in the morning, it can be an incredible energy booster.
- When you're having trouble digesting food, or you've just eaten a bad meal out at a restaurant, drink licorice tea to help the digestion process along.
- Feel free to use licorice as an herbal tea or in its alcohol-free tincture form.

CINNAMON LICORICE ROOT TEA

Makes 4 cups

The rich flavor of this fragrant tea is sure to conjure warm feelings. As you take each sip, imagine yourself as a child eating sweet licorice candy, and let the memory lighten your heart and bring you joy.

2 tablespoons dried licorice root
1 teaspoon orange zest
1 teaspoon ground cinnamon
½ teaspoon whole cloves

Mix all the ingredients together in a small bowl. Boil 4 cups of water. For each serving of tea, use 1 teaspoon of the blend in 1 cup of hot water.* Steep for 5 minutes or more.

*If a stronger, more medicinal tea is desired, use 2 teaspoons or up to 1 tablespoon of the tea blend per serving.

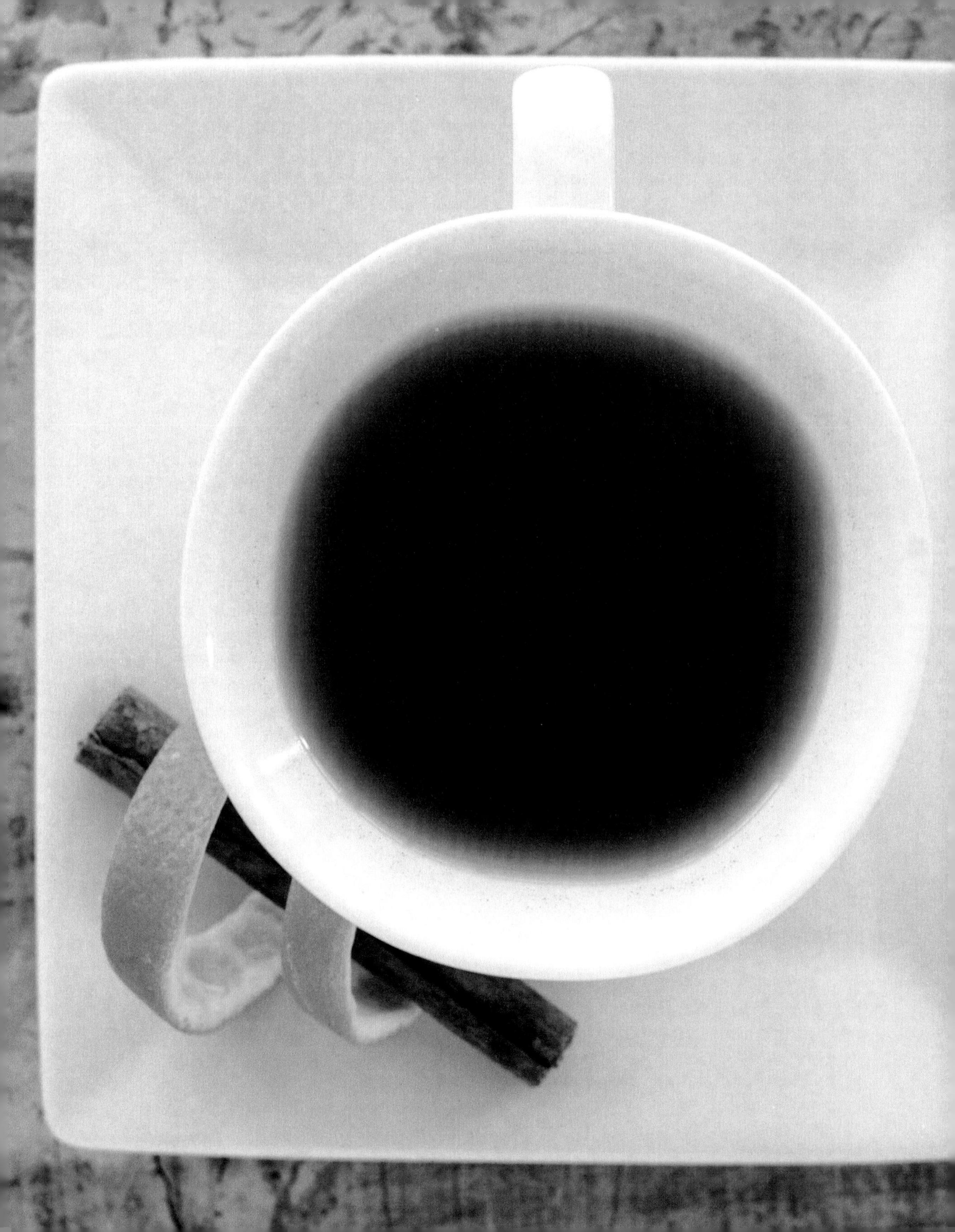

Parsley

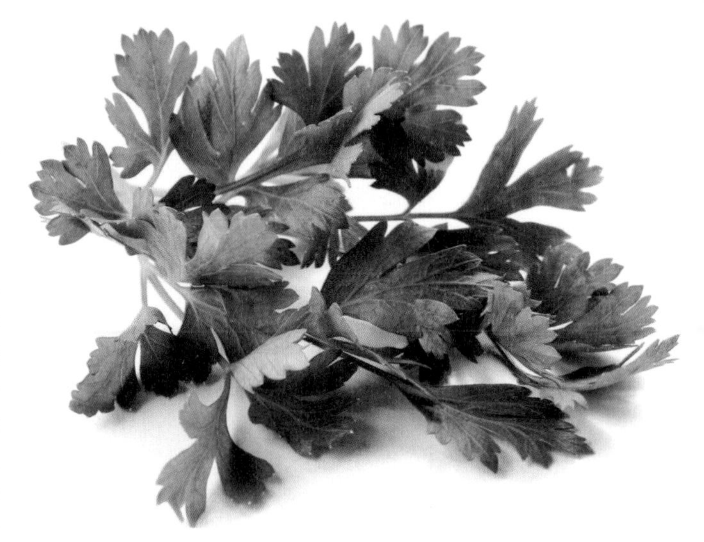

Though it could technically be grouped with the other aromatic herbs, parsley is in a class of its own because of its skill at alkalizing all the body systems. You've no doubt heard of the concept of body acidity and alkalinity—that when the body becomes acidic, disease can occur. Well, wherever parsley is sold, it should come with a sign that says, "Fights acidosis more than anything else." Normally, alkalizing foods only have the ability to promote alkalinity in one or two body systems, so other systems can remain acidic. Used appropriately and on a regular basis, parsley can alkalize the entire body, crossing body systems and driving out acidity across the board. (Note that pH strips don't give you the feedback on body acidity that you may think they do. For more on this, see the "Harmful Health Fads and Trends" chapter.) Mineral salts are a large part of what makes parsley so alkalizing—parsley's specialized mineral salts bind onto unproductive acids in the body to drive them out. This alkalizing skill makes parsley helpful for preventing and battling every type of cancer.

The herb is an all-purpose pathogen-fighter; it keeps bacteria, parasites, and fungus at bay. Parsley is amazing for anything mouth-related such as gum disease, tooth decay, and dry mouth, as it impedes the growth of unproductive microorganisms there. It's also a fantastic anti-DDT weapon—it has a great chelation effect that pulls out stores of herbicides and pesticides such as DDT that you never knew were hiding in your body and holding you back.

Parsley is full of nutrition, including B vitamins such as folic acid, traces of B_{12} coenzymes, and vitamins A, C, and K. It's also a highly remineralizing food, especially for those low in trace minerals; parsley provides magnesium, sulfur, iron, zinc, manganese, molybdenum, chromium, selenium, iodine, and calcium. Parsley is practically a wild food, as it doesn't need much tending to fare well and provide for you; it can even handle some colder weather, meaning that it has an adaptogenic nature. When you eat it, parsley passes this will to survive and thrive along to you. Parsley is an excellent herb to replenish you when you're depleted and exhausted. Like licorice root, though it doesn't usually make the lists of top adrenal boosters, parsley most definitely should.

CONDITIONS

If you have any of the following conditions, try bringing parsley into your life:

All types of cancer (especially blood cell cancers such as multiple myeloma), torn cartilage, phobias, anxiety, depression, gum disease, salivary duct problems, thrush, adrenal fatigue, Epstein-Barr virus (EBV)/mononucleosis, amyotrophic lateral sclerosis (ALS), migraines, thyroid disease, urinary tract infections (UTIs), Addison's disease, Parkinson's disease, dementia, Alzheimer's disease, arthritis, arteriosclerosis, atrial fibrillation, cardiovascular disease, chronic obstructive pulmonary disease (COPD), endocrine system disorders, hepatitis C, human immunodeficiency virus (HIV), bipolar disorder, Lyme disease, narcissistic personality disorder, fatty liver, ringworm, Sjögren's syndrome

SYMPTOMS

If you have any of the following symptoms, try bringing parsley into your life:

Nausea; lightheadedness; dizziness; acidosis; loss of smell; loss of taste; malaise; abdominal pain; tremors; gum pain; dry mouth; headaches; weight gain; nosebleeds; tooth decay; gum recession; cavities; all neurological symptoms (including tingles, numbness, spasms, twitches, nerve pain, and tightness of the chest); mineral deficiencies (including trace mineral deficiencies); chemical sensitivities; inflammation of the uterus, ovaries, and/or fallopian tubes; memory loss; poor circulation; pre-fatty liver; shortness of breath; brain lesions; spinal lesions; tooth pain

EMOTIONAL SUPPORT

When you feel like you're on an emotional roller coaster, turn to parsley. The herb grows in such a way that the stems and leaves on the outside mature first, and new growth continues in the center—so it's a very centered and centering herb. If you feel like you're being dragged along on someone else's emotional roller coaster, offer her or him a dish with parsley in it. When a person gets enough of this herb, you'll notice a more balanced state of mind and being.

SPIRITUAL LESSON

Too many people miss out on the health benefits of parsley because they're not wild about the flavor. It's not an allergy or an intolerance—they just decide to stick with what they know and love. When we don't like something, even if we know it's good for us, we tend to avoid it. What experiences, conversations, situations, responsibilities, and actions are you avoiding in your life that would ultimately help you? What valuable lessons are you missing out on? What benefits would you reap if you put aside your initial aversion and approached something you usually think of as unpleasant as an opportunity instead?

TIPS

- One excellent way to enjoy and benefit from parsley is to juice it with celery. The mineral salts in these related herbs work in tandem, with the parsley's salts binding onto acids such as lactic acid in the body and driving them out while celery's salts bind onto other sorts of toxins while also feeding and helping to form neurotransmitter chemicals (of which there are many varieties as yet undocumented by medical research).
- You can also make a tea from parsley, using the herb fresh or dried (though preferably fresh). The infusion process is a great way to extract the maximum amount of trace minerals and phytochemicals hidden deep within parsley, so that you can absorb these nutrients.

- For maximum benefit, seek out flat-leaf parsley. (Curly-leaf parsley still has great value, so don't skip it if flat-leaf isn't available.)
- Get into the habit of adding parsley to everything, whether you like the herb or not. At a certain point, habit will take over, and in the end, you'll at least be using parsley in one meal a day. If you're averse to parsley, experiment with it in various preparations (juiced, chopped and sprinkled on salad, blended into a smoothie, made into tea, and so on) until you find one you can tolerate. Then you can reap parsley's nutritional benefits while it also pushes out what shouldn't be in your system.

PARSLEY TABBOULEH

Makes 1 to 2 servings

This salad is the perfect addition to a big meal eaten around the table with family and friends. It pairs perfectly with hummus and a platter of roasted cauliflower. Traditionally, tabbouleh is eaten inside tender lettuce leaves. Serve it in a huge bowl and use your hands to scoop it up with lettuce cups. Enjoy the tradition of gathering together around this beautiful meal.

¼ cup almonds
4 cups parsley, tightly packed
⅛ cup mint, loosely packed
2 cups quartered tomatoes
2 cups quartered cucumber
½ cup chopped red onion
¼ teaspoon sea salt
1 teaspoon olive oil
½ lemon, juiced

Pulse ¼ cup almonds in a food processor until roughly chopped. Set aside.

Place 4 cups parsley in a food processor and pulse until finely chopped. Set aside.

Place the remaining ingredients in a food processor and pulse until chopped and well combined. Transfer the mixture to a large bowl. Add in the parsley and almonds and mix together. Serve and enjoy!

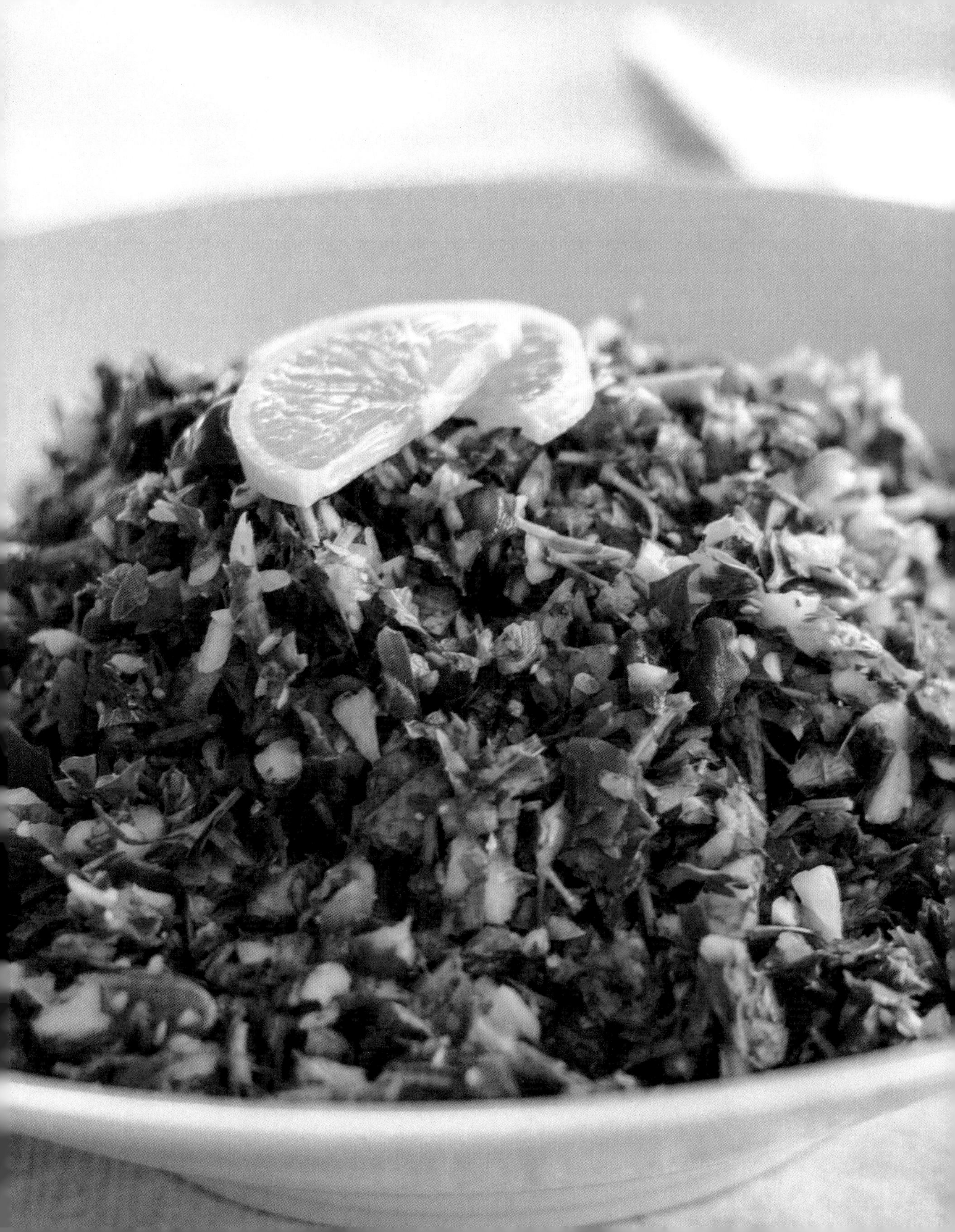

Raspberry Leaf

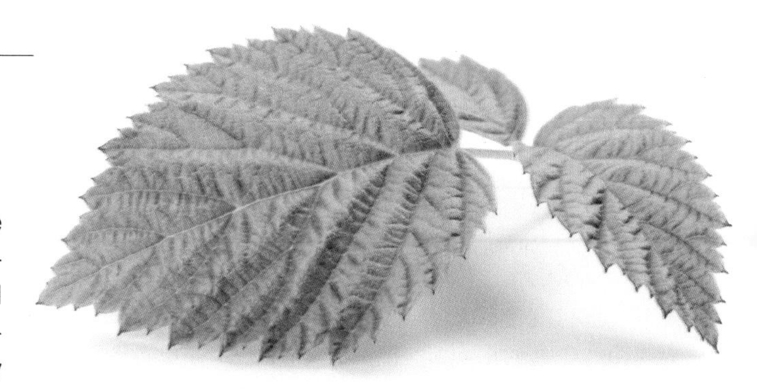

We often think of raspberry plants for one reason: the delicious and health-promoting berries it produces. The leaves, however, should receive equal credit. When it comes to balancing a woman's reproductive organs, raspberry leaf can't be beat. It is the ideal reproductive system reorganizer and protector. Raspberry leaf is also an overall hormonal balancer—for example, it supports adrenal gland production of estrogen, progesterone, and testosterone, and it feeds the thyroid gland with critical nutrients for replenishment. Raspberry leaf supports the entire endocrine system in hormone output.

All of this reproductive and hormonal support means that raspberry leaf brewed as tea is one of the most profound tonics to address infertility and prepare a woman's body for pregnancy. It is useful to help prevent miscarriages, and it is a secret tool to address exhaustion following childbirth and postpartum depression. Raspberry leaf is known to enhance production of breast milk. What doesn't get attention is that raspberry leaf also fortifies the mother's milk with vitamins and minerals, making it more nutritious for baby.

Raspberry leaf is also beneficial for men, mostly as a blood cleanser and overall detoxifier. For anybody, raspberry leaf's phytochemicals, including antioxidant compounds such as anthocyanins and polyphenols, make it an all-purpose anti-inflammatory, specifically for the organs and glands. It is also amazing for those with iron deficiencies, helps grow hair when needed, and because it helps strengthen the pancreas, those who are dealing with pancreatitis can do very well on this herb. Though it garners very little attention for its adaptogenic qualities, raspberry leaf should be classified as a top adaptogen.

CONDITIONS

If you have any of the following conditions, try bringing raspberry leaf into your life:

Infertility, miscarriage, fibroids, postpartum depression, anemia, urinary tract infections (UTIs) such as bladder infections and kidney infections, thyroid disease, pancreatitis, gum disease, low reproductive system battery, Graves' disease, Hashimoto's thyroiditis, uterine polyps, polycystic ovarian syndrome (PCOS), uterine prolapse, bladder prolapse, human papilloma virus (HPV), endocrine system disorders, bacterial vaginosis

SYMPTOMS

If you have any of the following symptoms, try bringing raspberry leaf into your life:

Low breast milk supply; gastritis; ovarian cysts; food allergies; fatigue; stomach upset; iron deficiency; hair loss; abnormal Pap smear results; inflamed uterus, ovaries, and/or fallopian tubes; hormonal imbalances; hypothyroid; hot flashes; inconsistent vaginal bleeding; vaginal discharge; vaginal burning; cramping

EMOTIONAL SUPPORT

For the person seeking comfort, serenity, compassion, consolation, warmth, affection, and a touch of admiration thrown in for good measure, raspberry leaf is an amazing herb. Use it for self-soothing, or offer it to a friend in need.

SPIRITUAL LESSON

A raspberry patch can overtake the garden if you don't tend it. It is controllable, though, if you have a little bit of time, patience, and education about which canes to cut back. Ultimately, this process results in a healthier, more fruitful plant. In our lives, we encounter other situations that border on chaos. Some of them are outside of our control—not all of them are, though. Raspberry plants teach us to keep an eye out for those situations that we can nip in the bud if we brave the thorns and bring a discerning eye. What in your life, if you tend to it now, could become more fruitful over time?

TIPS

- Make a cup of raspberry leaf tea if you feel a low point in the day. It can help take the edge off.
- For the most profound effect of restoring the reproductive system and balancing hormones, make a tea with raspberry leaf and nettle leaf together.
- Drink extra raspberry leaf tea during the full moon. This enhances its potency, because raspberry plants grow 25 percent more on full moons—and the dried leaf is still connected to these rhythms from its days attached to the cane.

RASPBERRY LEAF TEA

Makes 4 cups

Seeds, leaves, and petals align in this delicious tea. As you sip it, envision an alignment of your own, where your reproductive system and the rest of your body become one.

2 tablespoons raspberry leaf
8 cardamom pods
1 teaspoon rose petals or buds

Mix all the ingredients together in a small bowl. Boil 4 cups of water. For each serving of tea, use 1 teaspoon of the blend in 1 cup of hot water.* Steep for 5 minutes or more.

*If a stronger, more medicinal tea is desired, use 2 teaspoons or up to 1 tablespoon of the tea blend per serving.

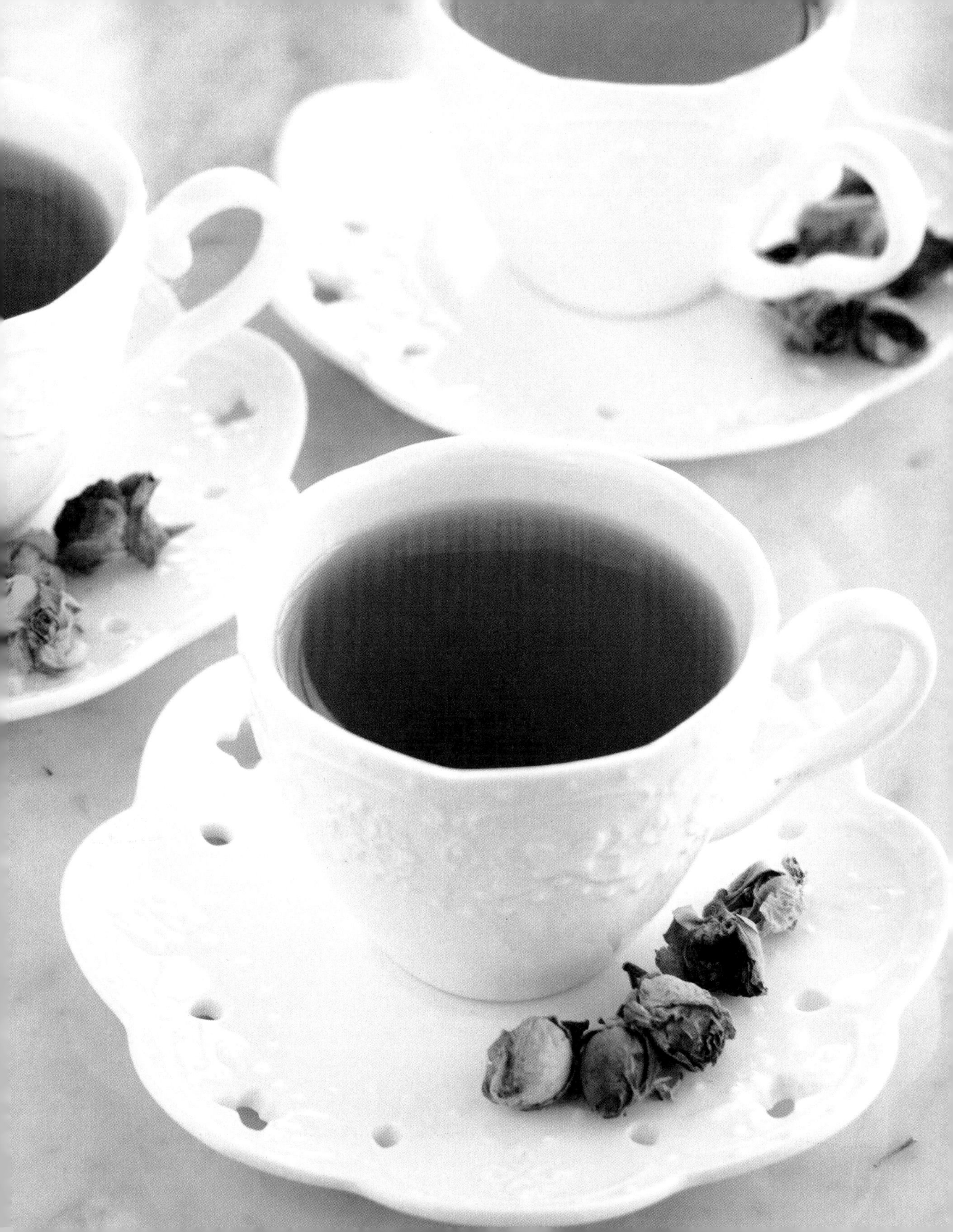

Turmeric

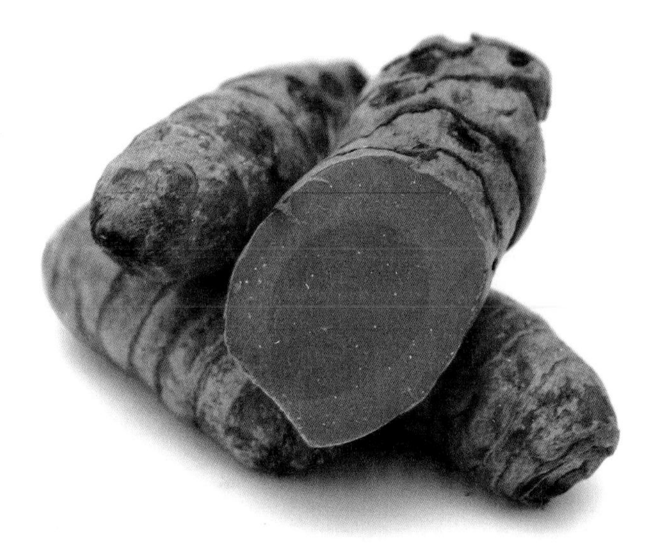

Turmeric is great for just about every aspect of our well-being. Famous for containing curcumin, a phytochemical with anti-inflammatory properties, turmeric is a particular asset for conditions such as lupus, in which the body can get stuck in a habitual cycle of reaction, even after the invader (in the case of lupus, the Epstein-Barr virus) is no longer present. Note that inflammation in chronic illness is due to the body's immune response to a foreign presence such as a virus—not, as many sources mistakenly say, due to the body turning against itself. Sometimes, though, once a cycle gets started, the body needs an ally to come in and break the pattern. Turmeric is ideal for this job, because it contains natural and very beneficial steroidal compounds from the curcumin as well as other aspects of the turmeric that are critical to calm down outsized inflammatory responses to pathogens.

This makes turmeric great for anything in the body that's inflamed and causing pain, from nerves to joints to the brain. Speaking of brain inflammation, many people walk around with undiagnosed mystery low-grade viral encephalitis, a swelling of the brain on such a minute scale that it's not detectable by medical testing, though its symptoms are sometimes diagnosed as myalgic encephalomyelitis/chronic fatigue syndrome (ME/CFS). (This is a tag for a mystery illness that's the result of brain inflammation from Epstein-Barr.) Undiscovered enchephalitis results in mystery pressure in the head, dizziness, deep headaches, blurry eyes that can't be fixed with a glasses prescription, confusion, severe anxiety, and panic. Turmeric is the ultimate antidote.

At the same time that it attends to inflammation, turmeric's powerful agents and compounds increase blood supply to areas of the body that need enhanced circulation, which makes this an ideal spice for those who have chronic histamine reactions, or toxic blood due to a sluggish liver or poor circulation. Turmeric's high level of manganese combined with its curcumin make it great for the cardiovascular system—it lowers bad cholesterol, raises good cholesterol, helps inhibit tumors and cysts, and can prevent virtually any type of cancer, especially skin cancers. Plus, the manganese activates curcumin's ability to extract toxic heavy metals from your system.

CONDITIONS

If you have any of the following conditions, try bringing turmeric into your life:

Allergies, lupus, encephalitis, anxiety, high cholesterol, tumors (including brain tumors), polycystic ovarian syndrome (PCOS), fibroids, all types of cancer (especially skin cancers), small intestinal bacterial overgrowth (SIBO), influenza, colds, sinus issues, chronic fatigue syndrome (CFS), Epstein-Barr virus (EBV)/ mononucleosis, multiple sclerosis (MS), rheumatoid arthritis (RA), amyotrophic lateral sclerosis (ALS), lymphoma (including non-Hodgkin's), eczema, psoriasis, heavy metal toxicity, bacterial pneumonia, bursitis, carpal tunnel syndrome, celiac disease, cerebral palsy, chronic bronchitis, eating disorders, electromagnetic hypersensitivity (EHS), emphysema, endometriosis, heart disease, insomnia, lipoma, adrenal fatigue, glaucoma, Lyme disease, Graves' disease, migraines, obesity, arthritis, Parkinson's disease, parasites, Raynaud's syndrome, seasonal affective disorder (SAD), sciatica, Hashimoto's thyroiditis, yeast infections, worms

SYMPTOMS

If you have any of the following symptoms, try bringing turmeric into your life:

Rashes, hives, congestion, brain inflammation, joint inflammation, nerve inflammation, poor circulation, cysts, sluggish liver, liver heat, mineral deficiencies, dandruff, back pain, neck pain, knee pain, foot pain, hyperthyroid, inflammation, pressure in the head, dizziness, deep headaches, blurry eyes, confusion, panic, congestion, sore throat, cough, body aches and pains, body stiffness, calcifications, enlarged spleen, chemical sensitivities, depersonalization, disorientation, dyskinesia, emotional eating, excess mucus, frozen shoulder, histamine reactions, hormonal imbalances, low hydrochloric acid, intermittent vaginal bleeding, jaw pain, outbursts of anger, leg cramps, low cortisol, menopause symptoms, muscle spasms, muscle stiffness, roving aches and pains, sinus pains, hypothyroid, weight gain

EMOTIONAL SUPPORT

For those who have trouble acknowledging their own self-worth, turmeric is ideal. If you find that you downplay your contributions to projects or relationships, are constantly down on yourself, or have trouble accepting compliments, bring turmeric into your life to help you appreciate just what a valuable, shining human being you are, and all the positives you have to offer.

SPIRITUAL LESSON

Turmeric's anti-inflammatory properties are so potent that they're meant to give us pause and consider what else in our lives could use calming. Inflammation doesn't just occur on a physical level. We can also become inflamed mentally, emotionally, and even spiritually. This often takes the form of judgment, blame, rage, or perpetual dissatisfaction. Like physical inflammation, it can feel very uncomfortable. It could be that the reason for your initial distress is long past, and you're stuck in a habitual feedback loop that makes you relive your pain over and over. The next time you feel a bout of existential inflammation coming on, honor whatever past experience has brought out this reaction, then take a cue from turmeric and gently try to end the cycle.

TIPS

- If you're dealing with congestion, cough, sore throat, cold, flu, and/or sinus problems, try juicing fresh turmeric and ginger together to make a small dose of concentrated serum. Periodically throughout the day, take tiny sips. The juice will act as an expectorant and help speed up the healing process.
- After a workout or any heavy labor, try to consume turmeric. It doesn't matter in what form—whether as a spice on food, juiced, as tea, or as a supplement—just as long as you get some into your body. Turmeric can shorten recovery time for muscles, ligaments, and joints after exercise, and it also acts as an anti-inflammatory for any minor injuries you might not have noticed that have the potential to turn into trouble otherwise.

TURMERIC-GINGER SHOTS

Makes 2 to 4 servings

These fiery, immune-boosting shots are a tasty variation on the turmeric-ginger serum I mentioned above. A go-to option for the first sign of a cold, these shots will help your body fight back against anything that tries to come against it!

4 inches turmeric
4 inches fresh ginger
2 oranges
4 garlic cloves

One at a time, run each ingredient through the juicer, keeping the juices separate. Combine 1 teaspoon turmeric juice, 1 teaspoon ginger juice, ¼ teaspoon garlic juice, and ¼ cup of orange juice in a small glass. Stir to combine and drink immediately.

Note: the amount of ingredients necessary will vary greatly based on the juicer that is used.

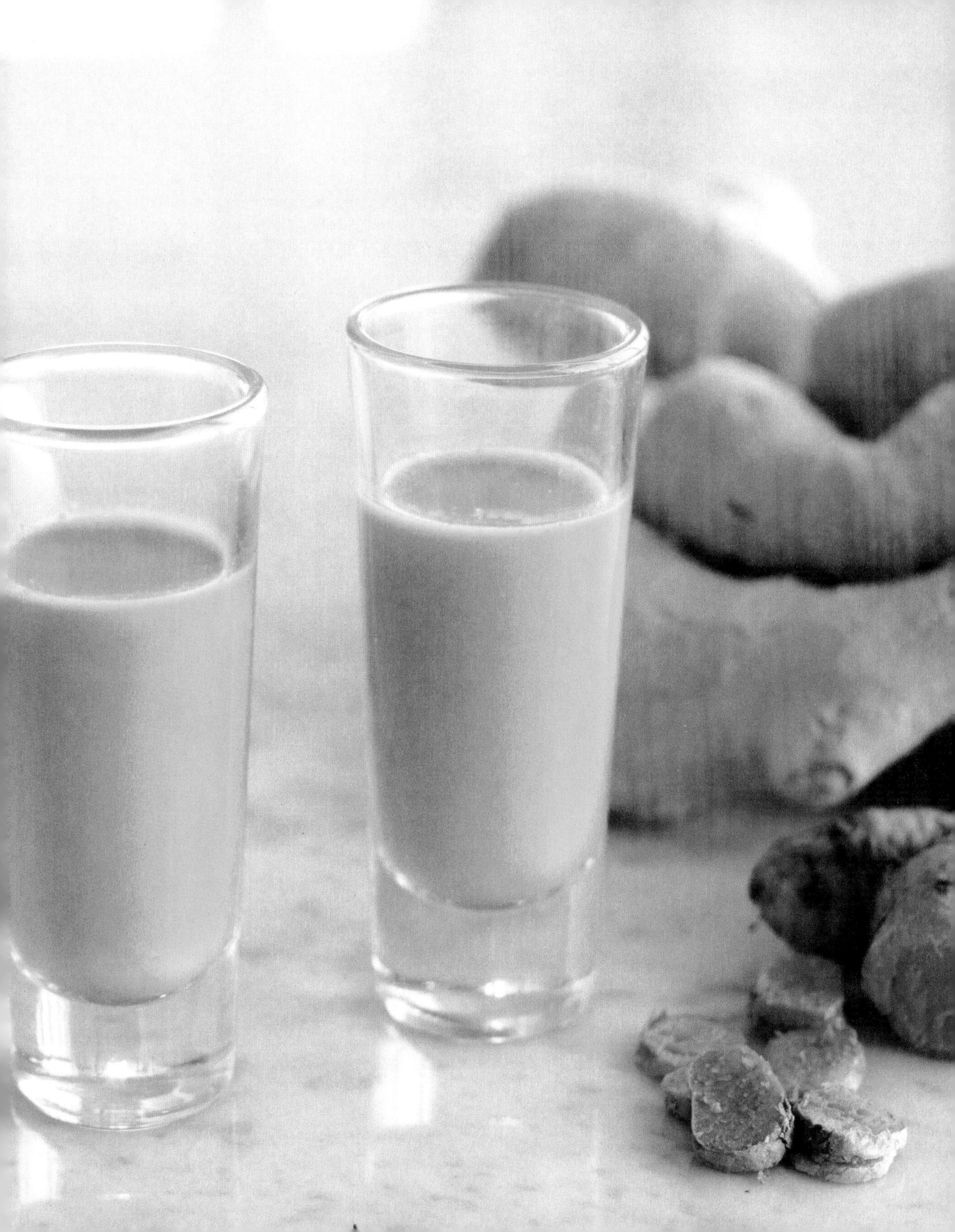

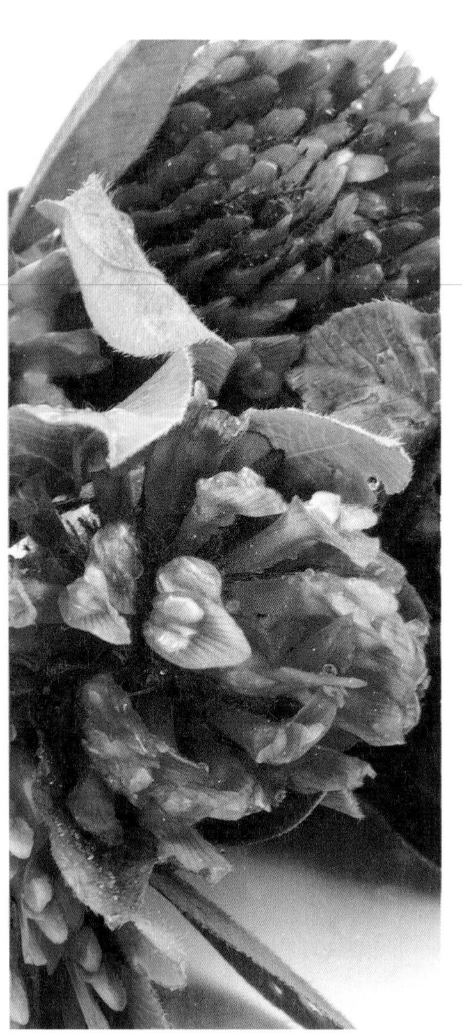
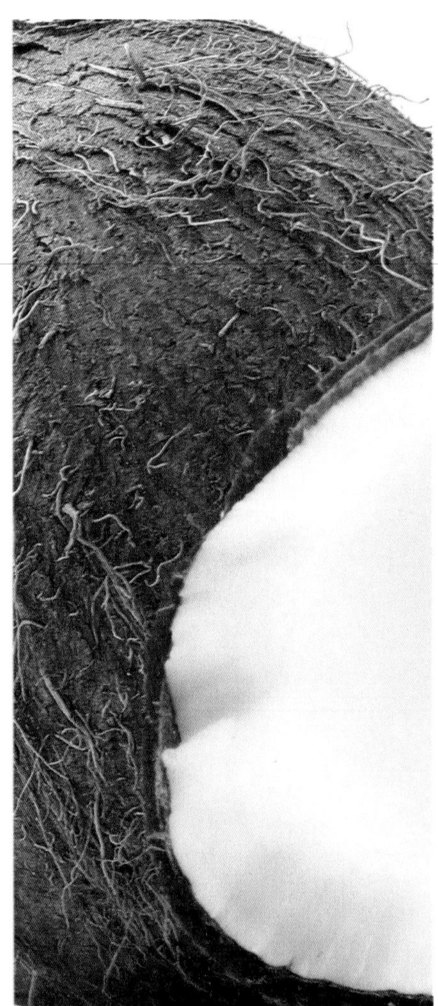
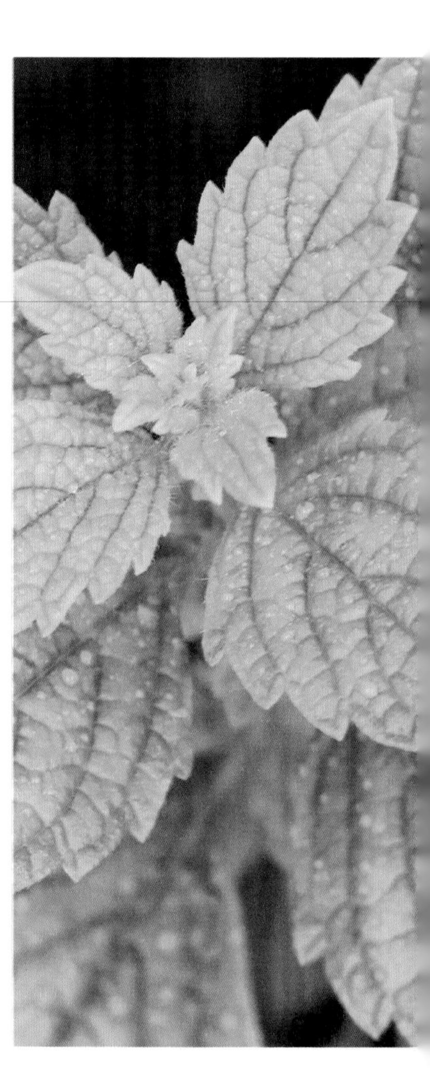

WILD FOODS

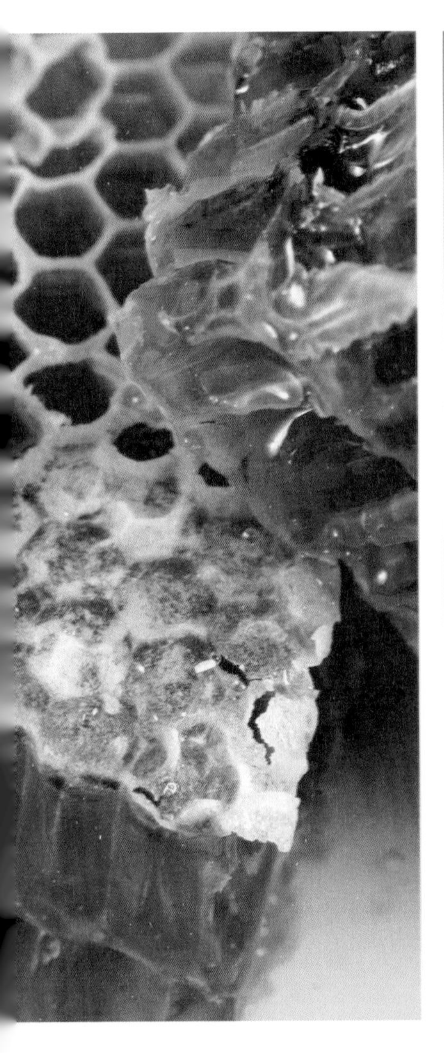

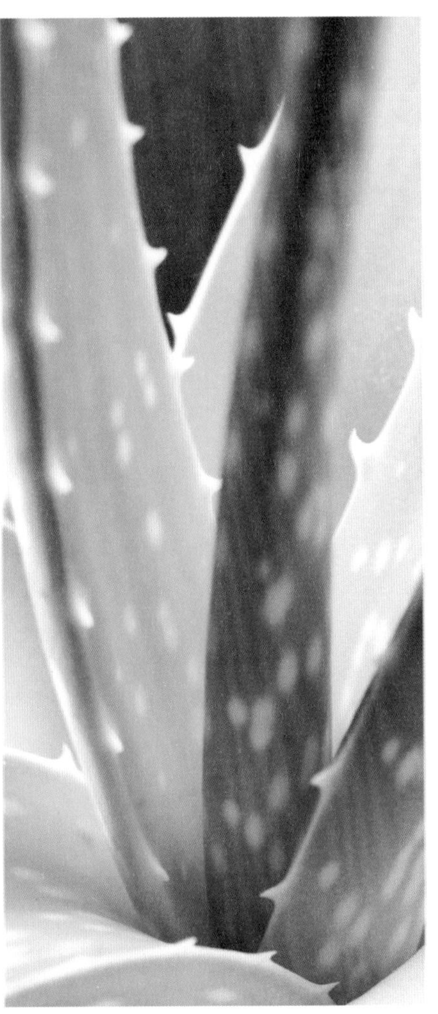

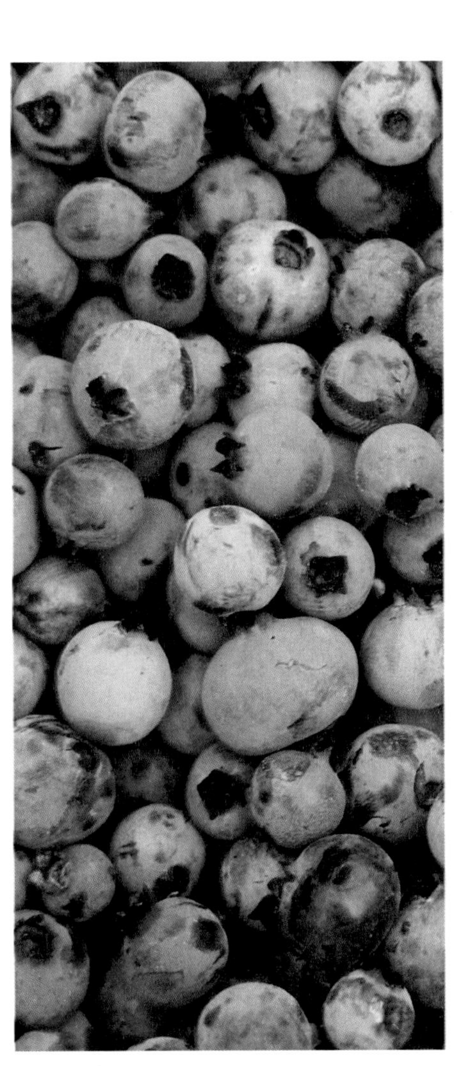

Aloe Vera

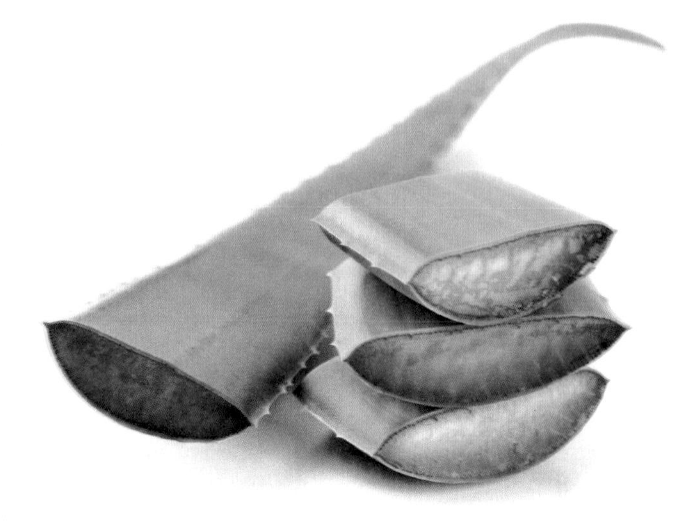

Aloe vera is famous for its soothing properties when applied on the outside of the body to burns, cuts, scrapes, bruises, bug bites, and most especially sunburn. Taken internally, though, fresh aloe has a much broader spectrum of potency. If you're drawn to enemas and colonics, make aloe vera a part of your life—consuming it offers a colon cleanse all on its own. Aloe is wonderful for relieving constipation.

Aloe vera also possesses more than 70 trace minerals that are grouped into undiscovered medicinal alloys. These alloys work together with the phytochemical aloin to calm inflammation in the gut, which makes it a top aid for IBS, Crohn's, and colitis. This anti-inflammatory nature rejuvenates the appendix, as well as the ileum—a critical portion of the intestinal tract, because that's where the body produces vitamin B_{12} when the digestive system is functioning as it should. That's not all—as aloe rehabilitates the ileum, it also delivers a very bioavailable form of B_{12}, making aloe an all-around B_{12} enhancer.

Aloe vera is antiviral, antibacterial, antifungal (including anti-mold), and anti-parasitic (including anti-worm). It is incredibly useful for killing off the pathogens that create colon cancer, stomach cancer, and rectal cancer, as well as eliminating *H. pylori* and supporting the pancreas. It also has the unique ability to stop the growth of polyps and reduce the growth of hemorrhoids. And if you're concerned that you've been exposed to radiation, turn to aloe—it has beta-carotene combined with lignins that remove radiation from the body.

CONDITIONS

If you have any of the following conditions, try bringing aloe vera into your life:

Irritable bowel syndrome (IBS), Crohn's disease, colitis, any other type of inflammatory bowel disease, colorectal cancer, stomach cancer, pancreatic cancer, Barrett's esophagus, small intestinal bacterial overgrowth (SIBO), stomach ulcers, urinary tract infections (UTIs) such as bladder infections and kidney infections, bacterial vaginosis, plantar fasciitis, Morton's neuroma, sciatica, Epstein-Barr virus (EBV)/mononucleosis, sunburn, bruises, cuts, scrapes, hemorrhoids, polyps, diverticulitis, acne, amyotrophic lateral sclerosis (ALS), eczema, psoriasis, all autoimmune diseases and disorders, *E. coli* infection, *C. difficile* infection, *H. pylori* infection, food poisoning, Barrett's esophagus, fatty liver, hiatal hernia, herpes simplex 1 (HSV-1), herpes simplex 2 (HSV-2), hepatitis A, hepatitis B, hepatitis C, hepatitis D, human papilloma virus (HPV), jaundice, liver disease, megacolon, MRSA, shingles, strep throat, PANDAS

SYMPTOMS

If you have any of the following symptoms, try bringing aloe vera into your life:

Inflammation, acid reflux, fatigue, constipation, bloating, anxiousness, dark under-eye circles, food allergies, abdominal distension, stomachaches, upset stomach, abdominal cramping, abdominal pressure, dysfunctional liver, stagnant liver, liver heat, pre-fatty liver, hormonal imbalances, appendix inflammation, intestinal inflammation, low hydrochloric acid

EMOTIONAL SUPPORT

Aloe is perfect for the person who's just gone through a major transition, such as moving to a new home, and is left feeling empty, nostalgic, alone, and a little lost. This wild food helps you feel at peace with your surroundings.

SPIRITUAL LESSON

Aloe has been in our world since ancient times, yet we often remain unfamiliar with all its uses. Becoming acquainted with aloe inspires us to take a fresh look at the world around us. What else in our lives could serve multiple purposes, if only we pioneer and explore its different facets?

TIPS

- Large, culinary aloe leaves are available from many grocery stores. Once you take one home, cut off a four-inch section from the middle of the leaf (discard the base and top of the leaf) and fillet it, removing the green skin and scooping out the clear, gelatinous flesh. You can then eat the flesh as is, blend it with water, or add it to smoothies.
- Even when aloe is from the grocery store or your own garden or windowsill, its wild nature is still intact.
- If you're dealing with dark under-eye circles, or if you're unhappy with the state of your skin and want to get back a youthful glow, consume fresh aloe on a daily basis. Aloe actually helps skin more from the inside out.
- For pets, aloe gel fresh from the plant (that is, not processed and combined with preservatives) is incredible for applying externally to scratch rashes, tick and flea bites, and areas of hair/fur loss.

ALOE COOLER

Makes 1 serving

In this beautiful drink, the flavors of orange juice and coconut water combine with aloe gel to create a delicious, bright cocktail. Enjoy this drink first thing in the morning, as it wakes up your whole body with hydration and a dose of citrus sunshine.

2 oranges

1 cup coconut water

¼ aloe leaf

Slice the oranges and juice them, which should yield about 1 cup of juice. Transfer the orange juice to a blender. Add the coconut water. Slice the aloe leaf open and scrape 2 tablespoons of the clear flesh into the blender with the orange-coconut mixture. Blend until smooth and foamy. Pour into a glass and enjoy right away.

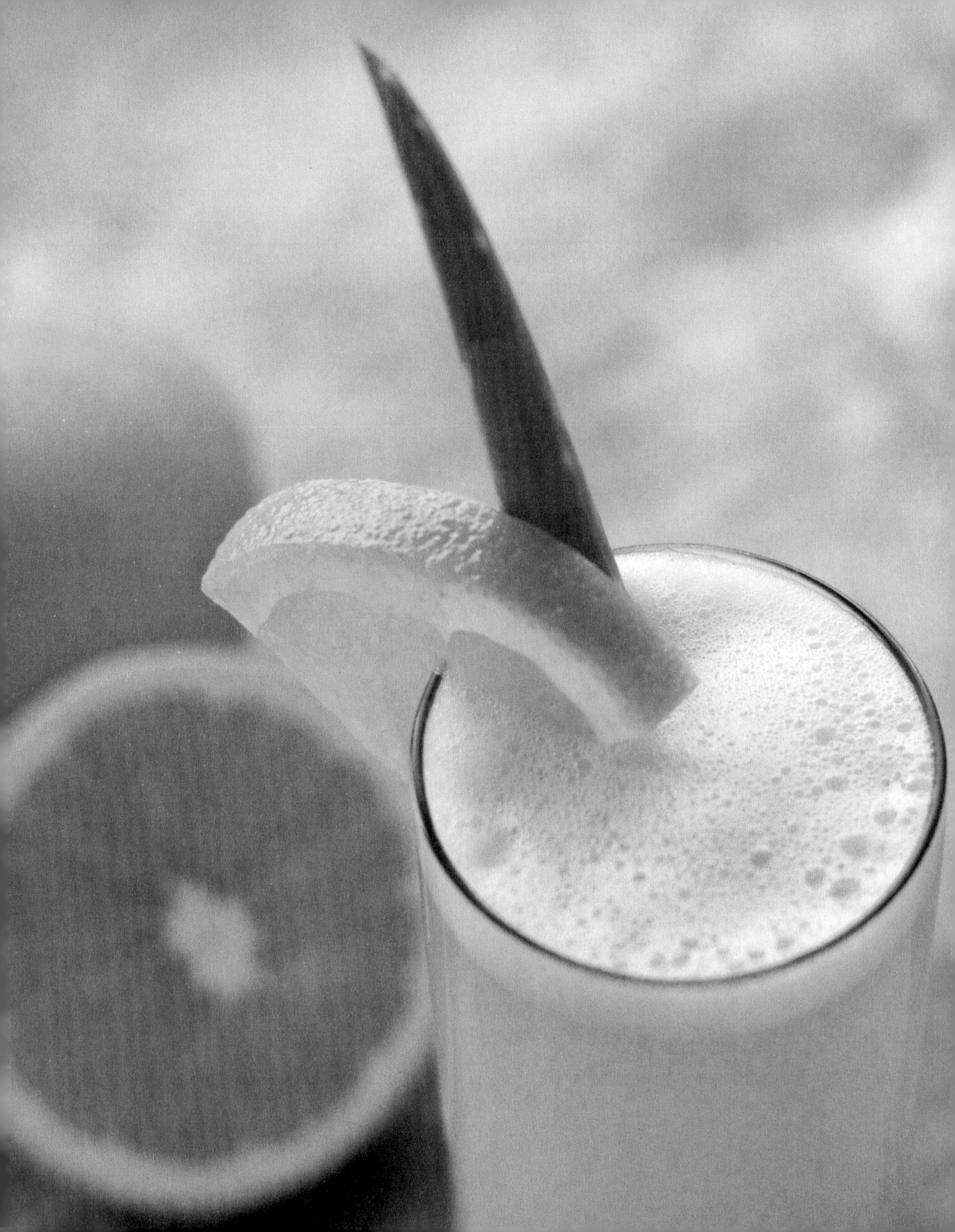

Atlantic Sea Vegetables

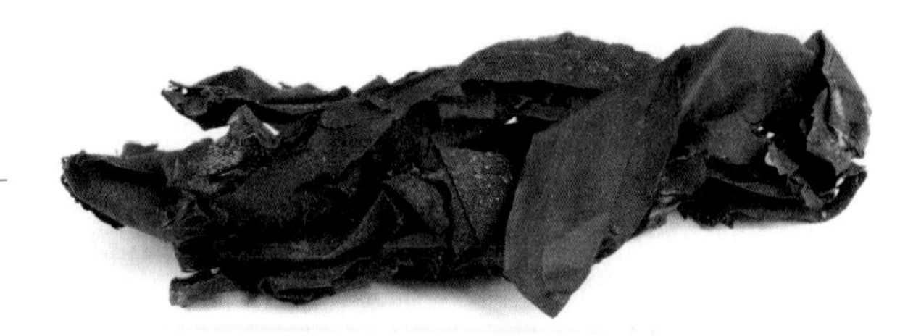

Sea vegetables (that is, seaweeds) from the Atlantic Ocean are extremely powerful at ridding the body of toxic heavy metals. One of the reasons certain heavy metals are so damaging to our bodies is that they're neuro-antagonists, which means they disrupt and diffuse electrical nerve impulses and cause nerves themselves to deteriorate. In the process, neurotransmitters burn out and blow out as if they were lightbulbs—which can result in anxiety and depression.

In the ocean, the sea vegetable's job is to absorb toxic heavy metals, radiation, and other toxins, and render them harmless. When dulse, bladderwrack, kelp, alaria, sea lettuce, laver, Irish moss, or rockweed encounter poisons in seawater, they continuously sponge them up, deactivate their destructive frequency, then release them back into the ocean, where the onetime pollutants can no longer cause additional harm because the seaweed has rendered them inactive.

When we consume sea vegetables, they bring that same miracle sponge-like ability to work for us—with a twist. Instead of releasing the inactivated toxic heavy metals, radiation, dioxins, pesticides such as DDT, and other poisons back into our systems once they've absorbed and disarmed them, the sea vegetables' bioactive phytochemicals lock onto the toxins and don't allow them to disperse while they're still in the body (because they're not in their natural environment). If sea vegetables have any traces of toxins when they enter our bodies, they stay bound to them, collect more along the way, and exit without passing along any contamination to us. They also serve as an emergency backup in the colon, grabbing onto and helping to ensure that any metals (carried along by other detox foods, such as cilantro) actually leave the body.

As they drive out poisons, the only thing that Atlantic sea vegetables leave behind in our bodies is nutrition—in particular, 50 health-promoting minerals. These minerals are ultra-bioavailable and assimilable, helping to nourish whichever body systems have deficiencies. As these minerals help bring you into balance, they also create electrolytes for stress assistance.

This wild food is helpful for any type of illness. It reconstructs damaged DNA, plus seaweed carries the grounding nature of the ocean—grounding that's transferred to us and can eliminate diseases of all kinds. Sea vegetables are particularly amazing for the endocrine system, because they absorb radiation that can in some cases be responsible for hypothyroidism (low activity of the thyroid) and disruption of the hypothalamus, pituitary gland, and pineal gland. Plus, sea vegetables are an excellent source of active iodine to protect the thyroid from radiation and viruses such as Epstein-Barr. Sea vegetables are also especially beneficial for the bones, tendons, ligaments, connective tissue, and teeth, and wonderful for addressing any toxic heavy metal–induced illness or symptom such as Alzheimer's, ADHD, epilepsy, or brain fog.

CONDITIONS

If you have any of the following conditions, try bringing Atlantic sea vegetables into your life:

Endocrine disorders, osteopenia, osteoporosis, bone fractures, injuries, epilepsy, Alzheimer's disease, dementia, migraines, Hashimoto's thyroiditis, Graves' disease, thyroid cancer, bipolar disorder, autism, attention-deficit/hyperactivity disorder (ADHD), radiation exposure (from dental work, medical X-rays, or cancer treatment), epilepsy, anemia, leukemia, bone cancer, brain cancer, bladder cancer, kidney cancer, liver cancer, lung cancer, stomach cancer, intestinal polyps, multiple chemical sensitivity (MCS), obsessive-compulsive disorder (OCD), depression, anxiety, Parkinson's disease, reproductive cancers (such as ovarian, uterine, and cervical), Asperger's, endometriosis, glaucoma, immune system deficiencies, seasonal affective disorder (SAD), lupus

SYMPTOMS

If you have any of the following symptoms, try bringing Atlantic sea vegetables into your life:

Brain fog; hypothyroid; memory loss; tics; spasms; grand mal seizures; blurry eyes; hair loss; balance issues; nausea; migraines; headaches; constipation; mineral deficiencies; all neurological symptoms (including tingles, numbness, spasms, twitches, nerve pain, and tightness of the chest); inflamed uterus, ovaries, and/or fallopian tubes; inflamed gallbladder, stomach, small intestine, and/or colon; Bell's palsy; outbursts of anger; sluggish liver; tremors

EMOTIONAL SUPPORT

For the person whose behavior is unpredictable—someone who frequently swings from up to down, from hot to cold—sea vegetables are an incredible tool. Often when somebody is hypersensitive, rocked easily, or emotionally unstable, she or he is ungrounded. Atlantic sea vegetables are the most grounding food possible. When we eat them, we get the energetic essence of going for a swim in the ocean, a very grounding activity.

SPIRITUAL LESSON

So often in life we absorb the worries, fears, and other stressful emotions of those around us. Left unchecked, these poisonous feelings can eat away at us and interfere with our well-being. Sea vegetables teach us the miraculous art of taking something that is energetically toxic and processing it in a way that disarms it and releases it back into the ether, so it can't harm anyone else.

TIPS

- To get more grounding from a meal, put a strip of kelp into your rice cooker, add a strip of it to a simmering pot of soup, or enjoy it with any other savory dish.
- For a supercharged toxin-removing elixir, put a handful of dulse into a smoothie made with wild blueberries, cilantro, spirulina, and barley grass juice powder.

NORI ROLLS WITH CREAMY AVOCADO DIPPING SAUCE

Makes 1 to 2 servings

These beautiful maki rolls are fun to make and have endless possibilities. Don't be afraid to get in the kitchen and start rolling your own. Fill them with the veggies below or come up with your own options. Just make sure to roll tightly, and they'll turn out great. Alongside the creamy avocado dipping sauce, they make the perfect lunch, snack, or light dinner.

4 carrots

3 zucchini

1 jicama, peeled

1 bunch scallions, ends trimmed

½ cup dulse pieces

8 nori sheets

FOR SAUCE:

1 avocado

1 lime, juiced

¼ cup cilantro

¼ jalapeño

½ medjool date

½ cup water

Slice the carrots, zucchini, and jicama into thin strips or "noodles" using a julienne peeler, spiralizer, or knife. Assemble the rolls by layering the carrots, zucchini, jicama, scallion, and dulse across the bottom of each nori sheet. Maintaining firm tension, roll up the nori sheet. Dip 1 finger in water and run it across the edge of the nori sheet to help the roll stick together. Slice into bite-size rolls, if desired.

For the sauce, blend all the remaining ingredients until smooth. Pour and enjoy!

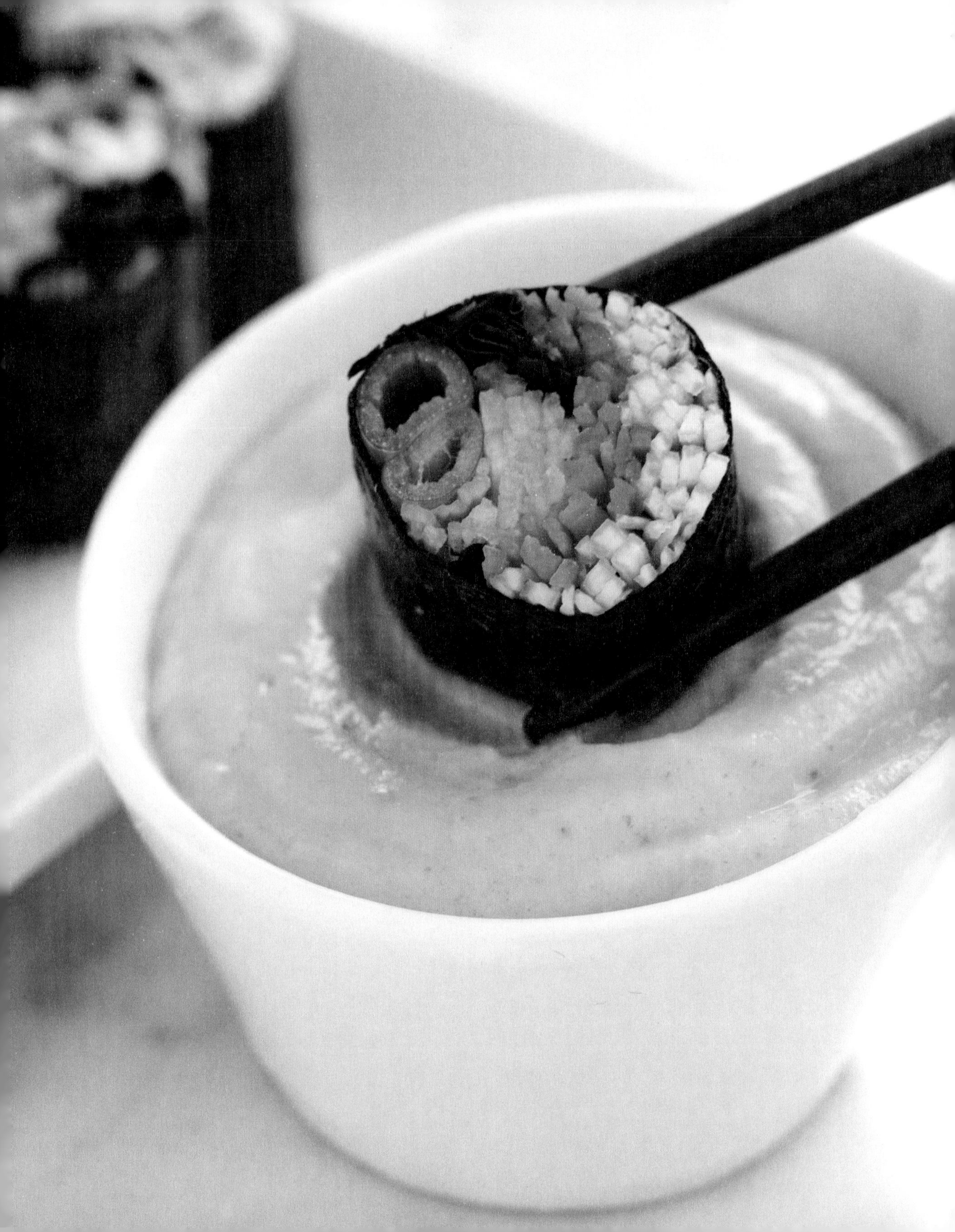

Burdock Root

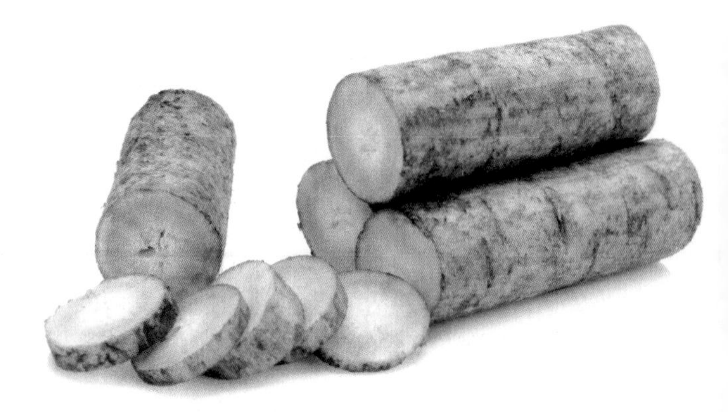

Burdock root is a force of nature to rehabilitate the liver. Burdock root has a grounding ability that comes from driving deep into the earth. When the liver is filled with viruses such as Epstein-Barr, shingles, HHV-6, and cytomegalovirus, or with unproductive bacteria, worms, fungi, or other pathogens, the liver loses its grounding, negative charge—because these pathogens operate on a positive charge that drains the organ. (For more on this concept of positive and negative charge, see "Garlic.") Fifty times more grounding than any other root vegetable, burdock reestablishes the liver's grounding mechanism, which in turn restrengthens and revitalizes the liver so it can push off pathogens.

Over time, if not attended to, the liver loses its sponge-like abilities and becomes dense and hard. Burdock's dense quality is exactly what's needed to soften a dense, stagnant liver. Phytochemicals in burdock also support the liver in reducing growth of cysts and adhesions and repairing scar tissue in the liver, plus its vigor at cleansing liver lobules is unmatched. Burdock also has the ability to detoxify the densest core of the liver, and to remove toxic hormones there that have come in from outside sources such as metals, plastics, herbicides, and fungicides, ultimately giving the liver a chance to breathe.

The nutrients in burdock root range from almost every trace mineral in the spectrum to traces of B vitamins, plus vitamins A, C, and K. This wild food also has a unique gift for cleansing the lymphatic system and the blood, enhancing white blood cells and killer cells to keep the lymph nodes strong so they can do their work of killing off pathogens and cancer cells. Plus the enzymes in burdock are highly active, and they work in combination with burdock's abundant amino acids as heavy metal detoxifiers.

CONDITIONS

If you have any of the following conditions, try bringing burdock root into your life:

Gout, liver disease, liver cancer, kidney stones, gallstones, lymphoma (including non-Hodgkin's), chronic infections, breast cancer, lung cancer, pleurisy, lupus, chronic fatigue syndrome (CFS), fibromyalgia, multiple sclerosis (MS), migraines, gum disease, acne, hepatitis C, adrenal fatigue, diabetes, bursitis, celiac disease, all autoimmune diseases and disorders, thyroid cancer, eczema, psoriasis, kidney infections, Lyme disease, worms, yeast infections

SYMPTOMS

If you have any of the following symptoms, try bringing burdock root into your life:

Scar tissue in the liver, liver adhesions, liver cysts, lesions in the liver, stagnant liver, sluggish liver, gallbladder spasms, food allergies, inflamed appendix, headaches, stomach pain, bloating, constipation, back pain, abdominal cramping, abdominal distension, accelerated aging, blood sugar imbalances, mineral deficiencies (including trace mineral deficiencies), myelin nerve damage, food sensitivities, sensations of humming or vibration in the body, blood toxicity, chemical sensitivities, digestive discomfort, enlarged spleen, inflammation, neuralgia, torn cartilage

EMOTIONAL SUPPORT

If you're looking to cleanse your body, mind, soul, and even the space around you from the ghosts of past experiences, bring burdock into your life for an emotional clearing.

SPIRITUAL LESSON

If you brush against a burdock plant that's gone to seed, you're likely to find later that you have burrs stuck to your socks, pants, shoelaces, sweater, hair . . . anything that those tiny hooks could attach themselves to. Burdock burrs stay with you for the length of your journey, until you're finally where you need to be. This is the burdock plant's method of preparing for the future—it sends out its seeds with any passerby, so that new plants can take root far and wide. Burdock teaches us to send along our own seeds of hope with each encounter, and to recognize the messages others have sent along with us to disseminate. As our loved ones and acquaintances navigate life, what kernels can we give them to one day plant in the world? And what seeds have we been given to disperse?

TIPS

- After a massage, drink burdock root tea or dine on burdock root soup to enhance lymphatic drainage.
- Try juicing fresh burdock root into your favorite fresh vegetable juice. It has a sweet, earthy taste that combines well with other flavors, and drinking it freshly juiced gets its minerals directly into your system without delay.
- If you like munching on carrots, try preparing burdock root in the same way: peel it with a carrot peeler, then cut it into sticks for snacking. Its antimicrobial properties and fibrous nature help clean the teeth, keep the mouth free of unproductive bacteria, and stave off gum disease.
- Offer a cup of burdock root tea to a friend who you think might be dealing with emotional or physical toxins and in need of some cleansing.

BURDOCK SOUP

Makes 2 to 4 servings

This soup is perfect for quiet afternoons and even early mornings. It's warm and clean and so simple to prepare. It feels like a gentle hug for your whole body. Make a big batch at the start of the week, and enjoy it all week long. Sip it out of a mug or eat it out of a big bowl—enjoy it as a gift to your body and soul.

2 cups sliced burdock root
2 cups sliced carrots
2 cups sliced mushrooms
2 cups sliced bok choy
1 yellow onion, diced
1 tablespoon minced garlic
1 tablespoon grated ginger
½ teaspoon sea salt

Place all the ingredients in a large pot. Cover with water and bring to a boil. Reduce heat and keep at a rapid simmer for 30 to 40 minutes, until vegetables are tender.

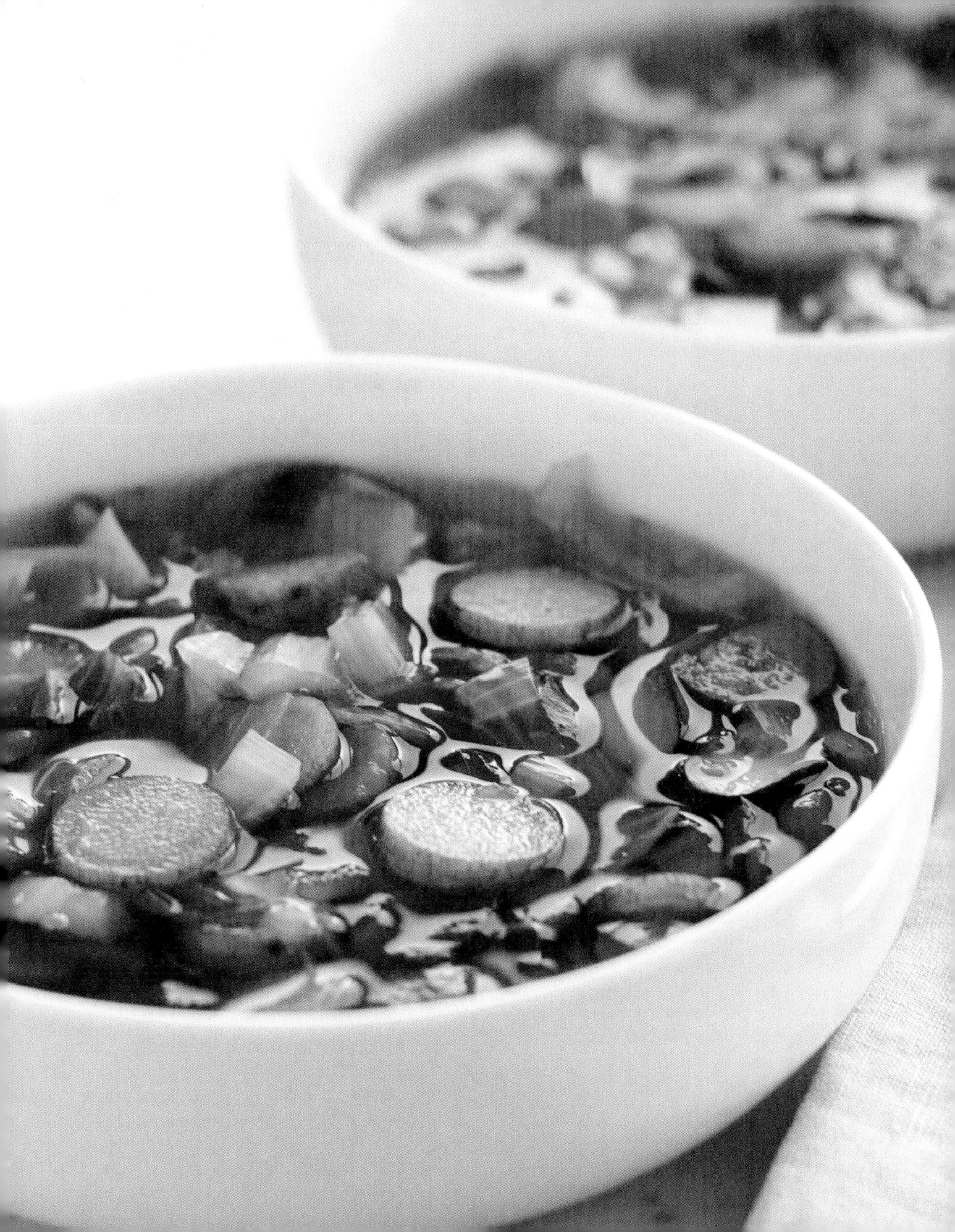

Chaga Mushroom

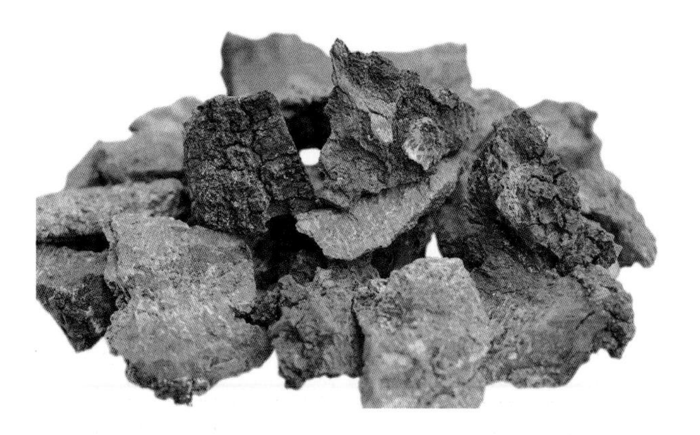

Chaga mushroom is all about building immunity—something we all want in our lives. Chaga (not technically a mushroom but rather pre-mushroom growth) possesses immune-system-enhancing nutrients that revitalize white blood cell count by increasing the production of lymphocytes, monocytes, neutrophils, basophils, and eosinophils, so that your body can battle invaders such as toxins, viruses, and bacteria, as well as fungi such as yeast and mold. This incredible wild food also strengthens red blood cells and bone marrow, balances blood platelets, and staves off cytokine storms, which are the result of the body overreacting to a pathogen or toxin. This type of reaction occurs because the immune system is racing to die out a fire. As when putting out a real fire, attending to the emergency can come at a cost; cytokine storms can result in blood vessels expanding (which can lead to hemorrhaging), hives, rashes, and fever. With chaga on your side, the body is much better equipped to deal with pathogens and toxins.

Chaga is one of the most medicinal tools and overall tonics of the century. The phytochemicals in chaga are wonderful for fighting cancer, regulating blood sugar, boosting the adrenals while regulating the rest of the endocrine system, breaking down and dissolving biofilm (that is, a jelly-like substance that's a by-product of certain viruses and fungi; more on this in "Rose Hips"), and destroying unproductive fungus in the intestinal tract. Speaking of which, there's a trending misconception that mushrooms and other edible fungi are bad for you, because people fear that ingesting fungus results in fungal overgrowth in the body. This couldn't be further from the truth. Mushrooms are some of the best fighters of unproductive fungus that we have.

CONDITIONS

If you have any of the following conditions, try bringing chaga into your life:

Bladder cancer, bone cancer, breast cancer, liver cancer, leukemia, ovarian cancer, prostate cancer, autoimmune diseases and disorders, Lyme disease, lupus, multiple sclerosis (MS), amyotrophic lateral sclerosis (ALS), carpal tunnel syndrome, tendonitis, bursitis, sciatica, fibromyalgia, chronic fatigue syndrome (CFS), small intestinal bacterial overgrowth (SIBO), hypertension, fatty liver, pneumonia, psoriasis, eczema, Graves' disease, immune system deficiencies, human immunodeficiency virus (HIV), Hashimoto's thyroiditis, Epstein-Barr virus (EBV)/mononucleosis, shingles, adrenal fatigue, mold exposure, migraines, anemia, multiple chemical sensitivity (MCS), electromagnetic hypersensitivity (EHS), celiac disease, gum infections, rosacea, thrush, vaginal strep

SYMPTOMS

If you have any of the following symptoms, try bringing chaga into your life:

Inflammation, shoulder pain, frozen shoulder, neck pain, back pain, headaches, head pain, pre-fatty liver, iron deficiency, joint pain, muscle fatigue, Bell's palsy, sluggish liver, stagnant liver, fever, rashes, hives, fingernail and toenail fungus, body fungus, hypothyroid, all neurological symptoms (including tingles, numbness, spasms, twitches, nerve pain, and tightness of the chest), jaw pain, body stiffness, bruising, dark under-eye circles, eye floaters, foot pain, joint inflammation, liver heat, hyperthyroid, swelling, fluid retention, neuralgia, poor circulation, sore throat

EMOTIONAL SUPPORT

For those who feel like they're missing out on something, who feel trapped in their life's direction, emotionally stagnant and numb, and can't make decisions—even when there's only one decision to make and they don't like the choice they've been handed—chaga is an invaluable tool. Bring it into your life when you need help envisioning what you want for the future, and how to make it happen.

SPIRITUAL LESSON

Chaga lives in harmony with the trees it grows on. Once it takes up residence on a tree, it grows very slowly so as not to disrupt its host. Chaga offers strength to its tree during times of storm and deep freeze, because it provides a living frequency of loyalty. Chaga possesses patience and intelligence of survival, knowing that if its host tree goes down, it does too. We can all learn about loyalty from this wild food. If you believe in someone or something, chaga teaches not to let go. To help our loved ones survive and thrive, we must do the same. When a situation warrants it, go all in and meditate on chaga's nature to support you. Like the chaga-tree relationship, we must all stay strong for each other—and for the greater good.

(If you've heard that chaga has a reputation for harming its host tree, note that irresponsible harvesting of chaga—not the chaga itself—is what so often damages the tree, ultimately taking both down.)

TIPS

- Look for chaga that's been ground into a very fine powder. This is the best form for nutrient absorption. You can use chaga powder in smoothies, or make a tea with it.
- To make chaga mushroom tea, stir the powder into hot water until it dissolves. For best results, add raw honey—this add-in will help drive the medicinal properties of the chaga deeper into hard-to-reach places, enhancing body system functions. Chaga-honey tea makes an excellent afternoon pick-me-up.
- Respect chaga. Before consuming it, honor its loyalty and the stoic nature it upholds. This will enhance your body's reception of its immune-enhancing phytochemicals.

CHAGA TEA LATTE

Makes 2 cups

This warm and creamy variation of chaga tea is just the thing when you need both strength and comfort. As you enjoy it, think about all that it's doing for your body as chaga helps you live to your full potential.

2 teaspoons chaga powder
½ teaspoon cinnamon
1 teaspoon raw honey
⅛ to ¼ cup coconut milk

Boil 2 cups of water. Divide the chaga powder and cinnamon evenly between 2 tea cups; pour 1 cup of hot water into each. Stir in the honey, using more if desired. Stir the coconut milk into each cup or use a frother to create coconut foam on top.

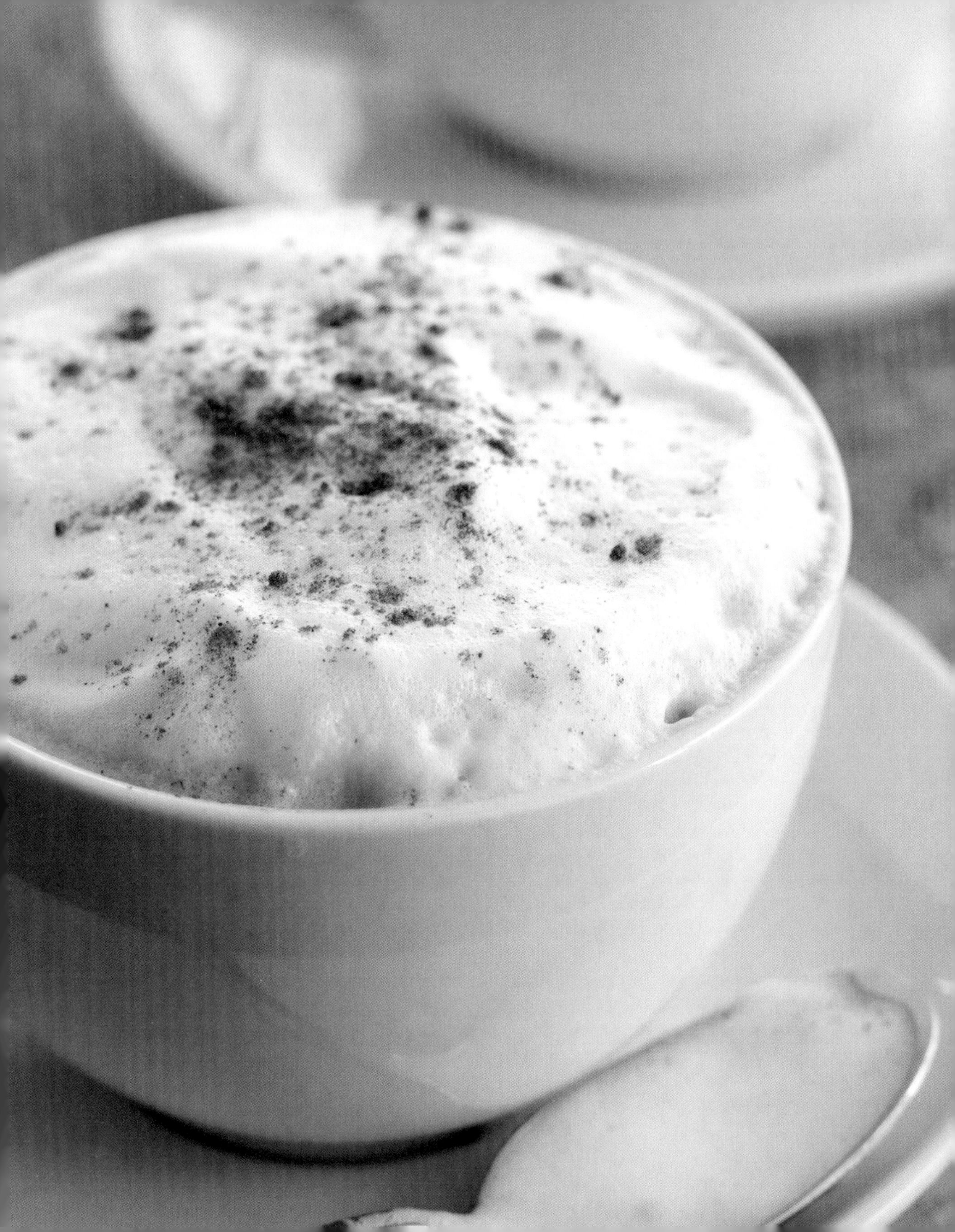

Coconut

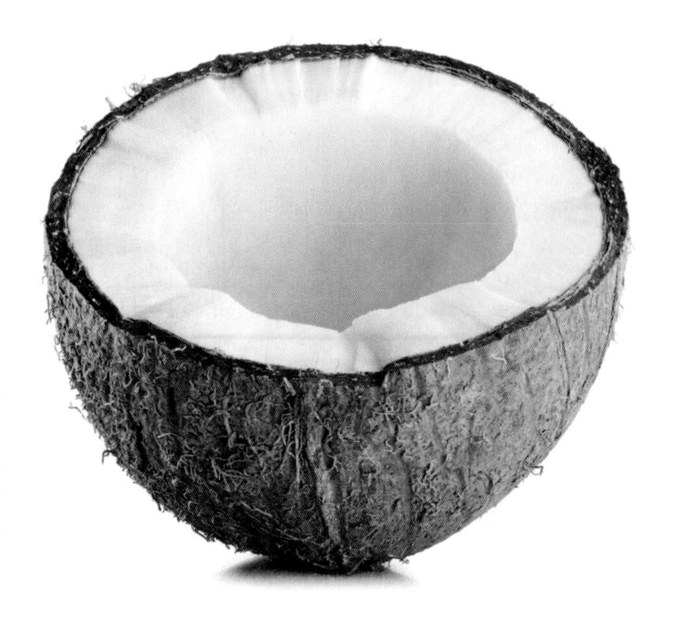

Coconut, especially in the form of coconut water and coconut oil, has enjoyed some time in the sun in recent years. We hear stories about how coconut water was used as IV fluid for wounded soldiers in World War II, and about health miracles people have experienced by incorporating coconut oil into their diets. Everywhere you turn, it seems, there's a positive claim about coconut—and rightfully so.

Now let's get down to what hasn't yet been discovered: that coconut enhances the power of anything it touches. It has an incredible reach. When combined with any healing food, coconut gets in touch with those benefits and supercharges them. For example, if you add coconut water to a smoothie with parsley, that coconut water increases the parsley's ability to remove unproductive acids from your body by 50 percent and dramatically improves the effects of parsley's already beneficial trace minerals. Or if you add coconut meat to a salad, everything else in the salad—cucumbers, lettuce, tomato, spinach, anything that has healing properties—becomes more nutritious and life-changing. Coconut drives a food to fulfill its highest purpose by igniting amino acids, vitamins, and other nutrients, and in doing so, nourishes you so you can perform your life's purpose and then some—your purpose-plus.

Though you wouldn't look at a coconut palm tree and think it has much in common with a human, we're more connected to these plants than you may realize. For one, as that IV story teaches us, coconut water is remarkably similar to human blood. Secondly, coconut palms are tropical—they need warmth. Though humans are scattered all over the globe, we really are tropical beings at our origins. You won't find someone surviving in a snowy climate without protective body gear and some source of heat. Coconut puts us in touch with that foundational essence of who we are.

Coconut water provides vital glucose and critical mineral salts, including potassium and sodium, to the bloodstream. This is a fundamental component of our neurotransmitter chemical production. If we don't have the neurotransmitter chemicals we need, it can lead to insomnia, neurological sleep apnea, and other sleep disturbances. The best thing you can do to avoid these issues is to drink coconut water—it is the best tool of all time for neurotransmitter support.

For those who struggle with infertility or other disorders of the reproductive system, take note that coconut water's trace minerals and electrolytes nourish your reproductive tissue. Coconut water is also incredibly important for people with hypoglycemia and other blood sugar disorders, including diabetes. It's critical for people with over- or underactive adrenals. It's good for every single brain and neurological disorder. Coconut water can greatly benefit people with Parkinson's, and it's also a must for those with Alzheimer's or other forms of dementia. It's incredible for helping to prevent the onset of seizures and offers special support for eye conditions.

Coconut meat (and the oil derived from it) is antipathogenic due to its lauric acid content combined with other antioxidants present in it, so turn to coconut when you're in need of an antibacterial and antiviral food. When coconut drops from the stomach into the intestinal tract, it kills off any pathogen it touches. Plus, its medium-chain fatty acids break loose other fats and aid in pushing them out of the body.

CONDITIONS

If you have any of the following conditions, try bringing coconut into your life:

Postural tachycardia syndrome (POTS); Addison's disease; Raynaud's syndrome; adrenal fatigue; hypoglycemia; diabetes; thyroid cancer; tachycardia; atrial fibrillation; depression; anxiety; bipolar disorder; Asperger's syndrome; insomnia; seizure disorders; optic nerve conditions; glaucoma; migraines; Parkinson's disease; Alzheimer's disease; dementia; Epstein-Barr virus (EBV)/mononucleosis; HHV-6; HHV-7; HHV-8; HHV-9; the undiscovered HHV-10, HHV-11, and HHV-12; thyroid disease; shingles; attention-deficit/hyperactivity disorder (ADHD); autism; thyroid nodules; urinary tract infections (UTIs); infertility; low reproductive system battery; sciatica; bacterial pneumonia; Lyme disease; mycoplasma; *Chlamydia pneumoniae*; parasites; carpal tunnel syndrome; depression; anxiety; hypertension; human papilloma virus (HPV); norovirus; pancreatitis; small intestinal bacterial overgrowth (SIBO); sunburn

SYMPTOMS

If you have any of the following symptoms, try bringing coconut into your life:

Heart palpitations, grand mal seizures, arrhythmia, anxiousness, brain fog, blurry eyes, Bell's palsy, memory loss, weight gain, food allergies, frozen shoulder, jaw pain, neuralgia, all neurological symptoms (including tingles, numbness, spasms, twitches, nerve pain, and tightness of the chest), back pain, blurry eyes, confusion, chemical sensitivities, mineral deficiencies, fatigue, listlessness, malaise, dehydration, headaches, difficulty swallowing, difficulty breathing, connective tissue inflammation, ear pain, foot pain, high blood pressure, sleep disturbances, low platelet counts, nervousness, ringing or buzzing in the ears, urinary urgency

EMOTIONAL SUPPORT

Do you know anyone who travels through life reacting to everything with the response, "But how does this affect me?" If so, offer her or him coconut in any form. Coconut is for that person who's narcissistic, self-consumed, and completely saturated in her or his singular worldview. Coconut opens the emotional channel for someone to let go of the self-addiction and weigh others' needs and values alongside her or his own.

SPIRITUAL LESSON

Coconut palms are quick to drop their coconuts in a storm. This comes from the trees' wisdom of survival—they can either hold onto the coconuts and risk toppling as the winds whip through, or they can let go of them, and make themselves less vulnerable. It's a lesson we would all do well to take to heart. When life gets stormy, we sometimes have to let go of what's most precious to us, and it can feel like the end of the world. Coconut trees teach us that in the end, the sun comes back out, and what matters most is that you're okay.

TIPS

- When buying coconut water, only get it if it's clear or very slightly tinged with pink. It's a misconception that deep pink or reddish coconut water is beneficial—in fact, this is a sign that it's rapidly oxidizing and going bad. Also avoid any coconut water that contains natural flavors, citric acid, or sweeteners such as agave nectar or refined cane sugar.
- If you're able to get ahold of some young, green coconuts, try to consume them over the course of a few days. If they sit too long without refrigeration, they're liable to pop, and you'll end up with coconut water on your walls and ceiling.
- If you don't have access to fresh coconuts, some of the best forms to seek out include jarred coconut butter or frozen young coconut meat to use with dishes such as salads. For cooking, use coconut oil.
- Bring coconut into your life if you have a fear of swimming or open water. Coconut trees often grow on the coast, leaning over the water's edge and dropping their coconuts into the ocean. Coconuts are excellent swimmers; they stay buoyant for long stretches of time and miles upon miles of open sea, taking on knowledge of the ocean as they float, until they eventually reach a new shore where they can take root. When you consume coconut, you inherit this natural instinct for life on the water, which helps to strengthen you as it alleviates your aquatic anxiety.
- Coconut in the evening is ideal for those who have trouble sleeping during a full moon. The coconut provides extra mineral salts and electrolytes for your neurotransmitters and electrical impulses; this helps defend you from the full moon's subtle gravitational pull.

YELLOW COCONUT CURRY

Makes 6 to 8 servings

This rich, complex curry is the perfect dinner for meals around the table with family and friends. The recipe makes a big batch, so you'll have enough for a hungry crew, or for leftovers to be eaten throughout the week. Yellow curry is mild and warming, with the mingled flavors of ginger, garlic, and turmeric simmered in coconut milk and loaded with potatoes, carrots, and squash. This dish will become a favorite to return to over and over again.

1 small kabocha squash
8 potatoes
8 carrots
1 tablespoon coconut oil
3 onions, diced
8 garlic cloves, minced
2 tablespoons grated ginger
2 tablespoons yellow curry powder
3 cups coconut milk
2 teaspoons honey
1½ teaspoons salt
½ cup cilantro
1 lime
Red pepper (optional)

Place the kabocha squash in a large pot and cover with water. Bring to a boil and cook for 5 to 7 minutes, until squash softens slightly. Drain and set aside to cool. Roughly dice the potatoes and carrots and set aside. When the squash is cool enough to handle, slice it in half and remove the seeds. Roughly dice the squash and return to the pot along with the carrots and potatoes. Add 2 inches of water to the pot and bring to a boil. Cover to steam, stirring occasionally. Add more water if needed. Steam until the vegetables are just cooked through.

For the curry, warm the coconut oil in a large pot. Add the onions and sauté over high heat until they are soft and fragrant (about 5 minutes). If needed, add water to prevent sticking. Add the garlic, ginger, and curry powder to the onions, stirring frequently for 1 minute. Add the coconut milk, honey, and salt, and continue stirring. Add the vegetables and bring to a low simmer. Simmer for 10 to 15 minutes, until vegetables are tender. Serve the curry topped with cilantro, lime juice, and red pepper, if desired.

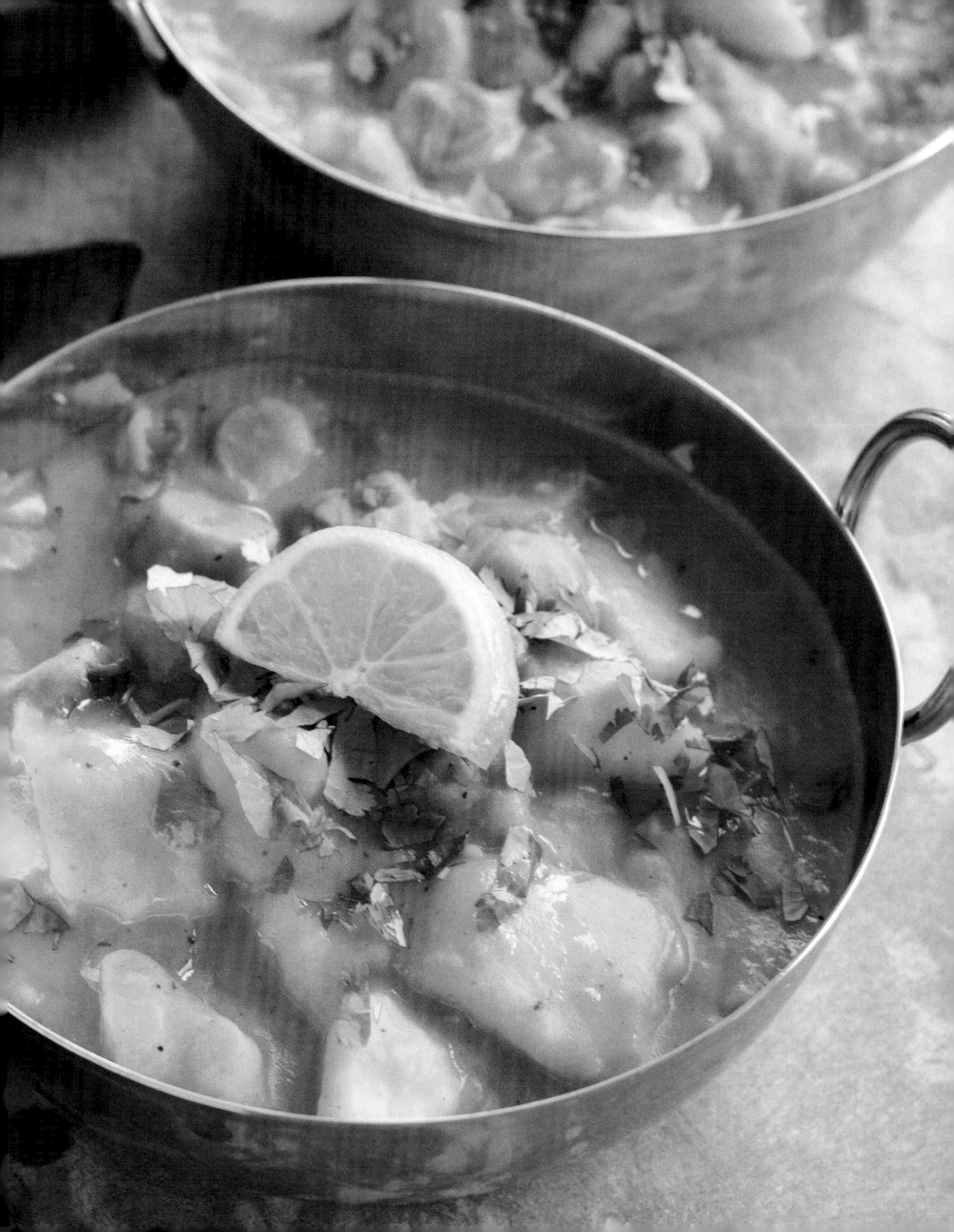

Dandelion

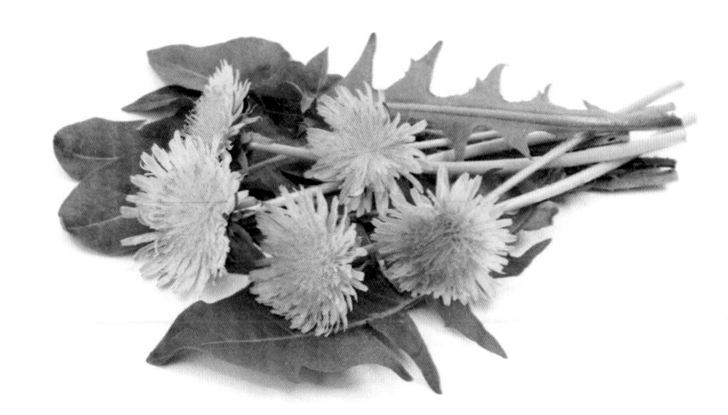

Dandelions come up in the early spring, just when our bodies are due for a spring cleaning. When consumed, the dandelion's defining characteristic is bitterness, and this is the very feature that lends it restorative properties. That bitterness is medicine derived from plant acids and healing alkaloids. Dandelions shake you out of hibernation, getting your blood pumping and your organs cleaning house from radiation, toxic heavy metals, DDT, and other poisons.

What makes the dandelion unique is that every part of the plant can be used: root, leaves, flower, and even stem. Each bit has a different degree of bitterness, and this corresponds with areas of the body that need different sorts of cleansing. To start with, the flowers (which have some bitterness yet are edging on slightly sweet) cleanse the hollow organs such as the stomach and intestinal tract, gallbladder, bladder, lungs, uterus, and heart.

Then there are the leaves. Phytochemicals in dandelion leaves purify blood and also help bring it to hard-to-reach places, so the leaves are a must for circulatory issues such as poor circulation. The leaves' bitterness is also geared to squeeze toxins out of the lymphatic system, making them ideal for addressing non-Hodgkin's lymphoma, swollen lymph nodes, and edema.

When you get to the stem of the dandelion, which is even more bitter than the flower and leaves, now you're in the world of cleansing the dense organs such as the spleen, liver, and brain—for example, by pushing out bile that's no longer useful. I've seen dandelion greens, eaten consistently, prevent splenectomies.

And when you get to the dandelion root, you're detoxifying even deeper into those dense organs. This is the bitterest part of the plant, and it forces the organs to purge on the deepest level for an intensified purification. When it comes to detoxing, dandelion root is not for the faint of heart.

Dandelion is not just a cleansing herb. It's like a housekeeping service at a fancy hotel that, after tidying up and gathering the trash, leaves a mint behind on your pillow. Dandelion's parting gift is better than candy, though—it leaves behind vital nutrients such as vitamin A, B vitamins, manganese, iodine, calcium, iron, magnesium, selenium, silica, and chlorophyll that give you energy and help your body stave off disease. Dandelion is a preventative for virtually any illness, and is especially great for the prostate.

CONDITIONS

If you have any of the following conditions, try bringing dandelion into your life:

Lymphoma (including non-Hodgkin's), edema, prostatitis, skin cancers, ringworm, rosacea, obesity, kidney stones, cirrhosis of the liver, hepatitis C, acne, amyotrophic lateral sclerosis (ALS), migraines, urinary tract infections (UTIs), blood disorders, blood cell disease, digestive disorders, fatty liver, celiac disease, kidney disease

SYMPTOMS

If you have any of the following symptoms, try bringing dandelion into your life:

Poor circulation; fluid retention; swollen lymph nodes; weight gain; hives; sluggish liver; stagnant liver; abdominal distension; abdominal pain; acid reflux; blood toxicity; congestion; constipation; liver cysts; digestive discomfort; dysfunctional liver; enlarged spleen; excess mucus; pre-fatty liver; fluid retention; high blood pressure; inflamed appendix; inflamed gallbladder, stomach, small intestine, and/or colon; histamine reactions; weak digestion

EMOTIONAL SUPPORT

We sometimes feel like we're missing pieces of ourselves, or our emotions cause us to act out and say things that we later regret and are not even sure why we mentioned in the first place. This is often because we're out of joint; our soul, spirit, and body are not working as one. For the person who wants to feel whole, dandelion is the perfect unifier, because it is truly all one with itself.

SPIRITUAL LESSON

So often, we get hung up on proving ourselves by being first, and it affects our sense of self-worth. This overachiever mentality starts at an early age: first in line, first to raise your hand, first to hand in an assignment, first one on the bus. Some people feel like they'll miss out forever on recognition and opportunity if they don't prove themselves in this way.

After dandelions' spring growth has died down in the heat of the summer, the plants aren't finished for the year—dandelions frequently reappear in fall. If you're someone who feels incomplete or less-than if you aren't the first on the scene, this is an important lesson to take to heart. Dandelions come back around again—and in this way teach us that we can find contentment and solace in not always being first, because there are new chances around the bend.

TIPS

- If you have an aversion to dandelion's bitter flavor, try roasted dandelion root tea. It's a wonderful detoxifying tonic, and the roasting takes the edge off the bitterness.
- Dandelion flowers are wonderful for making a cold tea. Pick fresh blooms and let them steep in cold water overnight to release their minerals, vitamins, and phytonutrients. To sweeten, add raw honey. This makes a delightful and powerfully invigorating drink.
- Any opportunity you get, pluck a dandelion leaf in the wild (for instance, from your pesticide-free lawn or on a hike) and eat it raw. Wild dandelion leaves grow with a fuzz that, while generally unnoticeable to us, is like a mecca for beneficial microorganisms such as elevated biotics. In fact, wild dandelion greens have one of the highest concentrations of elevated biotics available.
- If you don't have access to fresh dandelions, don't shy away from the dandelion greens you can find at the health food store—these are still wildly beneficial for your body and mind.
- Try the old pastime of blowing seeds off the head of a dandelion that's moved past flowering. This is a real and profound meditation.

DANDELION GREEN JUICE

Makes 1 to 2 servings

Dandelion greens' strong taste is tempered perfectly in this mild green citrus juice. Enjoy this refreshing drink as the perfect way to make dandelion greens a part of your day.

1 head of celery, stalks separated

2 cucumbers

2 medium oranges, peeled

10 dandelion leaves (with stems if you have them)

Run all the ingredients through a high-speed juicer. Add more dandelion according to taste. Pour into a glass and enjoy!

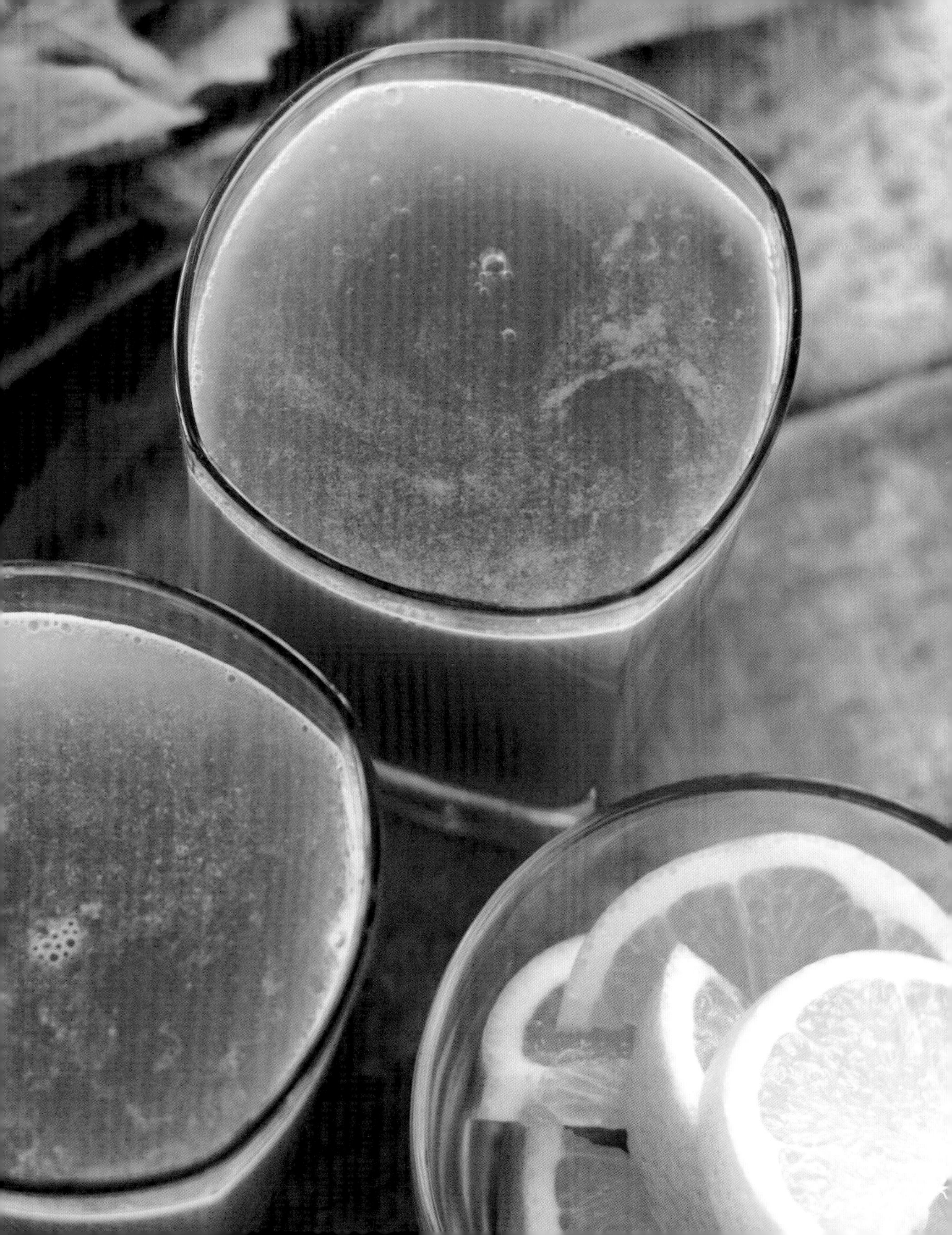

Nettle Leaf

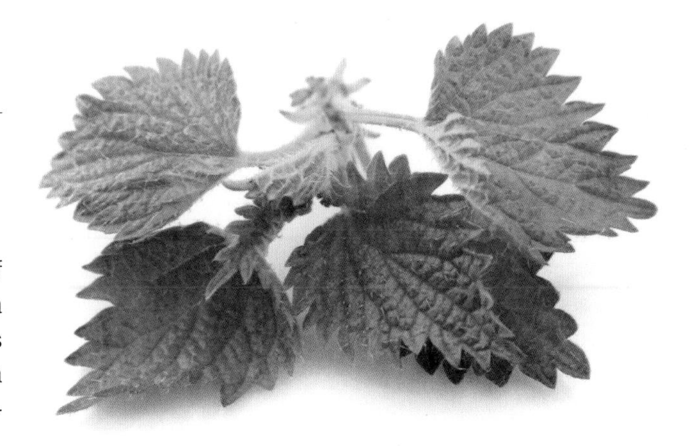

While you're not likely to find nettle leaf listed elsewhere as an adaptogenic herb, it is a star adaptogen, ideal for supporting our bodies through periods of stress. Nettle leaf contains a vast ocean of more than 700 undiscovered phytochemicals. It is life-giving and life-lengthening, an amazing anti-inflammatory for tired organs, and contains healing alkaloids yet to be discovered through scientific research.

In women's health, the ovaries get a lot of attention for producing the reproductive hormones. This means that when a test shows that a woman's hormone levels are deficient, health-care professionals tend to blame the reproductive system, which sometimes results in a prescription for unnecessary hormone replacement. In truth, the adrenal glands share the job equally of producing estrogen, progesterone, and testosterone in women. Low hormone test results often mean that the adrenals are either overactive (and therefore the excess adrenaline's corrosive nature is interfering with accurate readings) or underactive (and therefore they're not keeping up with production of sex hormones). The only way you can get an accurate reading from a hormone test of how the reproductive organs are doing is if the adrenals are perfectly healthy and balanced. So many women in their 20s and 30s are being told they've entered perimenopause, when the real cause of their suffering is adrenal fatigue. In countless cases where a woman's reproductive system is considered the problem, it's really the adrenals that need help—which is where nettle leaf comes in.

This anti-radiation wild food is amazing for pampering the adrenal glands and other members of the endocrine system that are overburdened, overworked, and overfatigued. And since the ovaries are part of the endocrine system, nettle is a win-win—it helps address multiple sources of hormone disruption at once. Nettle leaf is the ultimate reproductive herb of all time, especially for women. It enhances egg production by supporting the follicle-stimulating hormone that's integral to producing an ovum, and also rids the body of toxic estrogens that have entered from outside sources such as plastics and pesticides.

Rich with bone-building and bone-protecting herbs such as silica, nettle leaf also has more than 40 trace minerals in their most bioactive, bioavailable, and assimilable states. All of this, plus nettle is a potent pain reliever that enhances our ability to thrive.

CONDITIONS

If you have any of the following conditions, try bringing nettle leaf into your life:

Urinary tract infections (UTIs) such as bladder infections and kidney infections, interstitial cystitis, reproductive cancers, ovarian cancer, cervical cancer, uterine cancer, Epstein-Barr virus (EBV)/mononucleosis, rheumatoid arthritis (RA), shingles, posttraumatic stress disorder (PTSD), laryngitis, low reproductive system battery, acne, eczema, psoriasis, infertility, all autoimmune diseases and disorders, alopecia, anemia, anorexia, anxiety, depression, bladder prolapse, breast cancer, edema, endocrine system disorders, polycystic ovarian syndrome (PCOS), vaginal strep

SYMPTOMS

If you have any of the following symptoms, try bringing nettle leaf into your life:

Underactive/overactive adrenals, adrenal hormone imbalance, anxiousness, inflammation, reproductive hormonal imbalances, vaginal discharge, vaginal itching, vaginal burning, menstrual pain, menstrual cramping, premenstrual syndrome (PMS) symptoms, rashes, headaches, food allergies, menopause symptoms, abdominal cramping, accelerated aging, scar tissue, bloating, cold hands and feet, swelling, incontinence, irregular menstruation, low cortisol, mood swings, moodiness

EMOTIONAL SUPPORT

Nettle leaf is a wonderful centering herb for anyone who is highly distractible and scattered.

SPIRITUAL LESSON

When nettle first starts to sprout in the spring, it just seems like another bit of new growth in the garden bed or field—we tend to appreciate the bit of greenery and not think much more of it. Then suddenly, nettle shoots up, fills out, and makes its presence known. When we're not being mindful, it announces itself with a little sting when we brush against it. People who've had painful encounters like these tend to identify nettle as a weed, and that first nettle spotting of the season comes with a bit of dread. For those who've learned to approach nettle with respect, though, and who are tuned in to its many benefits, there's a little thrill that goes with seeing a new nettle plant take off—it's like reuniting with a long lost friend. Nettle teaches us to keep our eyes out for these sparks of gratitude everywhere. What else in your life have you treated with disregard, when really it's just a matter of learning to be open to it, work with it, and appreciate its true nature?

TIPS

- Even in its dried form, nettle resonates with a cycle of potency. Drink nettle leaf tea in the afternoon for its effects to be most powerful.
- For mosquito and other bug bites, scrapes, and minor burns, soak a cloth with nettle leaf tea, and apply the tea-soaked cloth to the area.
- Drink nettle tea prior to meditation to make the experience more centering.

NETTLE TEA WITH MINT AND GINGER

Makes 3 to 6 cups

Nettle's adaptogenic qualities help us get in touch with our intuition. As you sip this invigorating tea, reflect on your intuitive abilities—how they've served you in the past and what they're telling you right now.

2 tablespoons nettle leaf

2 tablespoons minced fresh mint

2 teaspoons grated ginger

Mix all the ingredients together in a small bowl. Boil 4 cups of water. For each serving of tea, use 1 teaspoon of the tea blend per 1 cup of hot water.* Steep for 5 minutes or more.

*If a stronger, more medicinal tea is desired, use 2 teaspoons or up to 1 tablespoon of the tea blend per serving.

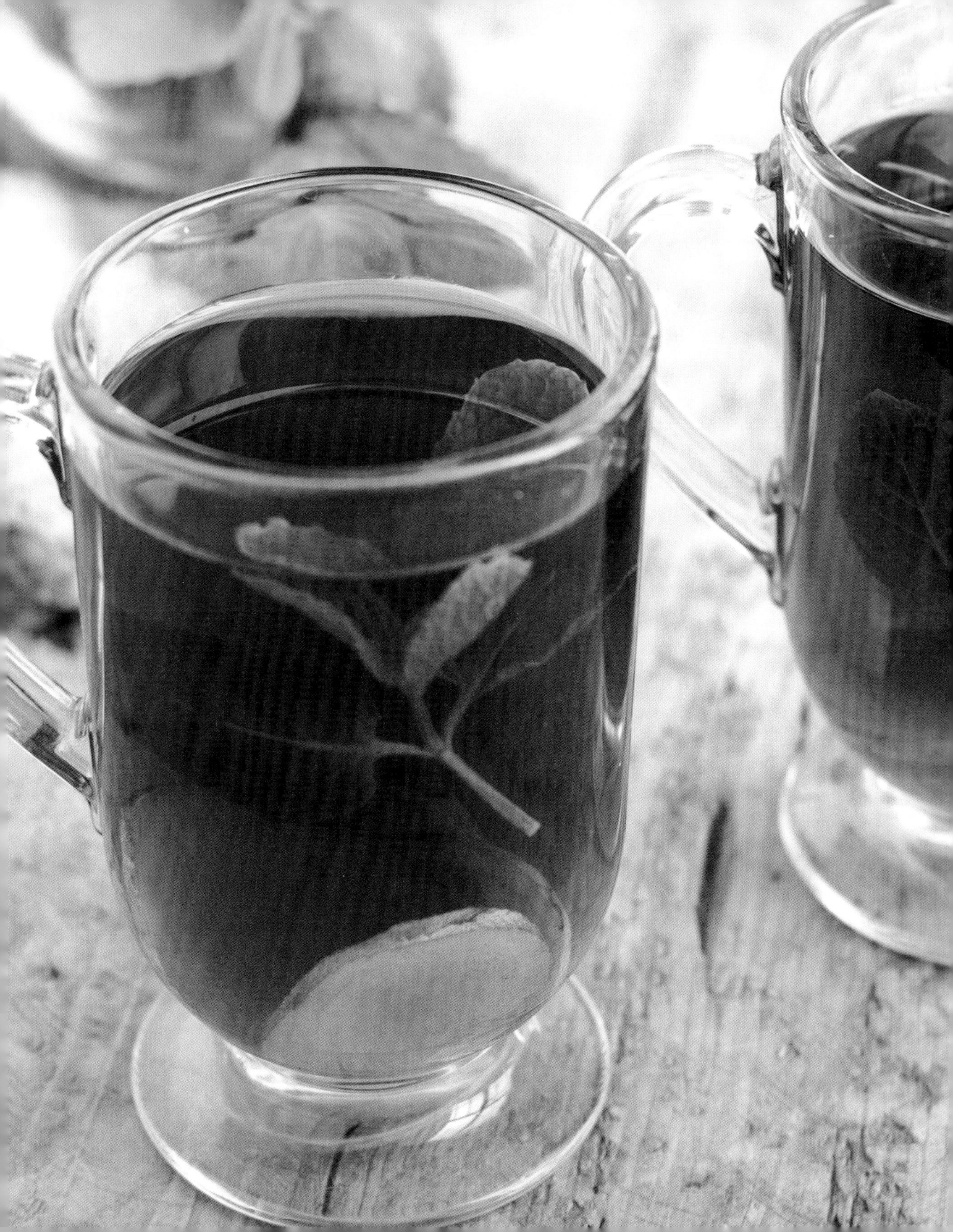

Raw Honey

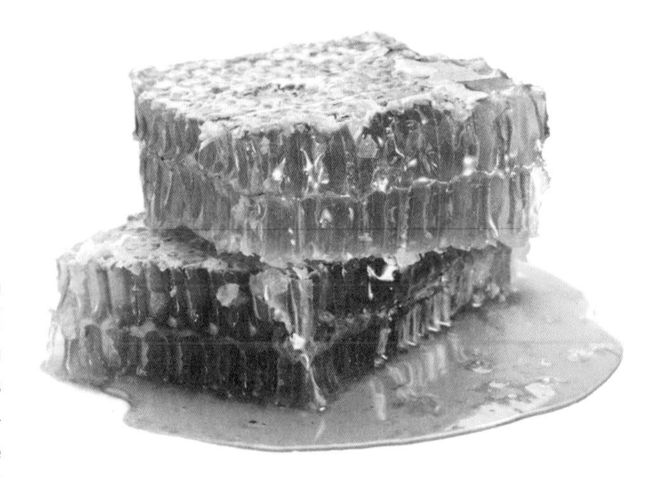

If you feel out of touch with miracles, then reacquaint yourself with honey. Unprocessed honey in its raw, living form is nothing less than a miracle from God and the earth. Honey has saved human life during drastic times of starvation, and it will become critical again in the future as a food for our survival. You don't need to be in dire circumstances to benefit from honey, though. Take a moment to think about what this wild food really is: nectar. It is liquid gold that can turn your life around.

For those who are afraid that honey is just pure sugar and therefore should be avoided, put your worry aside. If you turn your back on honey, you're missing out on its amazing health benefits. The sugar in honey is nothing like processed sugar—don't confuse it with table sugar or high-fructose corn syrup. Rather, because bees collect from plant species far and wide, the fructose and glucose in honey are saturated with more than 200,000 undiscovered phytochemical compounds and agents, including pathogen-killers, phytochemicals that protect you from radiation damage, and anti-cancerous phytochemicals. When drawn into cancerous tumors and cysts, this last class of phytochemicals shut down the cancerous growth process—meaning that raw honey can stop cancer in its tracks. Honey's highly absorbable sugar and B_{12} coenzymes make it one of the most powerful brain foods of our time. Plus, raw honey repairs DNA and is extremely high in minerals such as calcium, potassium, zinc, selenium, phosphorus, chromium, molybdenum, and manganese.

Our immune systems are constantly adapting to whatever microorganisms we encounter—which is why raw honey, one of the most adaptogenic foods on the planet, produced by bees, one of the most adaptogenic beings on the planet, is so important for supporting immunity. Honey in its raw form is a secret weapon against infectious illness. When you're dealing with weakened immunity and feel like you're extra susceptible to catching colds, flus, stomach bugs such as norovirus, and food poisoning, raw honey assists your body in keeping a strong first line of defense by strengthening neutrophils and macrophages so they can fight off pathogens. (It's not yet documented by medical science that these and other white blood cells feed off of immune-stimulating phytochemicals.) These properties also make raw honey anti-inflammatory—because it inhibits pathogens from procreating and thus releasing toxins that elevate inflammation. Honey is truly medicine for our planet.

CONDITIONS

If you have any of the following conditions, try bringing raw honey into your life:

Sinus infections, ear infections, diabetes, hypoglycemia, posttraumatic stress disorder (PTSD), allergies, sties, eye infections, MRSA, staph infections, mystery infertility, small intestinal bacterial overgrowth (SIBO), low reproductive system battery, insomnia, adrenal fatigue, colds, influenza, norovirus, all types of cancer, bipolar disorder, attention-deficit/hyperactivity disorder (ADHD), Alzheimer's disease, dementia, all autoimmune diseases and disorders, parasites, food poisoning, respiratory infections, colds, influenza, bronchitis, laryngitis, thrush

SYMPTOMS

If you have any of the following symptoms, try bringing raw honey into your life:

Sore throat, postnasal drip, inflammation, canker sores, sleep disturbances, bacterial infections in the gut, all neurological symptoms (including tingles, numbness, spasms, twitches, nerve pain, and tightness of the chest), body odor, dry skin, cysts, eye dryness, dizzy spells, earaches, ear pain, eye floaters, fever, headaches, hot flashes, joint pain, lack of energy, loss of libido, fatigue, memory issues, memory loss, sinus issues, shortness of breath, stomachaches

EMOTIONAL SUPPORT

Honey's sticky nature isn't just a physical trait; it also applies itself on an emotional level. If honey is in your life, then when you experience something good—something that lifts you up and feeds your soul—that memory sticks to you, and you don't lose it among the negative experiences that threaten to distract you.

SPIRITUAL LESSON

If you could trace your family lines back to their oldest days, you would find ancestors who subsisted on honey. Raw honey was not a survival food in the sense that it simply got people by until something better came along. Rather, it was (and still is) incredible medicinal nourishment. Honey is written into our lineage. Who we are—our souls, our DNA—in a sense derives from honey. This means that if we avoid honey, we're shutting off a part of ourselves that connects all the way back to the beginning of human life. Trends that cut us off from honey go to show how disconnected we can really become. Connecting with honey puts us back in touch with ourselves. It prompts us to ask what else we've turned a cold shoulder to that made us who we are today. What else deserves reevaluation?

TIPS

- Add raw honey to lemon water to enhance the honey's bioflavonoids and give the drink an additional immune boost.
- If you feel like you're coming down with something, take a teaspoon of raw honey before bed. This is also a good remedy to enhance a night's sleep.
- Use raw honey in place of all processed sugar and other sweeteners you normally use. Look for wildflower honey, if you can find it.
- Applied externally, honey is great for healing small wounds and revitalizing the skin. Try it on scars where you want to speed up the healing process.
- Consuming honey prior to meditation strengthens the mind and brings about happy sensations throughout the body.

HONEY-COCONUT ICE CREAM

Makes 2 to 4 servings

Fair warning: This ice cream recipe is dangerously good. It only takes a few minutes to prep with an ice cream maker, and in under an hour, you can have ice cream that is cleaner and way more delicious than anything available in the store. As a bonus, you'll have some leftover almond milk that you can use in smoothies or enjoy cold from the fridge.

1 cup almonds

2 dates, pitted

¼ inch vanilla bean, split lengthwise

1½ cups coconut cream (from approximately 2 13.5-ounce cans of refrigerated full-fat coconut milk)

⅛ teaspoon sea salt

⅛ cup raw honey

¼ cup chopped almonds (optional)

First, make the almond milk by blending the almonds, dates, and scraped seeds from the vanilla bean with 2 cups of water until smooth. Strain the mixture through a nut milk bag or cloth and set aside. Then, open the cans of coconut milk, being careful not to shake them. Separate off the heavy cream from each can. (See the Berries and Cream recipe for guidance.) In a medium bowl, mix the coconut cream with 1 cup of almond milk, sea salt, and raw honey until combined. Pour into the bowl of an ice cream maker and process according to the manufacturer's instructions.* Serve the ice cream topped with chopped almonds, if desired, and a drizzle of raw honey.

*Without an ice cream maker, freeze the mixture in a bowl and stir every 30 minutes until set.

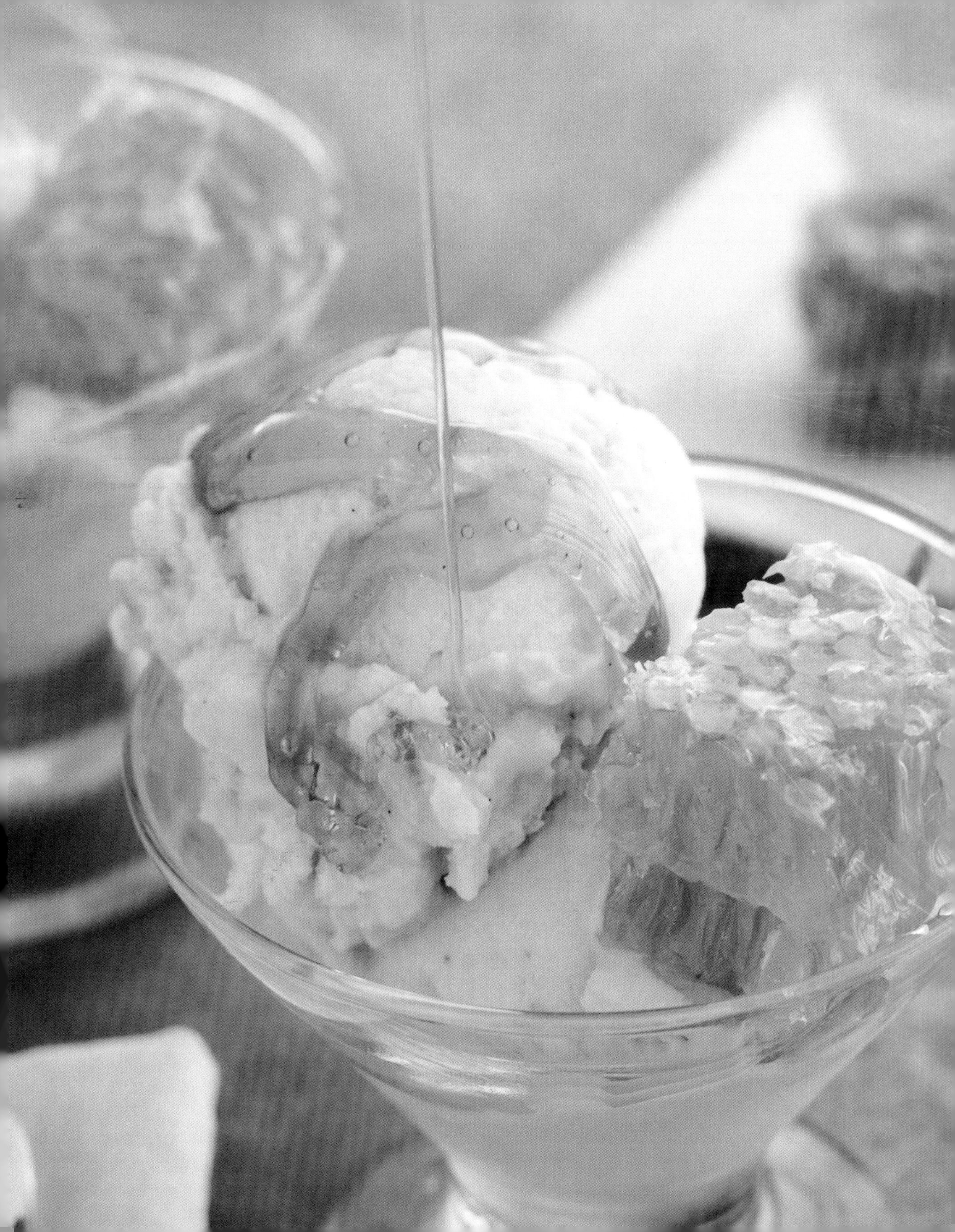

Red Clover

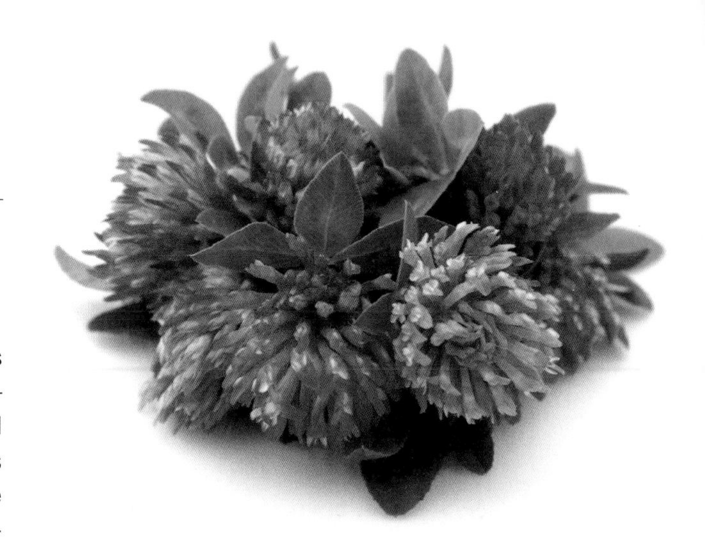

It's not just the rare and hard-to-find that has value. The very accessibility of some resources—think sunlight, air—makes them miracles in and of themselves. Red clover, one such wonder, is thought of as a common weed, when it should be heralded as a king. On top of red clover's generosity of spirit, it has a sympathetic energy; it actually cares about the person who's consuming it.

Red clover is the most powerful herb of all to support the lymphatic system and cleanse lymph fluid, and it can be effective for addressing any type of cancer. This generous wild herb—you can use both the flowers and the leaves—is a diuretic and the ultimate blood builder for those who are worried about virtually any type of blood disorder or disease, including leukemia, multiple myeloma, or just toxic blood overall due to the pancreas or liver not functioning properly.

Red clover is loaded with a bumper crop of nutrients and disease-fighting alkaloids. You can get more out of red clover than any multivitamin on the shelf. If you or your doctor are concerned that you have nutrient deficiencies, drink three cups daily of red clover tea. It is the ultimate tool for remineralization and an amazing replenisher of deficiencies specifically in molybdenum, manganese, selenium, iron, magnesium, vitamin A, B vitamins, cofactors of vitamins (phytonutrients that are not yet on the radar of medical research), and more. Plus, red clover's alkaloids work hand in hand with its amino acids to break up and reduce stored-up, unnecessary fat, so it can be flushed out of the body. It's one of the ultimate drivers of weight loss of our time.

Red clover also has an energizing effect, making it a stellar herb for someone who's feeling exhausted, fatigued, or depleted. You can have the best smoothie packed with fresh fruits, veggies, and superfood powders, and it likely won't match the replenishing nutrition contained in one cup of red clover tea. All of this combined with red clover's ability to cleanse toxic heavy metals and pesticides such as DDT makes this herb truly a must for survival in this century.

CONDITIONS

If you have any of the following conditions, try bringing red clover into your life:

Blood cell disease, B cell disease, leukemia, blood toxicity, hepatitis A, hepatitis B, hepatitis C, hepatitis D, blood cell cancers such as multiple myeloma, anemia (including sickle cell disease), liver disease, adrenal fatigue, low reproductive system battery, allergies, Epstein-Barr virus (EBV)/mononucleosis, acne, herpes simplex 1 (HSV-1), herpes simplex 2 (HSV-2), infertility, shingles, transient ischemic attack (TIA), salivary duct problems, celiac disease, eczema, psoriasis, Lyme disease

SYMPTOMS

If you have any of the following symptoms, try bringing red clover into your life:

High blood pressure, stagnant liver, sluggish liver, chronic diarrhea, chronic loose stools, constipation, hormonal imbalances, enlarged spleen, premenstrual syndrome (PMS) symptoms, menopause symptoms, food allergies, hives, rashes, blood sugar imbalances, melancholy, swollen lymph nodes, poor circulation, histamine reactions and sensitivities, dry skin, blood in the urine, calcifications, chemical sensitivities, body fungus, brittle nails, bruising, headaches, weak digestion, weight gain, sweets cravings

EMOTIONAL SUPPORT

Red clover is for people who live in the past, almost to their own detriment. When you find yourself trying to relive long-ago days because you're nostalgic for feelings of happiness and contentment you felt back then, turn to red clover. This herb helps bring these sustaining emotions into the present, so that you can feel joy and satisfaction in your current life.

SPIRITUAL LESSON

While red clover is used agriculturally in crop rotation, so often when we see it pop up in our lawns and gardens, we consider it a weed. Red clover can grow almost anywhere, and it doesn't care that it's stepped on, even though it should be considered royalty. It is a very forgiving plant that grows vigorously, with great tenacity. You can mow it, stomp on it, cut it down, and still it comes back over and over, providing hope and abundance. Where in your life have you been beaten down by adversity, and yet you still have so much to offer? Red clover teaches us to keep on going.

TIPS

- When you're seeking purification, try a cup of red clover tea in the evening. The herb's healing, cleansing properties will work overnight to find and discharge poisons from your system, making them readily available for your liver to process in the wee hours of the morning.
- Red clover usually blossoms in a cluster, giving off about 5 to 20 flowers at a time. To benefit from red clover's full medicinal effects, tune in to its natural rhythm with a regimen of one cup of red clover tea a day for 5 to 20 straight days. (There's nothing wrong with going past the 20 days. It's just like a new cluster of blossoms opening.)

RED CLOVER CHAMOMILE TEA

Makes 4 cups

When you wake up in want of a fresh beginning, drink a cup of this flower tea in the morning. You'll notice how the day starts to seem newer and brighter.

2 tablespoons red clover blossoms

1 tablespoons chamomile flowers

¼ teaspoon lavender flowers

Mix all the ingredients together in a small bowl. Boil 4 cups of water. For each serving of tea, use 1 teaspoon of the blend in 1 cup of hot water.* Steep for 5 minutes or more.

*If a stronger, more medicinal tea is desired, use 2 teaspoons or up to 1 tablespoon of the tea blend per serving.

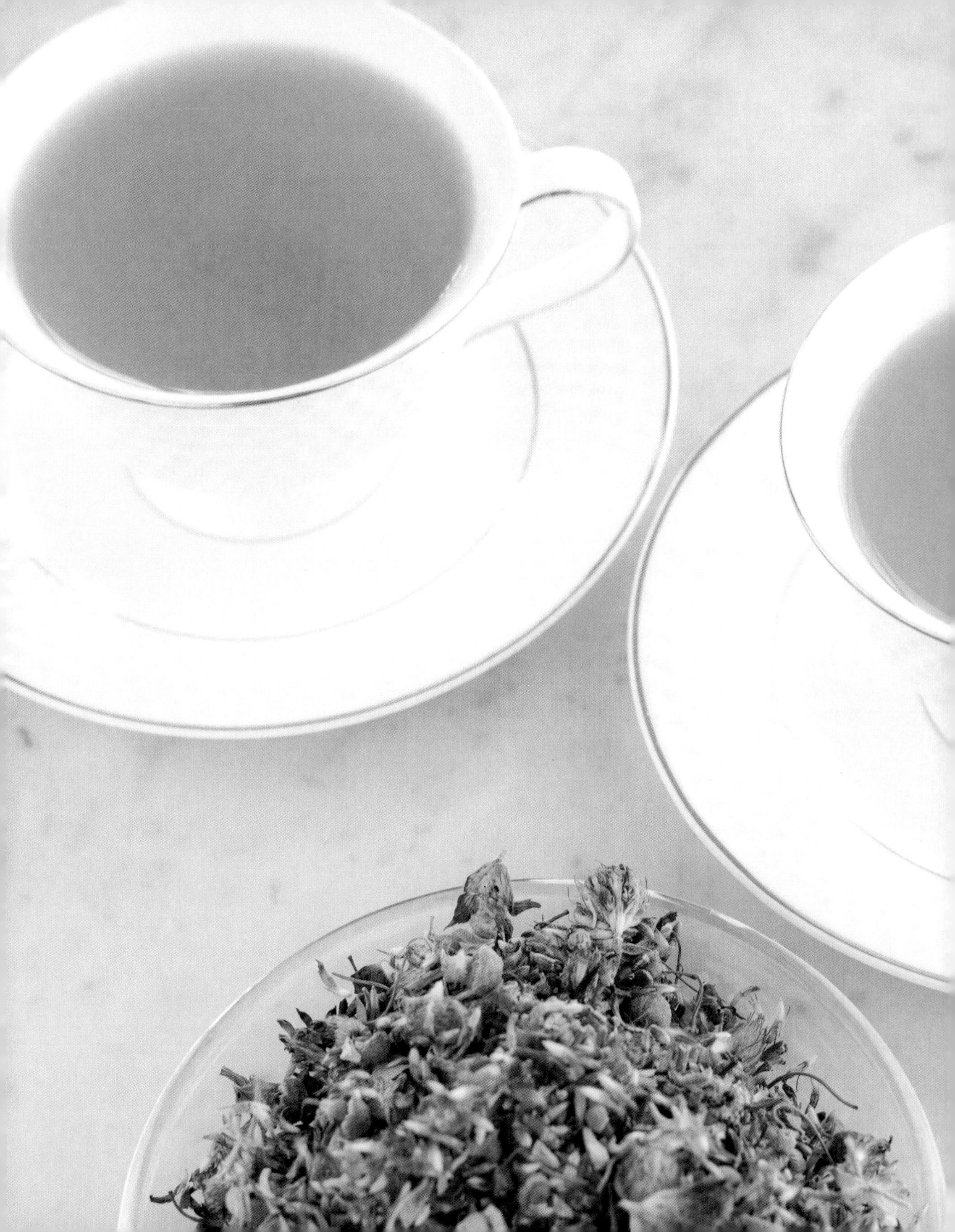

Rose Hips

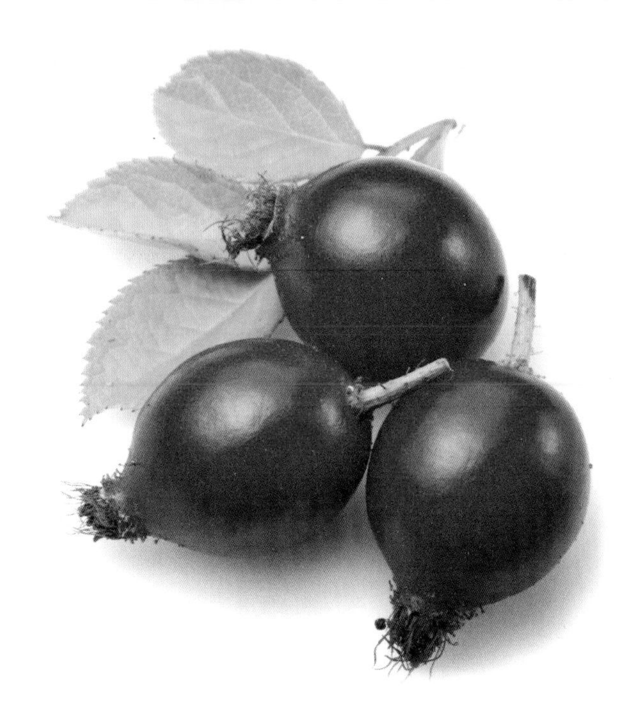

We tend to forget about vitamin C unless we're trying to fight off a cold. Even though we've read in the history books about sailors who used to contract scurvy on long voyages without fresh fruit—so we're familiar with the concept of vitamin C deficiency—it drifts off to the parts of our minds where we store information about DDT, mercury, and other dangers we think are set firmly in the past. Truth is, vitamin C deficiency is still a reality today, and it can contribute to almost any disease. Vitamin C is a critical part of how we survive here on earth—which is why you want rose hips in your life.

The vitamin C in rose hips is the most bioidentical, bioavailable form of vitamin C in existence—that is, the most usable form for our bodies. Plus, the vitamin C in rose hips has the power to transform other vitamin C found in the system from other foods you eat into something bigger and better. Vitamin C is anti-inflammatory (and the vitamin C in rose hips is more anti-inflammatory than from any other source); helps increase our blood's white count by strengthening our neutrophils, eosinophils, basophils, and macrophages; and generally boosts the immune system against viruses, bacteria, yeast, mold, and other unwanted fungus. Rose hips are a particularly helpful catalyst for battling virtually any type of infection.

When a virus such as Epstein-Barr is active in the body, it often gives off damaging neurotoxins and dermatoxins, and in the process, a jelly-like substance called biofilm forms from the virus's debris. This biofilm is not only like a petri dish for unproductive microorganisms such as bacteria in the body, it can also gunk up the works of critical organs. The liver acts as a sponge, absorbing this biofilm in an effort to protect the body, however the biofilm can break loose into the blood, and then, because the heart draws much of its blood from the liver, this sticky jelly residue can get caught in heart valves such as the mitral valve. This is a hidden cause of mystery heart palpitations, tachycardia, atrial fibrillation, and arrhythmia. The vitamin C in rose hips can stop this from occurring. It has a dissolving effect on biofilm, helping to break up deposits of it and ultimately give relief to the person who suffers from irregular heartbeats.

Rose hips are amazing for alleviating UTIs—much more powerful at the job than cranberries—and for healing skin conditions. They also have a higher ratio of antioxidants than most healing foods, and contain a wide variety of antioxidants (many of which are still undiscovered) in addition to vitamin C. Roses' roots go deeper into the soil than many other shrubs. Because of the depths to which they reach, they're able to work their way into clay and loam, and draw up nearly every type of mineral, including critical silica. Even when you grow roses in your backyard, the resulting rose hips are still a wild food. Grafting, hybridization, and cultivation cannot take the wildness out of the rose—these powers never waver.

CONDITIONS

If you have any of the following conditions, try bringing rose hips into your life:

Ear infections, dental issues, gum disease, gum abscesses, urinary tract infections (UTIs) such as bladder infections and kidney infections, diverticulitis, diverticulosis, small intestinal bacterial overgrowth (SIBO), laryngitis, tachycardia, atrial fibrillation, colds, influenza, sinus infections, acne, vitiligo, skin infections, staph infections, strep throat, sties, eye infections, MRSA, toenail and fingernail fungus, adrenal fatigue, herpex simplex 2 (HSV-2), all autoimmune diseases and disorders, chronic bronchitis, chronic fatigue syndrome (CFS), hemorrhoids, psoriatic arthritis, internal bacterial infections, seizure disorders, diabetes

SYMPTOMS

If you have any of the following symptoms, try bringing rose hips into your life:

Sore throat, canker sores, heart palpitations, stagnant liver, sluggish liver, constipation, rashes, excess mucus, fever, all neurological symptoms (including tingles, numbness, spasms, arrhythmia, enlarged spleen, twitches, nerve pain, and tightness of the chest), blurred vision, frozen shoulder, hot flashes, blisters, body pain, itchy skin, listlessness, brain lesions, mineral deficiencies, cough, dizzy spells, ringing or buzzing in the ears, dry skin, eye dryness, malaise, neck pain, nervousness, shoulder pain

EMOTIONAL SUPPORT

Have you ever felt like someone had it out for you? Like you were under psychic attack? Do others' negative opinions affect your state of mind? Rose hips are critical to protect you against this sort of ill will. Whether people are upset that you're pursuing natural approaches (such as natural childbirth or breastfeeding for a long period), laying down the law at work, or following your conscience when they wish you'd compromise your morals, bring in rose hips to block out the naysayers so you can pursue your path.

SPIRITUAL LESSON

The fleeting beauty of roses gets a lot of attention. What about when the petals drop away? It isn't cause for melancholy, or reflection on how we're at the mercy of time—it's cause for celebration. That big, showy, fragrant blossom was just the invitation; the party really gets started once the rose fades and the flower's fruit, the rose hip, begins to ripen. The same is true of people. Getting older isn't a reason to mourn—our younger years are just the beginning. As we age and our experience grows, we gain our real value: fruitful wisdom that we can share and use to nourish each other. What else in your life are you writing off as an end, when really, it's a beginning?

TIPS

- The rose hip is the rose's soul. Before you brew rose hip tea, set the serving of dried rose hips you intend to use in the sun for five minutes (no more). This will activate the rose hips' most powerful memory of swaying in the wind and basking in the sun on a perfect August day—which enhances the soul of the rose so it can pass on its maximum potency to you.
- Once you've made your tea, add a squeeze of lemon and some raw honey to make the vitamin C content highly active.

ORANGE ROSE HIPS ICED TEA

Makes 2 cups

When you have a spare moment to wind down, turn your mind to rose hips, and brew up a batch of this sweet, light, and refreshing iced tea. As you take time to enjoy it on your own or with a companion, bask in the drink's benefits and the simple pleasure of nourishing yourself.

2 teaspoons dried rose hips
½ cup orange juice

Boil 2 cups of water. Steep rosehips in 1½ cups of water for 5 minutes or more.* Place the tea in the refrigerator to cool. When cool, add ½ cup of orange juice. Serve over ice and enjoy!

*If a stronger, more medicinal tea is desired, use 2 teaspoons or up to 1 tablespoon of the tea blend per serving.

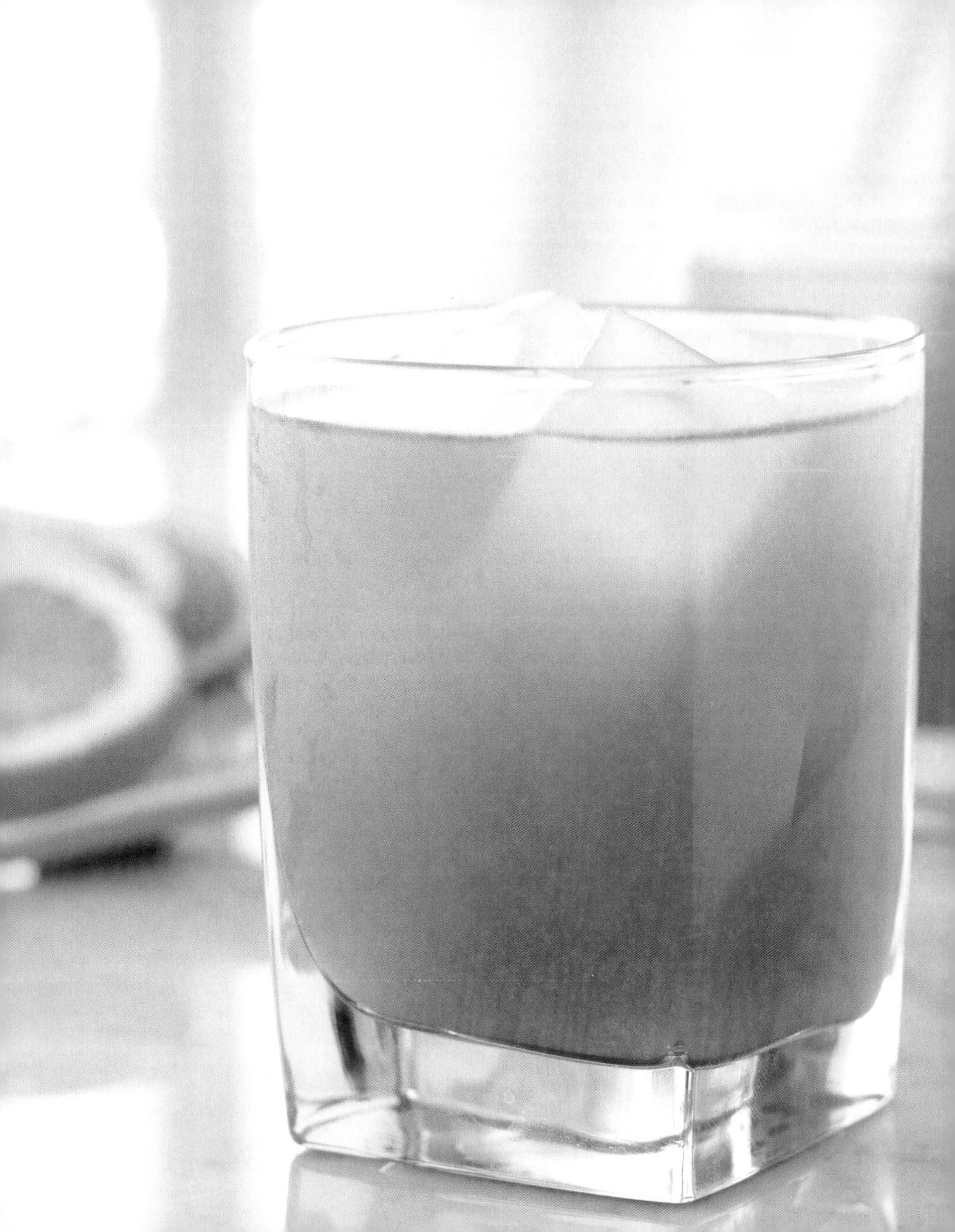

Wild Blueberries

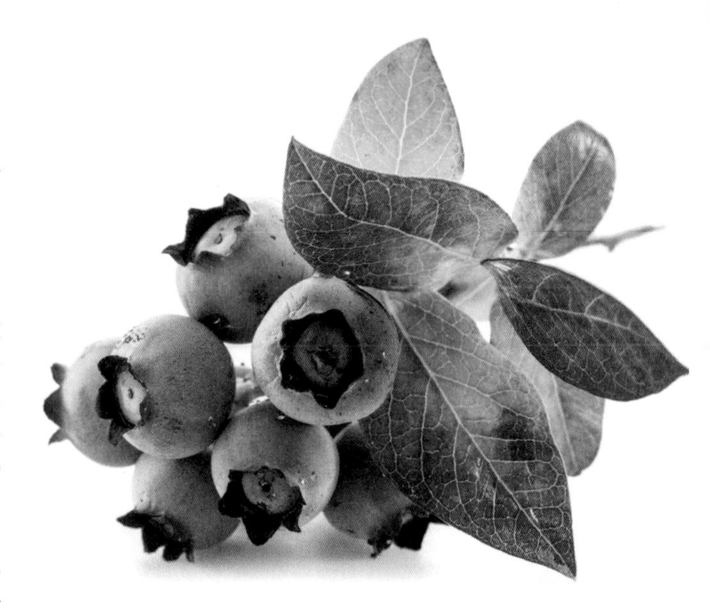

It's easy to get swept up in the belief that the ultimate healing food is hiding somewhere in the tropical wilds. We read about researchers who scour the jungle for miracle roots and berries, and we see exotic dried fruits for sale at the grocery store with packages proclaiming them "superfoods." Maybe one day, we tell ourselves, a true miracle food will be discovered out there in the rain forest—the root or berry or herb or nut that will save humanity.

While of course the rain forest has potent medicine to offer, that's not where scientists will find the most valuable food that can save us. The world's most powerful food is hiding on low, scrubby bushes in plain sight. I'm talking about the wild blueberry. There is not a cancer that wild blueberries cannot prevent, nor a disease known to humankind that wild blueberries cannot protect you from.

Do not confuse wild blueberries with their larger, cultivated cousins, which, while great for your health, don't offer even a fraction of wild blueberries' power. The difference between cultivated and wild blueberries is the difference between farm-raised salmon and wild salmon, or between industrial, grain-fed beef and free-range, grass-fed beef. Bringing cultivated blueberries into your life is like drinking from a paper cup; bringing wild blueberries into your life is like drinking from the golden cup that Jesus once drank from—the Holy Grail.

Wild blueberries hold ancient and sacred survival information from the heavens, going back tens of thousands of years. They have adapted to every fluctuation in climate over the millennia. Their innate intelligence has prevented them from accepting a monoculture; instead, they thrive with more than 100 variable strains that look similar yet have different genetic makeups, so that these plants can never be eradicated, no matter what comes in the future. While other food plants can only continue after a fire if their seeds survive and are replanted, wild blueberry plants can be burned to the ground, and they will come back stronger than ever. No other food on the planet has the ability to thrive in such trying conditions. It is the number-one adaptogen, period—even though it is not recognized as an adaptogenic food at all.

Currently, wild blueberries are acknowledged by nutrition experts for their sky-high levels of antioxidants. It goes beyond that—they have the highest proportion of antioxidants of any food on the planet. On top of that, these tiny jewels have a plethora of undiscovered qualities. For one, they're armed with dozens of antioxidant varieties that science does not yet know about, along with polyphenols, anthocyanins, anthocyanidins, dimethyl resveratrol, and as yet unknown cofactor adaptogenic amino acids. When you eat these berries, their innate intelligence reads your body, searches out potential disease, monitors your stress and toxicity levels, and figures out the best way to heal you—it is the only food that does that.

One of the most effective heavy metal detoxing foods, wild blueberries are fantastic at removing all other Unforgiving Four factors, too. Wild blueberries are also the most powerful brain food in existence, the most potent prebiotic there is, and a star at restoring the liver. Essentially, this fruit offers a benefit unobtainable from any other source for every part of the body. There is more information in one wild blueberry plant than there is on the entire Internet. If researchers had the technology to decipher what's inside wild blueberries and how to use it all, they would develop cures for every condition. One hundred years from now, medical science will use the wild blueberry as the key to unlock the secrets of how to heal disease.

This is the food you want in your life when you've been through the unthinkable and need the support to rise up again. It's also for anyone who needs a physical boost or strives athletically—wild blueberries in the system could mean the difference between life or death for a rock climber in a perilous situation. Wild blueberries are the sole food on the planet to contain the full power of the divine, the Holy Source, the universe, and they are revered by the angels as the key to keeping the human race alive in the coming times. Wild blueberries are, above all, the resurrection food.

CONDITIONS

If you have *any* condition, particularly if it's cancerous or related to the brain and/or nerves, try bringing wild blueberries into your life.

SYMPTOMS

If you have *any* symptom, whether emotional, spiritual, or physical, try bringing wild blueberries into your life.

EMOTIONAL SUPPORT

Wild blueberries have more inspiration to offer us than even the best motivational speakers on the planet, because they mend us on an emotional level. Wild blueberries strengthen the very fabric of who we are so that we won't be so susceptible to punishment, rejection, scorn, humiliation, devastation, and degradation. If you've struggled with feeling criticized, depreciated, discredited, mistreated, or neglected, this is a holy, healing food for you.

SPIRITUAL LESSON

I'm sure you've had an experience in life that leveled you. Something, whether an illness, troubled relationship, or tragic event, that brought you to your knees and practically annihilated your sense of self. Wild blueberries understand what you've been through. They know who you are, the damages you've dealt with, and how to help you rise again. Native Americans observed early on that when wildfire occurred, the only thing that would grow in its path afterward were wild blueberry plants—in fact, they would come back stronger and healthier than ever before. This is the source of the wild blueberry's power: not only can it rise from the ashes, it uses those ashes to its benefit.

And when frozen, because they are true adaptogens, wild blueberries don't lose their nutritional value as some fruits and vegetables do; their nutrition *increases*. The challenge of withstanding the freezing process pushes the fruit to perform at the top of its game, providing you with greater nutritional force and bioavailability.

On both ends of the spectrum, in fire and ice, wild blueberries don't just survive; they triumph. They take an adverse circumstance, meet it, and become better for it. When you eat this supernatural fruit, that indestructible essence becomes a part of you.

Lastly: We all hear a lot of talk about having the right mind-set to attract abundance, shaping our thoughts and actions to manifest the lives we want. This can be very helpful. A person who feels positive is more likely to make choices that lead her or him to more positivity. Sometimes, though, the subject tears us down. The last thing someone who's sick, suffering, or in otherwise unfortunate circumstances needs is to feel like they somehow created, attracted, or brought it upon themselves. If you want to know one of the secrets to manifesting abundance, it's the wild blueberry. I know, that's not what you'd expect! And yet it's true. These little berries are that powerful. When you are striving for anything, when you want to live a life of bounty and blessings, turn to wild blueberries and watch the magic happen.

TIPS

- Often the easiest place to find wild blueberries is in the frozen-food aisle at the local supermarket, in the cases that carry smoothie ingredients. As I said above, freezing makes the berries even healthier. To enjoy them, either whip them up into a frozen treat, or thaw and enjoy. Frozen wild blueberries blended with frozen bananas make a delicious and wholesome-beyond-belief ice cream.
- If you're in the United States, seek out frozen or fresh wild blueberries from Maine. If you're in Canada, seek out those from eastern Canada. If you live in another country, don't underestimate the wild blueberries that may be growing in your region; they hold miraculous benefits that far exceed those of any cultivated blueberry.
- If you know someone who's challenged by an illness, offer her or him wild blueberries to show your goodwill.
- When you eat wild blueberries, make a mindful note that they've been graced by God and the universe, that they are a gift from above.

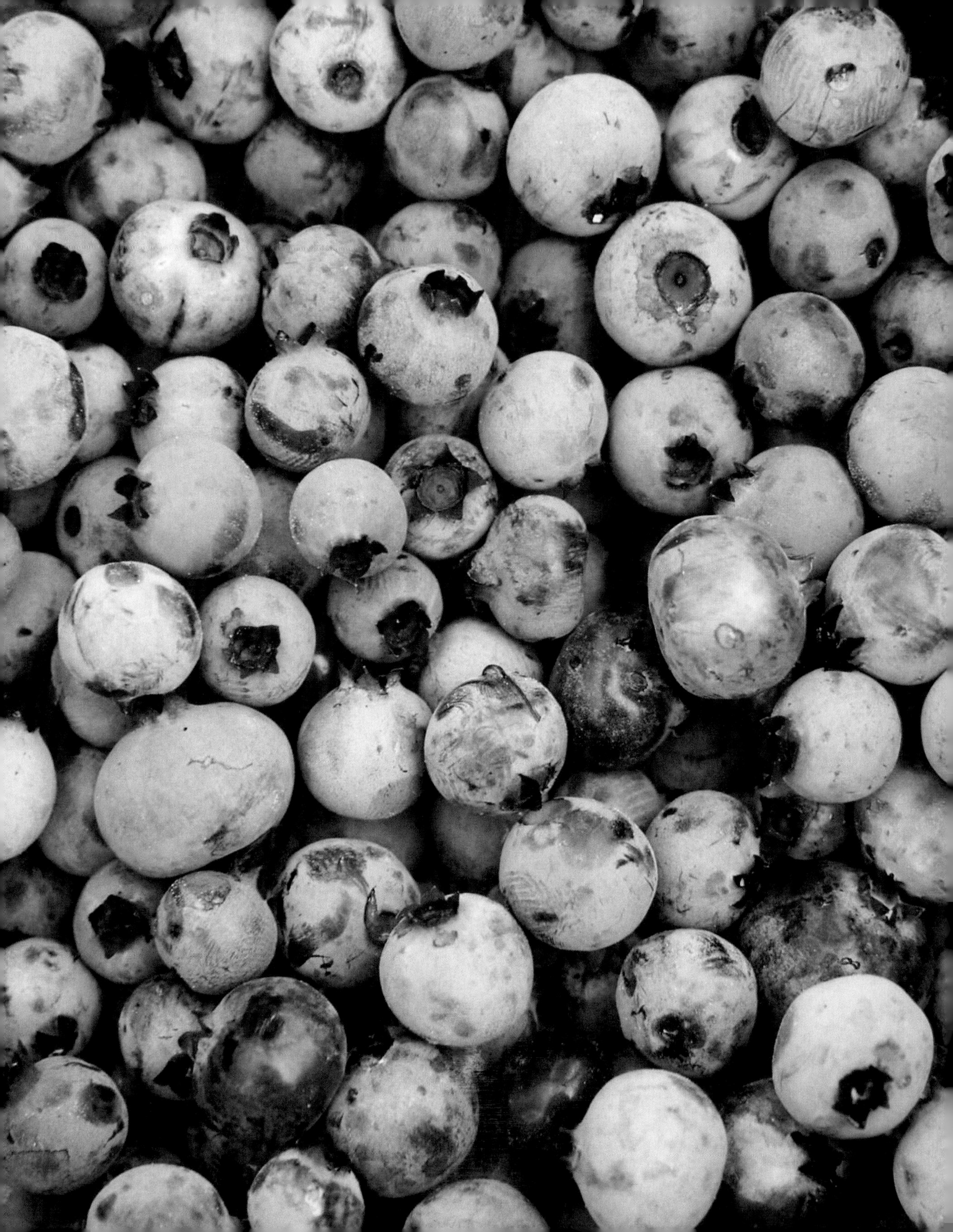

RAW WILD BLUEBERRY PIE

Makes 4 to 6 servings

Loaded with juicy wild blueberries that burst in your mouth and are piled into a sweet cashew crust, this pie is as simple and perfect as it gets. It takes only minutes to make—and about that long to disappear, too! Enjoy it for dessert, breakfast, or any time the urge strikes you.

- ⅓ cup cashews
- ⅓ cup unsweetened shredded coconut
- 4 cups dates, pitted
- 20 ounces frozen wild blueberries, thawed
- 1 mango, diced

For the crust, process the cashews, coconut, and 3 cups of dates in a food processor until thoroughly combined and smooth. Press the crust into a 9-inch pie dish. Cover and refrigerate.

For the filling, process half of the wild blueberries, the remaining cup of dates, and the mango in a food processor until smooth. Stir in the other half of the blueberries. Pour the filling into the pie crust and allow to set in the refrigerator for at least 40 minutes. Serve the pie cold and enjoy!

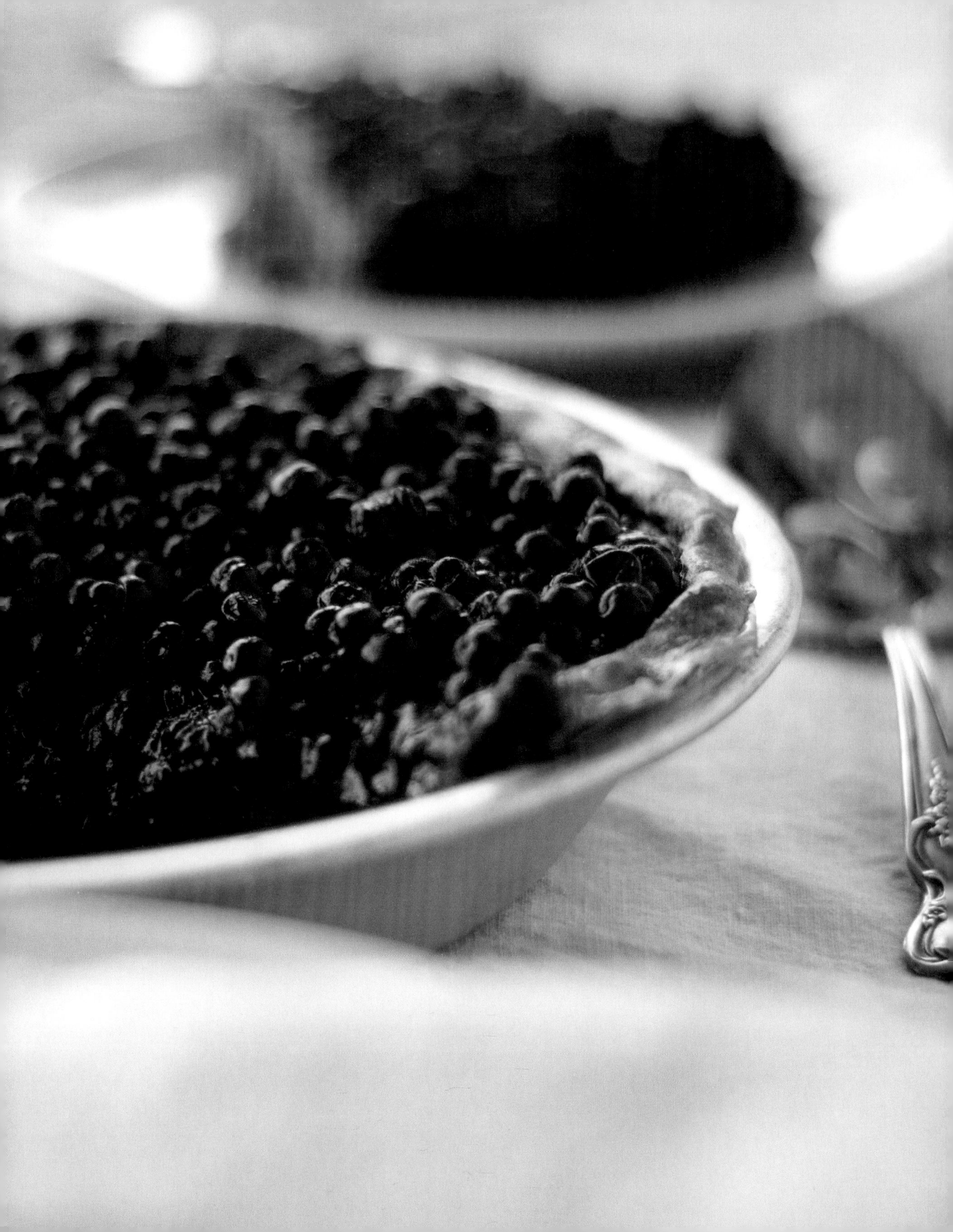

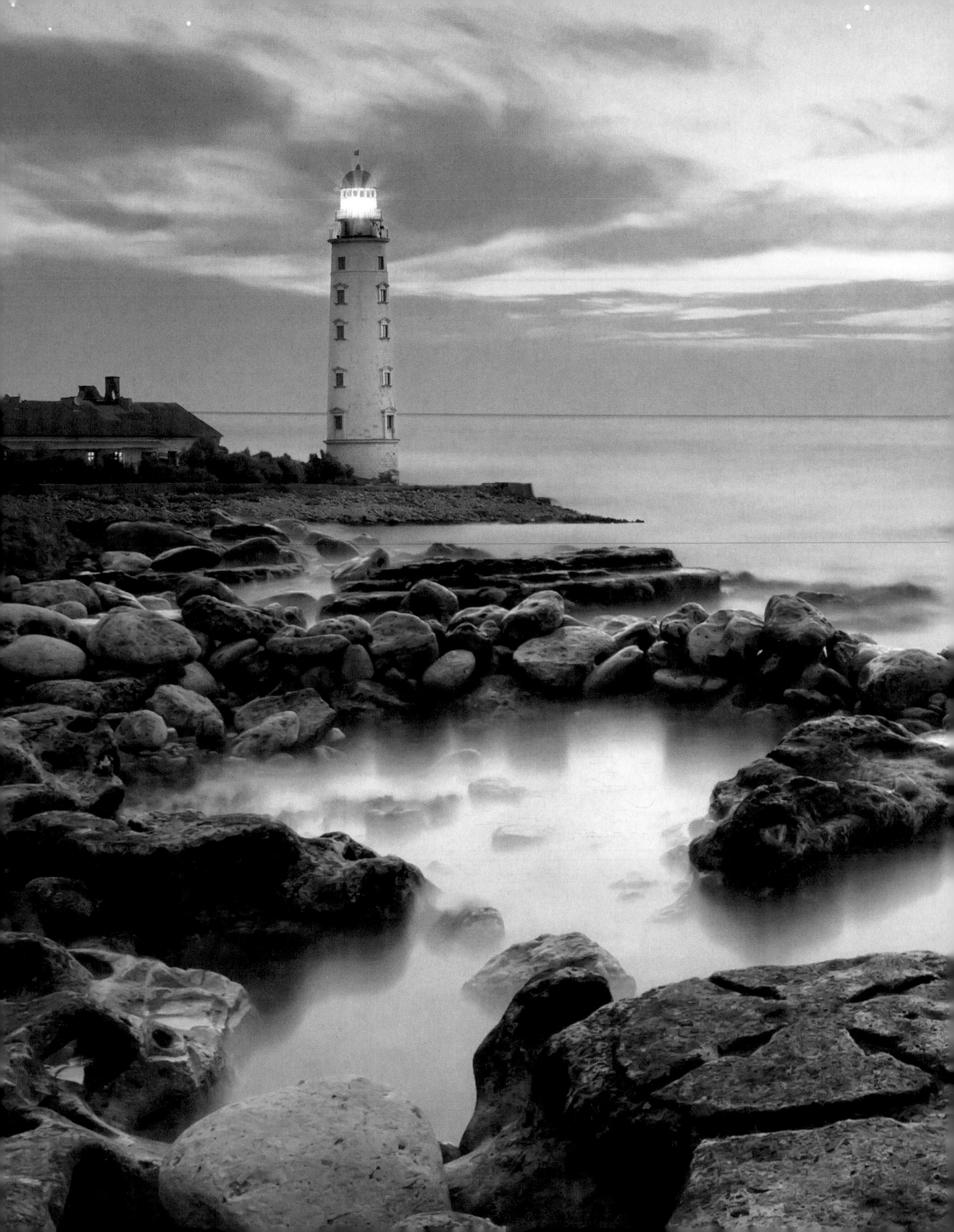

PART III

ARMING YOURSELF WITH THE TRUTH

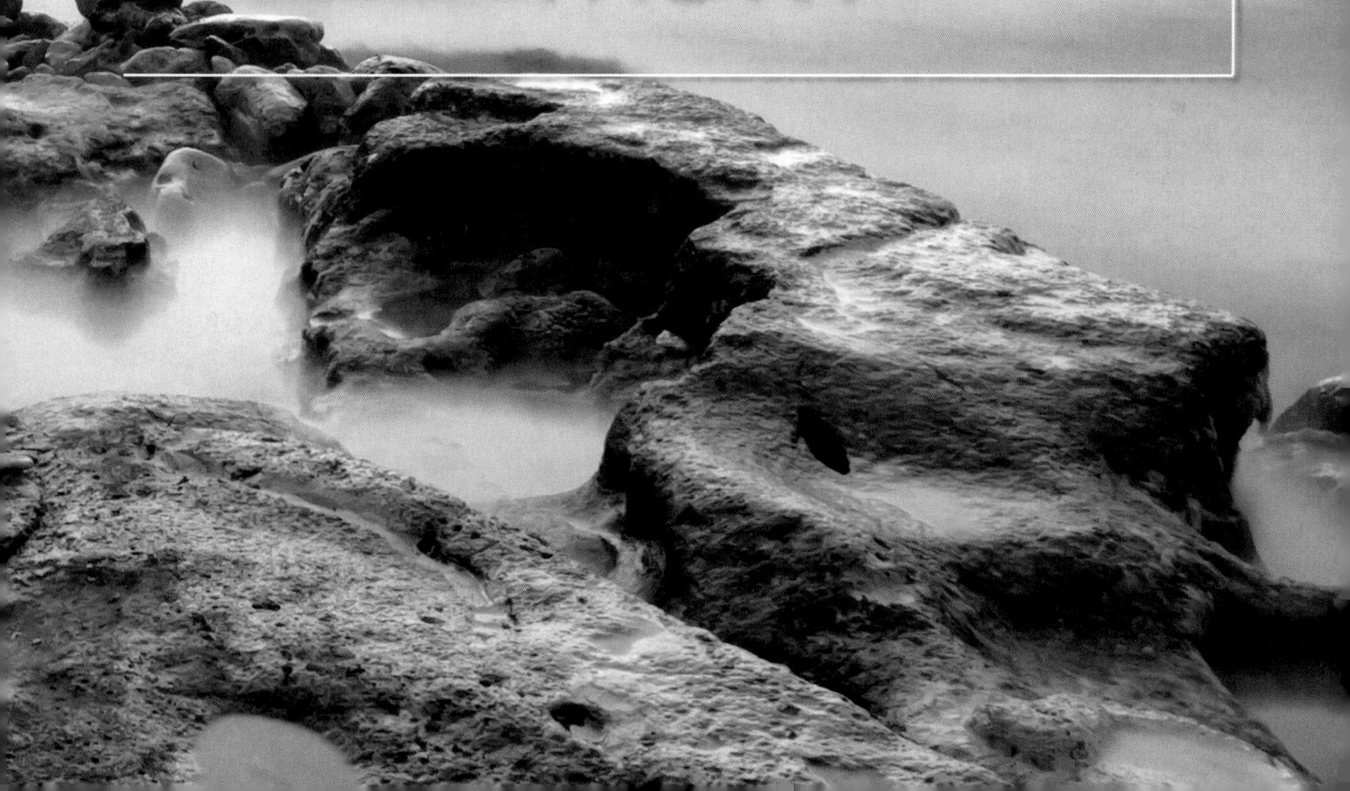

FERTILITY AND OUR FUTURE

When we're young, we so often picture ourselves having children when we grow up. As the years pass, we start to hear it from others: "When you have a daughter of your own . . ." or, "This will be a story to tell your son someday." We're brought up to see the family unit of parents plus kids as a given. It becomes an expectation, one that comes both from ourselves and others.

So if it happens that as an adult you decide that you would like to start a family, and then pregnancy becomes problematic, it can feel devastating on so many levels. At the foundation, there's that concept that's ingrained about what a family looks like—and suddenly this foundation is shaken. Then there are the emotions of loss—of both a person and a vision of the future—followed frequently by feelings of inadequacy or guilt. And then there's often the sense that you're letting others down, whether your partner was hoping for a daughter or son, or your parents were hoping for a grandchild.

It's gut-wrenching what people go through when they struggle with fertility. I'm sure you know someone who has struggled to have a baby. Maybe you've been that person hoping month after month to see a positive on the test stick, or praying not to miscarry again, and feeling let down time after time. Countless people have been there, tried every technique under the sun to boost fertility, only to face loss yet again.

These individuals can all confirm: Infertility is one of the great mysteries of our age. On the surface, it seems like a biological process that should unfold smoothly. In practice, it's often a source of frustration, confusion, disappointment, self-blame, and despair. While medical communities have pioneered methods to help some people have the families they dream of, the underlying issue remains: Why do so many who want to start a family encounter difficulty on that path?

Infertility is a sign of our times. Women and men alike are up against so much in our current era, from stress to pollutants to pathogens. The overload puts a strain on the body, sometimes with the heartbreaking outcome that someone is unable to conceive. Believe it or not, though, infertility isn't solely a result of changes for the worse; it's also a by-product of progress. It used to be that women were expected to start a family young, with limited alternatives to that prescribed norm. Much of a woman's focus went to conceiving at an early age, and because of the mind-body connection, this meant that her body's reserves went to her reproductive system.

Today, women have many more options. While females still don't get all the respect and freedom they deserve, a woman's role in society is much evolved from what it used to be. Conceiving from the get-go often isn't the priority anymore—and rightfully so. Many women choose instead to get an education, explore different career paths, and travel in early adulthood, rather than having children right away. They take the time to find the right partner, rather than settling for someone to conform with others' expectations. They aspire to live life, to truly become themselves before they start a family.

And so if the time comes when a woman's priorities shift and she's ready to get pregnant, her body isn't necessarily in gear. Sometimes that's due to antifertility actions, foods, or chemicals that a woman has unknowingly been exposed to in her life. Sometimes it's because of an underlying condition that until now she wasn't aware could disrupt her family plans. And often in play is a reproductive system that needs to be recharged with energy and attention. (Of course, sometimes it's none of the above, and we really need to look at the male side of the equation.)

A few years ago, a woman named Monica came to me in agony over her inability to conceive. She was 38 years old at the time, and felt that being a mother was one of her purposes in life. Yet every time she got pregnant, she soon miscarried. Monica felt fatigued, bereft, worried that her window of fertility was closing—and unwilling to give up hope. "I just don't get it," she told me. "I thought procreation was supposed to be the most natural process in the world. Why does it feel like a struggle?"

When I performed a read, Spirit revealed that an underlying viral issue was draining the "battery" of her reproductive system (a concept we'll explore soon), which prevented proper ovulation. All of her body's energy was going toward fending off the virus. Before she could be in the best possible shape to carry a baby to term, she had to heal and redirect her body's resources to her reproductive system. Following the guidelines in this chapter, Monica finally gave birth to a healthy boy one year later—and then three years later, a girl. With the proper care for her reproductive system, she saw her vision of motherhood through to reality.

The time has come for more people to experience healing like Monica's, to connect our society's progress with a true understanding of how fertility works. In this chapter, we'll cover all of the above, including principles of how a woman's reproductive system operates that are still unknown to science, as well as how to give your body the optimal care it craves for the best chance of delivering a healthy baby. If you've gone everywhere and tried everything, there is still hope. Infertility is not something you brought upon yourself. It's not a punishment, judgment, or life sentence. Your aspiration to expand your family is not only natural, it's noble: our survival as a species depends on caring and committed people like you to raise the new generations that will carry us into the future.

THE FUTURE OF THE HUMAN RACE

It's imperative for the survival of the human race that the planet's infertility rates start to move in the opposite direction. That may come as a surprise. As I mentioned in the "Save Yourself" chapter, you've probably heard that we're headed for a major population explosion. You may have drawn the conclusion that while infertility is heartbreaking on a personal level for the people it affects, it's not going to get in the way of world population numbers continuing to grow.

Truth is, we're headed for a very different future than growth models predict. Right now, yes, the number of people on the earth just keeps getting bigger. We're getting close to a plateau, though, as infertility rates skyrocket. Forty years from now, a full 50 percent of women of childbearing age will be unable to have a baby. Overall population numbers will start to head south.

If we're going stay afloat through the challenges ahead, the time to understand and address the infertility situation is right now. The future doesn't have to be bleak. There are measures you can take to protect your reproductive health, to ensure that there's a bright future ahead.

A HIDDEN CAUSE OF INFERTILITY

We're all familiar with the concept of a low battery. Since rechargeable batteries were invented, we've had to remember to keep them charged—with mixed success. Has your phone ever run out of juice midway through a day of errands because you forgot to plug it in the night before? We've all been there, watching that little battery icon wane to a sliver of red, knowing that our technology was struggling to draw power, and that before long, it wouldn't function at all—unless we charged it up again.

If the human body came with an indicator light, most women with infertility issues would see a low power warning. That's because a woman's reproductive system is like a battery: the proper care, forethought, and attention are required to charge it up and get it working at full strength. If you're a woman struggling with infertility, there's a good chance that your reproductive system needs a recharge.

Many women who've been trying to get pregnant for any period of time tell me that they pay loads of attention to their reproductive system, so their batteries should work at full strength. They eat well, keep track of their cycles, employ positive visualization—the whole nine yards. I always tell these women that these are excellent steps to take—they just need to know some secrets about how the reproductive system works in order to take their efforts to the next level.

Operating on Low Battery

First, it's important to understand how the reproductive system becomes drained. The major factor is birth control. These days, many women are on birth control medication with the hope of avoiding unwanted pregnancies until they're in a place in life where they're ready to conceive. As I said at the beginning of the chapter, it is, of course, a vital advancement in society for women to have the liberation to choose how they want their lives to unfold. You just need to be aware that if you've been on birth control, your body has learned to divert resources away from your reproductive system. Some women may start taking the pill (or whichever form of contraceptive medication) in early high school and continue on through the end of their 20s or beyond. Even someone who starts on the pill in her teens and cuts off the medication after college graduation in hopes of starting a family right away could already have been taking it for eight years. That's eight years of training her body not to have a baby. It doesn't mean that she's guaranteed to have trouble conceiving when she goes off the pill; it simply means that if she does have trouble, this is a likely factor.

Other forms of birth control, from abstinence to barrier contraceptives, can have a similar effect, because the more years a woman spends not getting pregnant, the less energy goes toward her reproductive system, and the more her body learns the pattern of withholding pregnancy. (Of course, low battery doesn't mean *no* battery; plenty of women can attest that they've conceived when they were actively trying to avoid pregnancy.)

This isn't to say that women should not put off having children—not at all. It's just important to understand that when making the transition from avoiding pregnancy to trying for it, the body may need some time and maintenance to adjust.

Recharging the Reproductive Battery

Have you ever left a car sitting in the driveway for a little too long? Life was busy, or maybe you were away, and when you finally got a chance to get back behind the wheel and turn the key, you could hear the engine sputter as it struggled to draw power from the battery? That's because, as we all know, a car needs time on the road for the alternator to keep the battery charged. Once you finally got the engine started—maybe with a jump-start—the only thing the car probably needed was a good, long drive, and then consistent road time afterward, to get back in working order.

Though the workings of a woman's body, especially her reproductive system, are of course much more intricate and enigmatic than those of an automobile, the mentality of maintenance is the same one to bring to your quest for fertility. A woman's reproductive system has a soul of its own, with its own specific set of needs. In addition to avoiding certain antifertility factors, bringing in a variety of life-giving, fertility-enhancing foods, and tapping into spiritual techniques—all of which I'll discuss later in the chapter—a critical piece of how to send your body the message that you're ready to have a baby is to learn how to consciously rewire so you're ready to form a new life.

This is different from dwelling on your desire to conceive. It's also not the same as the meditations you'll find at the end of this chapter. This is about physically making that mind-body connection so your body learns that it's time to start devoting resources to every last part of your reproductive system, to get it back in working order.

Here's the exercise: Imagine you're plugging a cord into your reproductive system to charge. Picture every last part of your reproductive system, from your uterus to your fallopian tubes to your ovaries, drawing power from this energy source.

It may sound simple or abstract, and yet it's very potent and real. In this day and age, our bodies are highly attuned to technology. Our eyes stare at screens from morning to night, gadgets wrapped around our wrists track our every movement, and our phones are always at our fingertips. From this nonstop exposure, our bodies truly connect to the concept of being plugged in.

The key is to perform the exercise regularly, to make it part of your daily routine. If you have a normal schedule for plugging in your phone—perhaps every night before bed—follow the same routine for visualizing your physical recharge. If you and your partner are struggling with infertility, if you've both visited the doctor and can't find any reason behind your difficulties, this technique, combined with the other healing tips in this chapter, could be the element that turns it all around.

MEN AND FERTILITY

To boost male fertility, it's all about getting back to basics. There are no magic bullets in this department, nor will an overly complicated approach help. Instead, you want to focus on the following simple steps to boost sperm count and motility.

First, it's important for men to lower their mercury levels. Mercury in the system is a huge reason why men's fertility drops, so if you're a man who's trying to start a family, it's important to add Hawaiian spirulina, frozen wild blueberries, cilantro, garlic, barley grass juice extract powder, and Atlantic sea vegetables such as dulse to your routine. I'm not just talking about a little of each here and there; you want to make this a daily protocol for a prolonged period.

Also, the same diet that promotes female fertility promotes male fertility, so men should take care to bring in an abundance of Holy Four foods. And the antifertility foods and chemicals listed below are just as important for men to avoid as women. Further, the herb ashwagandha can be very helpful for male fertility, as can nettle leaf, red clover blossoms, vitamin B_{12}, and zinc.

Zinc is actually one of the most precious minerals when it comes to the health of a man's sperm. It's not only important to eat foods rich in zinc (such as collard greens, radishes, artichokes, nettle leaf, parsley, and onions) and possibly to supplement with zinc; it's also important to preserve your zinc stores by abstaining from ejaculation that's not for procreation, because frequent emissions make it much more likely that the sperm will be docile, listless, and undernourished, both from being overused and because zinc reserves are lost with each emission. Instead, hold back so that you'll have the best chance of strong, healthy sperm.

ANTIFERTILITY FACTORS TO AVOID

If you're trying to have a baby, then you're no doubt already trying to limit exposure to toxins. And if you've read the first chapter of this book, then you also know that the Unforgiving Four are a threat to everyone's health. Radiation, DDT, toxic heavy metals, and the viral explosion have a direct effect on fertility rates, and the best way to combat the risk is with awareness and the healing power of food. It's also important to know that there are other hidden factors, including foods, chemicals, and actions, that can threaten fertility and drain the reproductive battery. For the best chance of conceiving and carrying out a healthy pregnancy, turn to the information below.

Antifertility Foods

If you've been struggling to conceive for no identifiable reason, it's a good idea to hold back adrenalized foods from your diet. Adrenalized foods are animal foods (such as chicken, turkey, lamb, other types of meat, fish, and dairy products) that are filled with adrenaline due to the animals' high stress at the time of slaughter or capture. Adrenaline is like an antifertility drug, and while many women are able to eat animal foods and still become pregnant, others are very susceptible to adrenaline's negative effects, even in trace amounts. You may want to try to limit your animal food intake by 50 percent, or keep your consumption to smaller animals such as birds, including pheasants and chickens, because they have such small adrenals. After you've given birth, you can go back to whatever way of eating you prefer.

Other foods that can instigate and worsen conditions such as PCOS, endometriosis, PID, uterine fibroids, and ovarian cysts—and in this way interfere with fertility—are eggs, corn, wheat, canola oil, dairy, aspartame, and MSG (look out for its hidden forms), as well as soy that's conventional and unsprouted. If you have PCOS or endometriosis and you hear recommendations that you should eat eggs for your condition, try not to get derailed. This advice could not be further from the truth. Rather than reversing these illnesses, eggs advance them, because eggs feed the pathogens behind these conditions. (For more on eggs and other hindering ingredients, see the chapter "Foods That Make Life Challenging.")

Antifertility Chemicals

When pregnant or trying to conceive, be aware that phytotoxic hormone chemicals—essentially foreign antifertility hormones found in pesticides, herbicides, and plastics—can bombard the reproductive system, sending it the exact opposite message of what you're aiming for. In whatever ways you can, try to limit your exposure to these chemicals. Also take care to avoid chlorine and fluoride.

Antifertility Actions

As I mentioned earlier in the chapter, spending years not wanting a baby, or searching for and not finding the right mate—and in the process taking measures to prevent pregnancy—can sometimes mean that the body becomes trained not to conceive. So if that's been your mindset in the past, and now you'd like to have a baby, you may need to take active measures, such as the recharging exercise above, to recondition your reproductive system for fertility.

Another major factor in women's struggles to have children is an overabundance of stress. Not only do adrenalized foods pose a problem; the excess adrenaline that the body produces when someone is under a lot of pressure can interfere with the reproductive system as well. That's because your body wants to protect you. If you undergo emotional upheaval or another form of extreme stress, your body's instinct is to prevent a baby from putting more stress on your body—so the excess adrenaline that is intended for fight or flight acts as an antifertility steroid. (Note that some steroids the body produces, such as the thyroid's thyroxine, are fertility-friendly.)

Adrenal fatigue can also get in the way of fertility, because much of a woman's progesterone, estrogen, and testosterone are produced in her adrenal glands. When the adrenals are under- or overactive, this means her reproductive hormones are out of balance and can interfere with fertility. If you've been dealing with adrenal issues and you want to have a baby, it's ideal to employ the technique of grazing (i.e., eating every one and a half to two hours), which prevents your adrenals from having to work overtime to fill in for dips in blood glucose levels. The foods to follow will also help balance your body's ability to deal with stress.

HEALING FOODS TO REGENERATE THE REPRODUCTIVE SYSTEM

When you're trying to conceive or to support an existing pregnancy, make this your mantra: "Eat fruit to produce fruit." That's because forming a fruit is exactly what you're doing when you foster a new life within. It sounds a little clichéd (and cheesy) to compare a woman's reproductive system to a flower, and yet that's really the case. If you've ever studied botany, then you know that flowers have an ovary, and that the ovary contains the ovules that become fertilized and eventually form fruit. Sound familiar? That's because it's very similar to human female anatomy.

You were once a tiny egg that became fertilized and formed into a miracle of a person. When you eat fruit, which was once a tiny egg that became fertilized and formed into the miracle of food, you join forces. The fruit's wisdom and life-giving properties become a part of you.

Which is to say nothing of the actual nutrition that fruit possesses. First and foremost, the reproductive system runs on glucose—and the best, most bioavailable source of glucose is fruit (and coconut water and raw honey). Our cultural obsession with high-protein diets works against you if you're a woman trying to become pregnant or to support a pregnancy, because a woman's reproductive system doesn't run on protein. In addition to glucose, it runs on minerals, trace minerals, electrolytes, micronutrients, phytochemicals, and other critical compounds found only in the Holy Four food groups of fruits, vegetables, herbs and spices, and wild foods. Your body uses these elements to protect itself by countering the poisonous hormone disrupters from plastics, pesticides, herbicides, pharmaceuticals, and GMO food.

When you think about a fertility-promoting diet, keep in mind the makeup of breast milk: high in sugar, with a lower amount of fat, and a comparatively small amount of protein. It's basically sugar water, in the best possible way. Because breast milk will be the first food for the baby you hope to have, it gets your body moving in the right direction if you start to adopt a similar approach to the overall composition of what you eat: highest on the list is natural sugar (in the form of fructose and glucose from whole food sources, most notably fruit), followed by some fat, and a much smaller portion of protein. Women on high-protein/low-carb diets, especially when they're over the age of 30, often have difficulty producing breast milk, because they don't have the right building blocks.

So if your main nutritional concern has been getting enough protein, shift focus to fruit. Spirit tells me that in the future, out of the thousands of hidden compounds, coenzymes, and phytochemicals that medical science will discover are present in fruits, vegetables, herbs and spices, and wild foods, one group will stand out: *pro-fertility compounds*. These powerful compounds will play a pivotal role in the future of procreation. Scientists will derive them from a particular variety of polyphenol, concentrate them, and use these concentrates to create new medicines to address the infertility crisis we'll be facing. For now, the way to get them is to consume Holy Four foods, particularly berries (including wild blueberries). The pro-fertility compounds in berries support the reproductive system by (1) balancing reproductive hormones, and (2) governing the reproductive system's absorption of the specific nutrients science has not yet discovered it needs in abundance to keep the reproductive battery charged.

Other ideal fruits for fertility are oranges, bananas, avocados, grapes, mangoes, melons, raspberries, cucumbers, cherries, and limes. And further powerful foods to regenerate the reproductive system—whether from "low battery" or conditions such as a history of pelvic inflammatory infections, endometriosis, fibroids, PCOS, or ovarian cysts—are asparagus, spinach, artichokes, kale, celery, butter leaf lettuce, potatoes, garlic, nettle leaf, raspberry leaf, coconut, sprouts, microgreens, red clover, and raw honey. You may want to go back to the middle section of this book to explore all that these foods do for you.

MEDITATIONS FOR FERTILITY

A woman's reproductive system has a soul of its own. This means that when you're trying to cultivate its fertility, it's essential to go beyond the physical steps above. There's a very real element of spiritual nurturing involved. Just as partners try to get in sync with each other when trying to conceive, it's important to get in touch, soul to soul, with your own reproductive system. The meditations that follow offer the chance to do that, plus they serve as powerful methods to adapt to stress.

Walking Meditation

On this meditative walk, tell your reproductive system that it's allowed to conceive now. You stand behind it 100 percent. Honor your reproductive system as a separate, sacred being, directly connected to the heavens, and acknowledge that it might have felt left out until now. It listens to you, and it wants to be respected. Don't shower it with demands; encourage it in a loving manner, the way you would a precious child who takes your guidance to heart, a child who's been afraid until now to blossom. For additional assistance, call aloud upon the Angel of Fertility. Make this walking meditation a part of your routine. By the end of each session, look within yourself for the feeling that you've truly granted your reproductive system the permission to move forward with a pregnancy, and that it's truly heard you.

Breathing in White Light

Lying on your back in a quiet room, take deep, gentle breaths with your eyes closed. Imagine that your mouth and nose are at your lower abdomen, and that with each breath, you're drawing white light directly into your reproductive organs. This is an exercise meant to amplify the recharging of your womb. When you're going a million miles a minute, forgetting to breathe as you move from stressor to stressor, your body learns that crisis management is the focus. Everything is happening up in your head, so that's where your physical resources are directed. By setting aside the time to perform this breathing meditation, you train your mind and body to lower that attention. As you take divine light into your reproductive system, you remind yourself physically and spiritually that your true focus right now is not the outside noise of what's taking place in your life on a daily basis; it's this sacred mission.

As you pursue this calling, know that it will have value for every area of your life. The intention behind conception is powerful. It expands, touches others, and changes your life, too, no matter what. If it turns out that even with everything you try, a baby does not come, don't lose faith in a greater good, or in your worthiness. Do not blame yourself. No matter the outcome, none of the time you put into trying for a baby is ever lost. So much in life is a process of conception and birthing—it's the story behind every great idea that becomes a reality, and every seed that grows into a sheltering tree. That energy you put into the hope for new life will shift and go into creating something else new and beautiful in our world. Whenever you make new life your focus, you bring yourself into divine alignment, and you make a difference on this earth.

HARMFUL HEALTH FADS AND TRENDS

Every day a new concept becomes popular in the health world. Suddenly what was once a niche interest turns into the latest craze. There's nothing inherently bad about fads and trends. Take the days of outsized shoulder pads, for instance: a few decades ago, they were everywhere in fashion. Shoulder pads weren't doing any harm—they were just something that people once liked that now they laugh about.

Certain health trends aren't doing harm, either, and they'll be nothing to be embarrassed about in a few decades' time. Farmers' markets and organic farming, for instance, are two movements in the right direction for our health. Thirty years from now, we'll look back at this as the moment when these ideas were finally starting to integrate into the mainstream, and we'll value this as a time of awakening.

And then there are the popular concepts that aren't so healthy, or can even be damaging. These are the theories that are like invasive weeds, threatening to take all the nutrients and attention away from their garden-mates and overshadow what's meant to grow there.

These fads and trends always sound convincing—at first. Whenever I hear about a new health concept that's gotten a lot of momentum, I'm ready to jump on the bandwagon with everyone else. Then I ask Spirit, and Spirit tells me the truth about whatever the health flavor of the month is—so that I can share it with others. This is inside information that has helped so many people protect themselves. This is inside information that you need, too.

Part of adaptation is letting go. In order to make progress, we have to make a break with what isn't working, and what in some cases is actually holding us back. So in the pages to come, I'll uncover the truth about top fads and trends that are leading people astray with their health, so you can protect yourself and your loved ones.

And remember, as new fads and trends crop up and cycle through popularity, always hold onto this enduring piece of ancient wisdom: The Holy Four of fruits, vegetables, herbs and spices, and wild foods are foundational for health. The importance of these foods will never be superseded by new discoveries. When you betray these foods for the sake of a convincing-sounding argument against them, you betray yourself. No matter what trends come along that make you fear fruit or cruciferous vegetables, or whatever other mistaken theories are to come, do not be swayed in the conviction that the life-changing foods are anything less than fundamental to our ability to survive and thrive here on earth.

ACIDITY, ALKALINITY, AND PH TEST STRIPS

Acidity and alkalinity have become a popular concept in health. It's based on a sound concept: when the body is acidic, it contributes to illness by feeding pathogens. However, the common method of testing for pH—test strips for urine or saliva—leads people astray. It's near impossible to get an accurate reading from a pH test strip.

For one thing, the results of test strips mean the opposite of what everyone thinks they do. When a person's urine gets an acidic pH reading, it means she or he is becoming more alkaline—because when you're detoxing and consuming alkaline juice and foods, you expel acids. People who are acidic, on the other hand, will get readings of elevated pH (that is, alkalinity), because when you're acidic internally, you excrete alkaline minerals such as calcium. So pH strips *can* be handy—if you flip the meaning of the results.

It's important to keep in mind, though, that we have different body systems. To name a few, there are the endocrine, digestive, nervous, lymphatic, and reproductive systems. Each one has a different acid-alkaline balance, and therefore a different pH. When one is more acidic, it can influence the overall test reading. Except then you have no way of knowing *which* body system is acidic, and if that acidity is a problem. Meanwhile, you could have plenty of body systems that are alkaline, and again, not know which ones. So along with not taking pH tests at face value, you have to understand that they're nonspecific.

A note on pH and dental health: You'll hear from some sources that an acidic pH in the mouth rots the teeth. This is a mistaken theory. In fact, acidity in the mouth is a good sign, as it indicates that your body is cleansing itself of acid. The sort of acid that makes saliva readings acidic does not cause dental decay. The true cause of teeth problems starts in the gut, where low hydrochloric acid levels (usually due to unproductive foods, pharmaceuticals, and/or excess adrenaline) contribute to putrefaction of food. When food sits rotting in the digestive system, it gives off ammonia gas, which seeps out through the intestinal lining and into other areas of the body. One of the places that the ammonia can end up is in the teeth. External acids such as coffee may wear down dental enamel; however, ammonia seeps into pores of the teeth and causes the real damage. (Not to be confused with the mistaken theory of leaky gut, this concept is called *ammonia permeability*, and it can cause other problems as well. For more information on what it is and how to prevent it, refer to the "Gut Health" chapter of my first book, *Medical Medium*.)

NIGHTSHADE FEAR

If you've heard that nightshade vegetables aggravate conditions such as arthritis, you can let go of this misconception. Potatoes, tomatoes, peppers, and eggplants, when ripe, have no negative effect on health. It's the opposite: These amazing foods enhance health with their nutrients and healing properties. They're exactly what you need when you're dealing with illness.

Modern-day nightshade fear is just a historical misunderstanding that's changed shape over the years. First, people were afraid of nightshades because their leaves and stems are toxic when consumed. (If that were a legitimate conclusion, then you'd have to avoid all sorts of other foods, too, including oranges and peaches, because that foliage will also make you sick if you eat it.) Once people caught on that the fruits (or tubers, in the case of potatoes) themselves were fine, tomato fear crept up again, because people were eating them off of pewter plates, and the tomato acid released toxic lead that poisoned tomato eaters. Finally, with the days of pewter plates gone, tomatoes were embraced once more.

However, fears like these tend to linger in the collective awareness. So in our current day, as mystery chronic pain has taken hold of more and more people, nightshades are there in the consciousness to be blamed. The modern-day theory goes that these foods are high in alkaloids that cause inflammation. It's not the alkaloids causing inflammation, though. It's *not* the foods that grow on nightshade plants that are the problem.

We have to look at the other ingredients served with these foods. In the case of ketchup and tomato sauce, there's often high-fructose corn syrup, and where there's tomato, you'll frequently find a wheat crust or slice of sandwich bread. With eggplant, there's the inevitable parmesan. Bell peppers get stuffed with sausage and Monterey Jack. Potatoes are so often deep-fat-fried or twice-baked and encrusted with bacon bits. Corn, wheat, high dairy fat, and frying are the real triggers to illness in these situations, because they feed pathogens. When people feel better by cutting out nightshades from their diets, it's because they've lowered their intake of these other ingredients.

Nightshades would have an entirely different reputation if the popular dishes were baked potatoes heaped with salsa and avocado, steamed eggplant drizzled with olive oil and lemon juice, red bell pepper sticks with hummus, and tomatoes stuffed with sundried tomato-tahini dip. If these were the norm, no one would have made a link between nightshades and inflammation, because there's no link to be found when unproductive foods aren't in the mix.

In the rare case where someone eats a juicy, ripe tomato on its own, or a plain steamed potato, and experiences the onset of symptoms, it's practically guaranteed that she or he has symptoms when eating other types of healthy fruits and vegetables, too. It's a sign that the person is dealing with an elevated pathogenic load—the fruits and vegetables are causing a detox reaction. Potato is an incredible antiviral, very high in the amino acid lysine, so if someone is compromised by any sort of viral infection (whether they're aware of its presence or not), she or he is likely to feel an effect in the body as the virus dies off. And tomato skins actually kill off unproductive bacteria, fungus, worms, and other parasites—so as they're eliminated from the intestinal tract, it can lead to detox symptoms. It's a classic case of Holy Four foods getting blamed when they're actually helping us all.

None of this is to say that you should go eating those dark nightshade berries in the woods—those *are* poisonous. Stick to known human food. Also make sure that what you're eating is fully ripe. Most green bell peppers that you'll see on the grocery store shelf are just unripe versions of the red bell peppers nearby. Opt for the red ones, because a green pepper or tomato (unless it's a variety that's green when ripe) is still in the nightshade realm and can be an irritant. (*Anything* at such an unripe stage can be irritating.) Once ripe, the fruit itself is no longer actually a nightshade.

"GOITROGENIC" FOODS

Cruciferous vegetables such as kale, cauliflower, broccoli, cabbage, and more have gotten a bad name lately. So have other completely innocent foods such as peaches, pears, strawberries, and spinach. Don't believe the hype that these foods that contain so-called goitrogens are harmful to the thyroid. The concept of goitrogens—that is, goiter-causing compounds—has been blown way out of proportion. In the first place, none of these foods contain enough goitrogens to even be a health concern. Secondly, the goitrogens in these foods are bonded to phytochemicals and amino acids that stop the goitrogens from doing harm. Even if you were to eat 100 pounds of broccoli in a day (which is humanly impossible), the goitrogens wouldn't be a concern.

What is a problem is if you avoid these foods. You will be doing your thyroid a major disservice, because they contain some of the nutrients that your thyroid gland needs most, including the bioactive trace mineral iodine. For someone with a goiter, these are the exact foods that will help that goiter heal. For someone with thyroid nodules or tumors, these are the foods with properties to fight them. Medical science does not yet have a full picture of what sort of nutrition the thyroid truly needs to thrive, and so a huge group of foods get wiped out of people's diets out of fear of one compound that has yet to be fully studied. Until medicine understands the multiple trace minerals, vitamins, phytochemicals, and other nutrients that the thyroid needs—which are all abundant in goitrogenic foods—goitrogens will continue to be misunderstood. Don't be one of the people who follows this trend and misses out on the opportunity for health.

VITAMIN D MEGADOSES

Everybody's talking about vitamin D lately. Across the alternative-conventional spectrum, practitioners are telling patients that they should be worried about their vitamin D levels. This universal agreement is a bit of a red flag. When everyone goes along with one idea, it's a sign that the concept is not getting enough of a healthy prodding to reveal whether or not it's true. Rather, widespread acceptance becomes like a law of our world—like electricity—and we think of it as unquestionable.

Of course vitamin D is important. It's great that it's getting its due credit these days, and that recent vitamin D awareness is encouraging people to get more sunlight—in part because sunlight offers so many other health benefits, too. I am in no way against vitamin D. It's safe to take (D_3 is best), and should be considered a normal, basic, and fundamental part of any multivitamin.

What we have to be wary of is the claim that intense megadoses of vitamin D supplementation is the key to health. The body does not like to be force-fed its nutrients in giant doses of 50,000 IUs—as so often happens with the vitamin D supplement trend. The result is that the body discards almost all of it on purpose, because it's deemed toxic when it comes in at such a high level. Most of us should not exceed 10,000 IUs daily of vitamin D on a regular basis.

Vitamin D should not be regarded as the Holy Grail for health. For the more than 200 million Americans who suffer with chronic symptoms and conditions, vitamin D is not the answer for healing. Vitamin D deficiency is not the reason why so many people are ill. While the long-term results of vitamin D deficiency aren't good, those problems (such as osteoporosis) aren't life-threatening, and they only develop in combination with many other factors. Other nutrients deserve more of our attention, because deficiencies in each on their own—regardless of other factors—*can* be life-threatening. A severe lack of B_{12} alone, for example, can lead to rapid deterioration of the nervous system, including conditions such as myelopathy, and eventual death.

If there's anything that should be closely monitored and diligently supplemented in the way that vitamin D is, it's zinc. This mineral does anything and everything that vitamin D is said to do. And while vitamin D is helpful on some levels, zinc deficiencies have a markedly damaging effect on all levels of quality of life. With a severe zinc deficiency, you can become gravely ill. A severe lack of vitamin D, on the other hand, while not ideal, does not result in death or grave illness. Eating plenty of zinc-rich foods and supplementing with zinc sulfate (at normal levels, not in megadoses) can offer so much relief for the person who suffers from chronic illness.

B_{12} DEFICIENCY

One popular trend focuses on the belief that becoming vegetarian or vegan makes you automatically B_{12}-deficient. The truth is that an escalating number of people across the globe are deficient in vitamin B_{12}, regardless of whether or not they eat meat. What's behind the deficiency is a lack of elevated biotics in people's diets. These microorganisms live on the skins and leaves of the Holy Four, and you get them from eating fresh, raw, *unwashed*, chemical-free produce from a trusted growing source. (For more on elevated biotics, see the "Adaptation" chapter.)

Note that a blood test that comes back with normal to high readings of B_{12} does not mean that the B_{12} is actually making a difference in someone's health, because the vitamin may not be in its most usable, bioactive form, and therefore the organs may not be absorbing it.

B_{12} SHOTS

Many people are curious about whether or not they should get vitamin B_{12} shots. The truth is that B_{12} shots do not usually have the right variety of B_{12} for them to be beneficial. Plus, B_{12} has to be taken orally to be effective. When we take oral B_{12}, it gets absorbed into the digestive system, where it's "tagged" and made active and bioavailable, so that when it enters the bloodstream, it's in a form that our nerves and organs accept. When the vitamin is injected, it bypasses this process, so the shots aren't as effective as oral B_{12} supplementation. The best kind to look for is a high-quality adenosylcobalamin-methylcobalamin blend. And of course, as I just mentioned, eating foods with elevated biotics on them helps your body create its own B_{12}.

FLOATING STOOL ANALYSIS

There's a widespread belief that a stool that floats in the toilet bowl is a sign of ill health—most notably an indication that you're not properly absorbing nutrients such as fat. You'll hear that a stool that sinks is supposed to be the sign of a digestive tract that's in top working order.

In fact, it's the reverse. "Floaters" are a good sign. (Although diarrhea is, of course, a different story. Any particles that float in that instance are pieces of undigested food, and an indication that something's amiss to cause the body to expel waste before it was finished with digestion.) Intact stools that rise to the top of the bowl, or are semi-submerged, are stools made of mostly fiber, and that's a great thing. It means that (a) your dietary fiber intake is high enough, and (b) your digestive tract is in proper working order, so that as food undergoes digestion, all the fats, proteins, sugars, carbohydrates, and other nutrients are being properly absorbed and assimilated, leaving behind mostly fiber in the waste matter. A fibrous stool is a wonderful scrubber of the intestines. As it travels through the digestive tract, it gathers old debris, including ammonia gas stored in pockets. This gives the stool its floating tendency.

On the other hand, a dense and heavy stool that sinks quickly to the bottom of the toilet bowl means it's full of undigested fats and proteins. This can be an indication that someone's liver is on overload—perhaps to the point of pre-fatty liver, sluggish liver, or the underproduction of bile—which means that it's not able to help the body break down and absorb fats or put them to proper use. These dense stools, also low in fiber and potentially full of unabsorbed proteins and carbohydrates, travel through the middle of the intestinal tract without making enough contact along the intestinal linings to sweep out ammonia gas and other debris.

Don't stress yourself out about sinking stools. Sometimes the liver intentionally gets rid of excess fat to protect you, not because it's having trouble. Other times, a dense stool does not have to do with your liver; rather, it's stress that's put your gut in knots and compacted waste matter. Just do your best to eat plenty of fiber and go easy on your liver whenever possible.

The real takeaway here is not to fear a floating stool. The healthier your diet gets—the more you incorporate the life-changing foods, and especially if you try the 28-Day Cleanse in my first book—the more likely you are to experience floaters and stools that are submerged but not sitting on the bottom, which I jokingly call sub-style stools (because if you can't joke about a subject like this, what can you joke about?). Passing these stools from time to time is an indication that your body is doing some much-needed maintenance.

FECAL MICROBIOTA TRANSPLANT

This practice has gone by a few different names, among them fecal microbiota transplant (FMT), fecal bacteriotherapy, and stool transplant. The idea is that fecal matter from a seemingly healthy person is transferred to a patient dealing with an illness, most commonly an intestinal issue such as *C. difficile* infection. The productive bacteria from the donor's stool is meant to enhance the flora of the patient, so that she or he can achieve balance in the gut and overcome infection.

The problem here is that there are so many varieties of unproductive bacteria, viruses, and rare strains of fungus that medical communities are not yet aware they should test for in the "healthy" person's stool. So regardless of how sterile the transplant procedure is, the person receiving the specimen could be exposed to pathogens in the stool that have eluded testing. If the recipient has an illness or weakened immune system to begin with, it's a risk that doesn't outweigh the benefits.

PREBIOTICS

The concept of prebiotics has taken off lately. This is one fad that's not harmful in any way; I just want you to understand what it really means. The term *prebiotics* refers to those foods that feed productive bacteria and other beneficial microorganisms in the gut. There's a lot of material out there that talks about which fruits and vegetables are prebiotics, and prebiotic supplements are on the market, too. What isn't understood is that every single fruit and vegetable in its raw state (at least, each one that can be eaten raw) is a prebiotic. Even some steamed vegetables can be prebiotics. So rather than getting wrapped up in the hype and worrying about yet one more nutritional to-do, all you have to worry about is keeping enough of the Holy Four foods in your diet, and making sure you eat some of them raw or steamed.

ALCOHOL IN HERBAL PRODUCTS

It's all too common to see alcohol on an herbal supplement's list of ingredients. The long-standing practice of including alcohol (sometimes called "ethanol") in these products is still going strong—and it's a problem. No one is at fault here. It's an old practice that hasn't yet been fixed and replaced. So while your loving doctor, herbalist, or other practitioner offers you so much other important care, and only intends to help by offering you herbal remedies with alcohol in them, it's best to ask for an alternative.

There are a few reasons why you should steer clear of alcohol in herbal products. In the case of herbal extracts such as tinctures, the presence of alcohol usually means that there's a lower concentration of the medicinal herb. Further, most alcohol in herbal products is corn grain alcohol, and therefore GMO-contaminated, even if it's organic—which herbal product manufacturers don't know. GMO corn feeds viruses, bacteria, fungi, and cancer, which defeats the intended purity of the herbs. The alcohol cancels out the herb's benefits.

The same goes for flower essences. These distillations are meant to be so carefully prepared, so delicate—and then the presence of GMO corn grain alcohol pollutes it. And in homeopathy, where you have a plant substance that's been diluted to enhance its potency, those administering it are often very careful about monitoring what other herbs, supplements, and pharmaceuticals someone is taking so as not to disturb the effects of this homeopathic process. Meanwhile, no one realizes that the alcohol used to preserve the dilution is a mutated, Frankensteined substance that's completely foreign to the body, and interrupts the intended healing effects of the herbal therapy.

Don't be fooled by assurances that the alcohol in herbal products burns off when you add hot water. For one thing, you have to add water that's boiling at an accelerated rate for the alcohol to truly burn off—and most people only use warm or hot water with their extracts.

For another, corn grain alcohol is not a phantom substance that disappears when heat is applied; the problem with the corn grain alcohol is not just the alcohol content itself. You can't get rid of whatever residue the alcohol leaves behind. Plus, by the time you use an herbal product such as a tincture, it's already been sitting in a bottle for months or even years, and in that time, the alcohol has saturated the herbal content in the bottle. Being soaked in corn grain alcohol has changed the herb in every way, shape, and form, and you can't burn off alteration to the herb itself.

To protect yourself, read the labels of herbal supplements very carefully and avoid any that list *alcohol* or *ethanol*. Actively seek out alcohol-free versions. If it's impossible to find alcohol-free, then a product made with grape alcohol should be your first pick, and brandy is the next-best preservative. While any alcohol in the herbal product is still not ideal, these two alternatives are light years ahead of the GMO options.

OIL PULLING

The concept of oil pulling—that is, swishing oil in your mouth for a prolonged period in order to draw toxins out of your body—is not a harmful trend so much as it's a waste of time. I'm sorry to report that oil pulling does not, in fact, pull out toxins, and the act of swishing is not enough for the oil to kill bacteria in your mouth. You can now have those 20 minutes a day of your life back.

To make a real difference in your oral health, put some coconut oil on your toothbrush and brush it into your teeth and gums (after you've brushed with toothpaste and rinsed). It takes this brushing action, rather than swishing, to make an impact. Use only coconut oil—no other oil will do. The compounds in coconut have powerful antibacterial, antiviral, and antifungal properties to help keep gum disease at bay.

FOODS THAT MAKE LIFE CHALLENGING

By now you know all about how certain foods can change your life tremendously for the better. There's another element to protecting yourself: In order to adapt to the ever-shifting demands we all encounter, we also want to avoid actively moving in the opposite direction of healing. When someone can't fend off the Unforgiving Four, one of the major reasons is that she or he is eating certain foods that get in the way of adaptation. These are foods that feed pathogens (which contributes to inflammation) and/or are inherently destructive to the body. I call these the *life-challenging foods*.

They're not always obvious ingredients. In fact, you'll hear arguments from other sources to defend most of the foods I list below. Most of them *were* helpful for your health, once upon a time. However, the astronomical increase in illness, along with human intervention with the genetic makeup of some of these foods, mean that we have to be much more careful about what we eat these days. Some ingredients are not what they once were. And sometimes, they're hidden. Not every item that you'll find at the health food store will help you with your health—it's not just a matter of avoiding fast food and other greasy, processed meal choices.

The life-challenging foods are ones that trigger the very symptoms and conditions that the life-changing foods help alleviate. The life-challenging foods also contribute to what I call *less-gevity*. They make life harder and shorter.

I'm not the food police. I know how much emotion, convenience, and fitting in are tied up with eating some of the foods below. I wish I could tell you that pizza with a fried egg on top is the best thing you can order if you're sick and looking for relief. Believe me, if that were the truth, that's exactly what you'd be reading about here. The reality is that if you're dealing with a health challenge, you will serve yourself much better by cutting back on certain foods until recovery.

It's not all sacrifice. After all, if you eat more of the life-changing foods from Part II, "The Holy Four," it means you'll have to cut back somewhere else—and the information below will make that choice easy. Like so many of the people I've helped, you're likely to find that when you remove life-challenging foods from your routine, life opens up in incredible ways.

DAIRY

Many people feel they can't live without dairy products, whether in the form of cream in coffee, a morning cup of yogurt, cheese in all its delicious forms, whey protein powder in smoothies, butter on toast, kefir with granola, milk and cereal, or the like.

Dairy can make life very challenging, though, because it bogs down the liver, which prevents toxins from leaving the body efficiently, and stresses the pancreas, which causes heightened insulin resistance. For those sensitive to dairy, it creates malabsorption problems (that is, trouble absorbing the nutrients in foods because the digestive tract is too inflamed), and for many people, it creates a heightened allergic response to any slight environmental stimulus such as dust and pollen. Further, dairy feeds the pathogens that are behind so many ailments.

If you're experiencing any of the conditions or symptoms below, you may want to consider cutting back on dairy, or cutting it out altogether while you attend to your health.

Conditions

If you have any of the following conditions, try taking dairy out of your life until recovery:

Celiac disease, Crohn's disease, colitis, irritable bowel syndrome (IBS), diverticulitis, any other type of inflammatory bowel disease, chronic sinusitis, sleep apnea, Epstein-Barr virus (EBV)/mononucleosis, Hashimoto's thyroiditis, Graves' disease, chronic ear infections, common colds, liver disease, fatty liver, gout, interstitial cystitis, acne, urinary tract infections (UTIs), yeast infections, eczema, psoriasis, seasonal allergies, Lyme disease, chronic fatigue syndrome (CFS), fibromyalgia, rheumatoid arthritis (RA), lupus, human papilloma virus (HPV), Raynaud's syndrome, diabetes, hypoglycemia, polyps, nodules, osteoporosis, bacterial pneumonia, brain lesions, polycystic ovarian syndrome (PCOS), endometriosis, small intestinal bacterial overgrowth (SIBO), *H. pylori* infection, all autoimmune diseases and disorders, gallstones, gallbladder disease, psoriatic arthritis

Symptoms

If you have any of the following symptoms, try taking dairy out of your life until recovery:

Constipation; inflammation; hypothyroid; hyperthyroid; stomach cramps; stomach pain; dizziness; pre-fatty liver; sluggish liver; fatigue; heart palpitations; menopause symptoms; tingling; numbness; poor circulation; inflamed gallbladder, stomach, small intestine, and/or colon; hair loss; postnasal drip; sweets cravings; *Candida* overgrowth; food sensitivities; hot flashes; body aches and pains; joint pain; joint inflammation; eye watering; eye dryness; blurry eyes; eye floaters; ringing or buzzing in the ears; emotional eating; hormonal imbalances; headaches; heartburn; brain fog; diarrhea; clogged ears; histamine reactions; flatulence; congestion; difficulty swallowing; hives; digestive discomfort; weight gain; premenstrual syndrome (PMS) symptoms

EGGS

You'll often hear that eggs are the perfect food. Eating them is ingrained in our culture, as they've been a staple for centuries. Problem is, the illnesses that are around today were not such a presence in the past. Eggs no longer work *for* us—they now work *against* us by feeding the viral explosion, especially those viruses that contribute to autoimmune disorders and cancer. This is true even when they're pasture-raised or free-range eggs.

Many people feel fine eating eggs. If you're not dealing with any symptoms or conditions and eggs work great for your body, or if they're one of the only foods you have access to, then by all means, keep eating them—just make sure they're pasture-raised. If, on the other hand, you are dealing with a health challenge, it is best to take a break from eggs at least until you're better. Otherwise, they will make it more challenging to heal.

Conditions

If you have any of the following conditions, try taking eggs out of your life until recovery:

Breast cancer, reproductive cancers, Alzheimer's disease, dementia, brain tumors, brain cancer, polycystic ovarian syndrome (PCOS), fibroids, Epstein-Barr virus (EBV)/mononucleosis, thyroid nodules, Hashimoto's thyroiditis and other thyroid disorders, all autoimmune diseases and disorders, inflammatory bowel diseases, acne, adrenal fatigue, migraines, hormonal imbalances, Raynaud's syndrome, insomnia, depression, anxiety, depersonalization, gallstones, gallbladder disease, Lyme disease, liver disease, endometriosis, interstitial cystitis, psoriatic arthritis, carpal tunnel syndrome, urinary tract infections (UTIs), vertigo, bacterial vaginosis, vaginal strep, yeast infections, tendonitis, human papilloma virus (HPV), small intestinal bacterial overgrowth (SIBO), adenomas

Symptoms

If you have any of the following symptoms, try taking eggs out of your life until recovery:

Heart palpitations, brain fog, memory issues, cysts, congestion, *Candida* overgrowth, body aches and pains, spasms, twitches, edema, food sensitivities, weight issues, hypothyroid, hyperthyroid, vaginal burning, vaginal discharge, vaginal itching, hair loss, constipation, hot flashes, loss of libido, menopause symptoms, premenstrual syndrome (PMS) symptoms

CORN

Corn used to be a wonderful part of our existence as a species. For more than 2,000 years, corn helped humanity not only survive; it helped us thrive. It has a great deal to do with why we've gotten as far as we have. Corn used to be nutritious, healing, and fortifying. Then in the snap of a finger, it was destroyed by GMO engineering. Because corn's DNA has been altered, it now has the ability to feed all manners of ill, giving fuel to the pathogens that contribute to our modern-day epidemic of chronic illness.

If you're trying to recover from a health challenge, try keeping corn out of your diet at least until you've recovered. Once you've gotten better, make sure that the corn you choose is organic, and preferably an heirloom variety—although unfortunately, neither of these is a guarantee that the corn hasn't been GMO-contaminated. Continue to keep limits on how much corn you consume.

Conditions

If you have any of the following conditions, try taking corn out of your life until recovery:

All types of cancer, all autoimmune diseases and disorders, multiple sclerosis (MS), amyotrophic lateral sclerosis (ALS), Addison's disease, Cushing's syndrome, Sjögren's syndrome, lupus, chronic fatigue syndrome (CFS), Epstein-Barr virus (EBV)/mononucleosis, colitis, irritable bowel syndrome (IBS), Crohn's disease, Lyme disease, vertigo, neurological asthma (an unknown condition), bacterial infection, acne, allergies, brain lesions, *Candida* overgrowth, immune system deficiencies

Symptoms

If you have any of the following symptoms, try taking corn out of your life until recovery:

Ulcers (including peptic), all neurological symptoms (including tingles, numbness, spasms, twitches, nerve pain, and tightness of the chest), bloating, abdominal cramping, food sensitivities, diarrhea, inflammation

WHEAT

I'm sure that most of you reading this have gone off wheat at some point in your healing process, or else you know someone who has. Many people feel a difference when they take wheat out of the diet—alleviation of specific symptoms as well as a general increase in well-being.

That's because yet again, wheat is one of those foods that's changed in usefulness over the years. What was once a staple of survival has altered since the 1950s due to human intervention. Recent tinkering especially has made wheat a highly inflammatory food, because it feeds pathogens in the body. It's not just gluten that makes wheat a problem for so many people. There are other compounds in it, too, that give fuel to pathogens, which in turn gives rise to all types of symptoms.

If you can eat wheat and feel fine, then chances are that you're free from the various viruses (and sometimes bacteria) that disrupt the body and cause the illnesses so often labeled as autoimmune disease, Lyme disease, and the like. If you do have health troubles, though, avoid wheat until your condition improves, then if you want to add wheat back into your diet, monitor how you feel as you reintroduce it.

Conditions

If you have any of the following conditions, try taking wheat out of your life until recovery:

Crohn's disease, colitis, celiac disease, irritable bowel syndrome (IBS), *H. pylori* infection, all other intestinal conditions, gastroesophageal reflux disease (GERD), sleep apnea, chronic sinusitis, interstitial cystitis, urinary tract infections (UTIs), yeast infections, depression, anxiety, bronchitis, small intestinal bacterial overgrowth (SIBO)

Symptoms

If you have any of the following symptoms, try taking wheat out of your life until recovery:

Clogged ears, overabundance of mucus (in ears, nose, throat, or stools), bloating, gastritis, fatigue, nausea, malaise, listlessness, acid reflux, swelling, itchy skin, joint discomfort, brain fog, chest tightness, food sensitivities, headaches, chemical sensitivities, histamine reactions, cough, congestion, inflammation, hives, hot flashes, mold exposure, sore throat

CANOLA OIL

One seemingly innocuous oil that has snuck into our lives is canola oil (also known as rapeseed oil). While awareness of canola's health risks is growing, there's a competing campaign that promotes its benefits. It has become a staple in restaurants, used mostly as a replacement for unhealthy lard, cottonseed oil, and corn oil, and as a cheaper, lower-fat alternative to olive oil. The irony is, canola has its own set of pitfalls.

Don't be fooled when you hear that canola oil is good for you. Whatever valuable components canola oil has are outweighed by the downsides. If you found out that the wholesome dinners you enjoyed at a friend's house every Friday night were laced with arsenic, would you still think they were wholesome? Or would you feel that any nutrition they contained were rendered obsolete? While you may not die by the end of the meal, the repeated exposure would still be extremely risky business. You would certainly experience a loss of vitality by the 100th meal. Be just as wary of canola.

Canola oil is severely damaging to the immune system, causing it to become dysfunctional and disruptive to organ and gut health. Canola oil not only feeds pathogens as the other foods above do; it also eats away at all linings in the body—from the stomach and intestinal tract linings to those of veins, arteries, the heart, kidneys, bladder, ureter, urethra, and, if you're a woman, the linings of the reproductive system.

Conditions

If you have any of the following conditions or want to avoid them, try taking canola oil out of your life:

Any kind of intestinal distress or disorder (including gastroesophageal reflux disease [GERD], pancreatitis, fatty liver, Crohn's disease, colitis, and irritable bowel syndrome [IBS]), any kind of neurological condition (including Parkinson's disease, multiple sclerosis [MS], chronic fatigue syndrome [CFS], psoriatic arthritis, fibromyalgia, and rheumatoid arthritis [RA]), Lyme disease, anxiety, depression, thyroid diseases and disorders, stroke, transient ischemic attack (TIA), amyotrophic lateral sclerosis (ALS), polycystic ovarian syndrome (PCOS), endometriosis, lupus, postural tachycardia syndrome (POTS), Raynaud's syndrome, adenomas

Symptoms

If you have any of the following symptoms or want to avoid them, try taking canola oil out of your life:

Hair loss, hypothyroid, hyperthyroid, nerve pain, ulcers, intestinal spasms, constipation, diarrhea, chronic loose stools, mucus in the stools, acid reflux, hormonal imbalances, all neurological symptoms (including tingles, numbness, spasms, twitches, nerve pain, and tightness of the chest), trigeminal neuralgia, myelin nerve damage

NATURAL FLAVORS

These hidden toxins invade our food under the guise of harmless additives. What's labeled as *natural flavors* (or *natural cherry flavor, natural fruit flavor, natural chocolate flavor, natural vanilla flavor,* and the like) is actually MSG—a neurotoxin that builds up in the brain and destroys neurons and glial cells. MSG is incredibly detrimental to the central nervous system and can wreak havoc on your life.

And yet it's becoming a trend for these so-called natural flavorings to be added to even the purest organic packaged foods, as well as herbal teas and nutritional supplements. If you want to avoid illness, be very discerning with food labels—if "natural" and "flavor" are anywhere near each other on an ingredients list, put the package back on the shelf. (Though don't be afraid of vanilla extract, as long as that's exactly how it's labeled.)

Conditions

If you have any of the following conditions or want to avoid them, try taking "natural flavors" out of your life:

Autism, attention-deficit/hyperactivity disorder (ADHD), migraines, Alzheimer's disease, dementia, Parkinson's disease, anxiety, depression, all other neurological conditions, Hashimoto's thyroiditis and other thyroid disorders, insomnia, stroke, amyotrophic lateral sclerosis (ALS), transient ischemic attack (TIA), sciatica, macular degeneration, Lyme disease

Symptoms

If you have any of the following symptoms or want to avoid them, try taking natural flavors out of your life:

Lack of focus and concentration, memory issues, headaches, fatigue, body aches and pains, jaw pain, tooth pain, ringing in the ears, restless leg syndrome, tingles and numbness, back pain, muscle spasms, leg cramps, frozen shoulder, Bell's palsy, bloating, hair loss, difficulty breathing, difficulty swallowing, joint pain, body stiffness, tightness of the chest, memory loss, brain fog, head pain, seizures, muscle tightness, neuralgia, hypothyroid, hyperthyroid, pinched nerves, trouble focusing, trouble sleeping

LIFE-CHANGING ANGELS

In the world we cannot see with our eyes—the spiritual world, where angelic forces reside—there is a complete understanding of the Quickening that we're experiencing here on earth. God's angels are alert to our need to adapt with the changing times in order to survive and thrive here. In fact, there's a special group of angels called the *life-changing angels* whose mission is to support us through this time. They see you. They work hard for you. They know how much you deserve to ride the wave of life today—not get swallowed by it.

The life-changing angels support us via our food supply. They are the reason the life-changing foods are life-changing. They are God's answer to our growing pains—because God has the deepest love for us, and compassion for what we're up against, and wants us to access the tools to cope. In some cases, the life-changing angels' job is to spread awareness. For example, these angels are the reason the organic and integrated pest management (IPM) movements have taken off. There's also a massive group of these angels working to disarm GMO food production.

Further, angels fortify fruits and vegetables from the ground up; they give angelic powers to every apple you eat, and every leaf of spinach. Angels coax plants to yield abundant harvests, direct food to the hungry, and control weather for the best outcomes of the crops—even going so far as to influence wind patterns to keep as many skyborne chemicals as possible from getting into your food. Angelic forces are involved in ripening, and in some cases will soften the fall of a ripened fruit so that it remains viable for someone to eat. As you read this, angelic forces are nurturing seeds in the earth, working hard to ensure that a meal you eat months in the future will be the most beneficial that it can possibly be for your health in that moment.

Angels understand that food is a matter of life or death, and not just for humans. The life-changing angels govern and support the yearly migration of animals, traveling alongside them to help provide nourishment on their journeys. These angels also influence pollinators, guiding hummingbirds, bees, and the like to the flowers of our food plants for mutual benefit.

The declining bee population is of particular concern—the angels know more than anyone the bees' critical role in pollination, and in production of one of the most ancient medicinal foods on the planet, honey. Throughout the ages, honey has been manna from heaven for human civilization. Entire societies have celebrated it, and it has saved whole settlements from starvation and malnutrition. Honey will play a critical role in the future of humankind—even though trends may convince you that it has no nutritional worth. Further, the end of bees would mean the end of agriculture as we know it. If it weren't for bees, it's very possible that we would not be here today, so the angels are doing everything in their power to look out for them, which includes influencing us to plant nectar sources and practice beekeeping.

Maple water is another survival food that the angels see us relying on in the future, so they work at all hours to preserve our maple trees. The angels empower some of the most adaptogenic fruits, vegetables, herbs, and spices, imbuing them with the very qualities that make them so valuable. Wild blueberries, for example, are a wonder food precisely because they are graced by God and the angels with the power of resurrection.

The life-changing angels want to help you. They understand that our lives are all changing, no matter what, and they want to make sure those changes are for the better. Just like fruits and vegetables are the most taken-for-granted foods, the life-changing angels are the most taken-for-granted angels in all of the Holy Kingdom.

We think of food's nutrition as a given, of basics like the water cycle as mundane clockwork, of stumbling upon a delicious heirloom tomato at the market as chance—when really, the life-changing angels have a role in all of it. None of this is to negate science. Of course there are scientific explanations for how biological and ecological processes work. Even well-regarded doctors and scientists, though, acknowledge that there are mysteries of the universe. Rather than pointing to science as an argument against God, they point to it as proof of God. It goes back to what I said in the introduction: there is so much we know, and *so much more to know.*

Consider for a moment the miracle of how a seed as small as the head of a pin contains the potential to unfurl into a tomato plant. Imagine how many factors had to go just right for even one perfect tomato to form—and then for it to make it to the market, for you to take it home, remember to eat it before it went bad . . . all of it culminating in that moment when you finally take a bite, and the salty-sweet-acid taste brings you an intense moment of pleasure, while its nutrients travel through your body to bring you the most vital nourishment.

I think of it like a symphony. All of those separate musicians are masters of their instruments and know their parts perfectly. Yet it still takes a conductor to make it come together into one perfect sound. The life-changing angels are the conductors, making sure that every element works in divine unison.

Many people are aware that angels are at hand. What's unknown is this full scope of angelic involvement in our day-to-day functioning. Since the moment you first came into this world and took your first breath, you've had this birthright of connecting to the angels (and even before you were born, you had a divine right to angelic help in utero through your mother). The life-changing angels have had a role in keeping you nourished for your entire life—and that's without you asking. And all along, you've supported these angels every time you buy from an organic farmer, plant a butterfly garden, or donate to a food pantry. This whole time, there's been this back and forth; the angels have looked out for you, and you've helped them as well. Now they want you to know how to call on them directly.

CALLING UPON THE ANGELS

The method for calling upon the life-changing angels is the same one that I described in my first book for calling upon the essential angels: you must ask for them, by name, out loud. Our minds are pinball machines of activity, with thoughts and emotions darting all over the place. It's too much noise for the angels to spend their time listening to when they have so much other work to do. It doesn't have to be a shout—it need not be above a whisper—the angels just need any vocal cue that you're receptive to their intervention. (If you are deaf or unable to speak, use sign language or a mental message to ask for the Angel of Deliverance. She will help you get in touch with the angel you have in mind.)

Angels and humans have a powerful trait in common: free will. It's what allows us to go about our lives with any sense of agency. It is the foundation of participation, communication, and freedom. The angels devote their free will to constant service. So another reason that it takes this special way of calling upon the angels aloud to receive their direct help is that they want to see us use our free will for good, too. Before they help with our specific requests, they want to feel that we are actively participating in our own lives and actively reaching out to them. Then the angels feel like their free will is well spent in working alongside us.

So you must take a moment to clear your mind and speak aloud, "Angel of Provision, please help me." (Or use the name of whichever life-changing angel below you're trying to reach.) This method for deliberately calling upon the named angels is the most powerful way to receive angelic aid.

THE 12 LIFE-CHANGING ANGELS

Here are 12 of the life-changing angels you can call upon to help you. Each of these angels is female and has an army of other angels working behind her on major tasks, such as trying to win the war on GMO crops. You can call on the named angel, though, and she will help you directly.

- **Angel of Disarmament:** When you have to eat produce you know has been sprayed with synthetic pesticides and/or herbicides, or may be contaminated by GMO crops, call upon this angel to disarm the chemicals so that they can have a minimal effect on your system and protect you from harm.
- **Angel of Abundance:** This is the angel you want on your side when you grow your own food and hope for bountiful crops.
- **Angel of Provision:** Her job is to route food to people who are undernourished or starving. If your food resources are very limited, or you work with a food bank or soup kitchen, call upon the Angel of Provision for help getting nourishment into hungry bellies.
- **Angel of Enrichment:** This angel enhances the nutrition of the Holy Four, amplifying the strength of phytochemicals, vitamins, minerals, and other nutrients and tailoring them specifically to your needs, so that food can truly be your medicine.
- **Angel of Harmony:** When you want to become one with your food and enhance mindful eating, this angel will heighten your appreciation for your meal and bring you in tune with what you take into your body. She will also help eliminate

food- and eating-related pain from your past, leave behind your fear over eating too much or too little, and bring you a fresh start.

- **Angel of Synchronicity:** Everything is about timing with the growth of plants, so this angel's job is to synchronize a host of disparate processes. She prompts the flower to open at just the right moment, leads a bee to the blossom, monitors water intake and temperature so the fruit can form yet not burst or burn out, and then signals the fruit to ripen. And that's just one small peek at her responsibilities. Call upon the Angel of Synchronicity when you need assistance to understand how to care for your food plants, or when you're foraging for wild food and want to find the best specimens.
- **Angel of Habit:** When you're stuck in a rut of eating certain unproductive foods you grew up on, or if you have a child or other loved one who's a picky eater, call upon the Angel of Habit to help break the pattern and expand interest in different, healthier food choices.
- **Angel of Addiction:** If you're addictively drawn to the wrong foods, or make a habit of overeating, the Angel of Addiction will help you free yourself from the misery.
- **Angel of Solidarity:** This is the angel to call upon when you want friends, family, co-workers, and even restaurants to support you in healthy eating habits. She will guide others to back you up and discourage them from tempting you with unproductive foods.
- **Angel of Honesty:** If you're uncomfortable about the source of a food you're buying or eating, and you want to know if it really is free-range, wild-caught, organic, gluten-free, or to be sure it's not genetically modified—or if you want assurance that a dish prepared at a restaurant is made with pure olive oil, not a canola oil blend—call upon the Angel of Honesty to help you get a straight answer.
- **Angel of Insight:** When you want to eat more healthful food, call upon the Angel of Insight to bolster your spirit and will, and to provide magical inspiration to stay on track. This is also the angel leading the organic, seed-saving, and health-food movements, and the resurgence of farmers' markets and heirloom food varieties.
- **Angel of Mother's Milk:** This angel protects a new mother's milk supply and allows for communication between mother and baby during breastfeeding. One of her responsibilities is to change the nutrient profile of the breast milk in order to suit the baby's needs in the moment.

THE LIFE-CHANGING ANGELS AT WORK

I once had a client named Amelia who couldn't make friends with food. She was a recent college grad living back at home. For as long as she could remember, she'd gone back and forth between binge eating and starving herself. She could never feel peace at the family dinner table, because her thoughts always turned obsessively to the serving dishes before her: Was the meal healthy enough? Was it filling enough? Would she be able to stop eating after one plateful? Would it make her gain weight? Would she regret having eaten at all?

When I spoke with Amelia for the first time, I advised her to call upon the Angel of Harmony to help her with mindful eating.

"I've tried mindful eating," Amelia said, "and I've studied meditation. It didn't help my eating problem."

I assured her that asking for help from an angel was different. When you practice meditation and mindful eating on your own, it all depends on you. It's like trying to move a heavy bureau on your own. When a friend helps, the burden becomes half as heavy—or maybe the friend even shoulders most of it, so that all you have to do is keep the bureau steady. When things are too much to lift by yourself, you have to ask for assistance. And when you need the particular assistance of making peace with food, the Angel of Harmony is the one to call.

Amelia agreed to give it a try. After we hung up, she spoke aloud: "Angel of Harmony, please help me become friends with food." Right away, she had a revelation: calling upon the Angel of Harmony was the first time she'd turned to an outside source for help and not felt like she would be judged for it. She'd never realized what a role that sense of judgment had played in making her feel crazy and perpetuating her food anxiety. When she visited her nutrition coach, she always felt like she was under a microscope. When she sat at the dinner table, she felt her parents' and brother's stares. This was the first time that she didn't feel weaker because she'd asked for help.

The next day, Amelia came downstairs in the morning, walked into the kitchen, and felt the familiar pit in her stomach and flush of her cheeks that accompanied her customary panic about what to eat. After her epiphany the day before, Amelia had expected smoother sailing. She wondered if her relief had just been a hallucination. Even so, she took a breath and spoke again to the Angel of Harmony. "Please help me," she whispered. The divine sense of relief came back. This time, she had the sensation of a cage door being opened to set her free.

And yet on the third day, Amelia was still struggling over food. She'd been home alone since the morning and had purposely starved herself all day—even though rationally, she knew this wasn't productive. When dinnertime came around, she finally felt that she'd earned a meal. Before she started to eat, she asked the Angel of Harmony to help her eat mindfully and appreciate what she was putting into her body.

Just then, Amelia heard a clink in the kitchen. She got up to check if her parents had come home without her realizing. Despite the fact that she had heard the distinct sound of a utensil hitting a plate, no one was there. Amelia stood still for a moment, puzzling it out. Suddenly, she realized the Angel of Harmony was there with her. Amelia felt the urge to return to the table, where she started to cry. Years and years of wounds over food, struggles with overeating and under-eating, and judgments other people made about what and how much she put into her body all started to surface and dissipate, as though they were coming out and leaving for good.

When the tears subsided, Amelia felt the Angel of Harmony leave her presence. A warm feeling overtook her, and she looked down at her plate. For the first time since she was a little girl, she started to eat in complete and total peace. She never wanted to blame food again, and she never wanted to blame herself, either, for what she'd been through with food. The usual nervousness, anxiety, turmoil, worry, and fear that accompanied mealtime were nowhere to be found.

From that day on, Amelia felt free and enjoyed food without hang-ups. She found herself less tempted by the foods that used to sway her to binge eat and motivated to eat healthier foods for the simple reason that she enjoyed them more. Amelia felt that her healing had been made possible by the Angel of Harmony's complete lack of judgment, and her ability to look past Amelia's quirks and see the truth of who Amelia really was.

This is just one example of a life-changing angel at work. Amelia believed in the Angel of Harmony; her life has changed. There is nothing like the unconditional love of the angels. It cannot be matched by anyone or anything—it's that powerful.

When calling upon the angels in your own life, it's important to remember to be open to how the angels will intervene. It's not all bolts of lightning or epiphanies. Sometimes angels provide guidance in your dreams, or present new opportunities. In the case of the Angel of Disarmament, her presence may not be anything you can feel—that doesn't mean she isn't protecting you. With the Angel of Solidarity, it's possible that instead of influencing your favorite restaurant to start serving healthier fare, she'll guide you to a better place to eat.

Also, the angels always have the greater good in mind. This means that if you ask the Angel of Abundance to bless your field of rapeseed, she's more likely to lead you in a different direction, because she knows that the canola oil made from that crop is a problematic food for people's health. (For more on canola, see the "Foods That Make Life Challenging" chapter.) Angelic aid hinges on you being receptive to it, too. Remember this as you call upon, for example, the Angel of Habit—you'll need to work alongside her if you want to break your nighttime cookie routine.

Depending on how busy they are, the angels may be able to help you within a few seconds, or there may be a bit of a delay. You can call on the angels individually, or in combination. For example, if you're stuck eating at a roadside diner while traveling, you can call on the Angel of Honesty just before the waitress comes to the table, then the Angel of Disarmament and the Angel of Enrichment together when your food arrives. (And again, all you need to do is whisper—this doesn't have to be an exercise that calls attention to you. Many people quietly pray over their food, so you'll fit in.)

The angels want you to ask for their help, no matter how busy they are, so don't worry that you're being a nuisance. Just continue to call for their help, keep a light heart, and be patient.

THIS IS YOUR TIME

When I talk about angels, I'm not talking about anything cutesy. Records throughout the millennia point to angels' existence. God's angels are not to be mistaken for fluff. I am talking about nothing less than full-force divine beings who have been with us since our ancestors first walked the earth.

Some people feel that it's silly, naïve, or even delusional to believe that God would grant spiritual support in the form of angels. If you've held yourself back from letting yourself believe in angels, I understand. We're taught to believe in what we can see, hear, touch, measure, and weigh. "I'll believe it when I see it," goes the common expression.

On the flip side, strict belief systems that are meant to elevate us above the need for proof sometimes let us down instead. That's because belief isn't enough on its own. Belief can be stressed and strained and broken down. Cracks can develop on its surface, plunging you into icy waters below.

Life can be so difficult at times that it feels random, or worse, cruel. Let me assure you: Whatever tragedies you've witnessed or traumas you've faced were not the judgments of a coldhearted, punishing God, nor were they the result of a divine vacuum. The problems in our world are attributable to the reckless decisions of humans who have lost faith in the good of others and made poor use of their free will, and who are influenced by fallen angels who no longer work for God. That's what is responsible for violence, war, and the destruction of the planet.

When we feel like there is no reason to have faith, that's when we need it the most—faith that there is a divine presence in this world, a presence that sees the same suffering we do, finds it senseless, and wants to offer us aid. Don't let the troublemakers and peace-breakers, those people overtaken by greed and rage, rob you of your faith. Do not let them rob you of a sense of peace amid the chaos. God's angels, such as the life-changing angels and the essential angels, are busy running around the globe dying out fires caused by the people who've lost faith and started listening to the fallen angels. And God's archangels are going head-to-head with the war machines. Faith is intricate, and belief is one piece woven through it. Belief in God's angels, coupled with faith that God has not abandoned or betrayed us, can be a lifeline if you let it.

If you once believed in angels, then felt like your efforts to make contact with them didn't work and therefore angels must not be real, you can now revise your thinking. After reading this book, you've entered into a different time in your life. You need not despair or live in the dark anymore. You've learned the secrets of how to change your life, and the key to contacting angels. You can ask for their support, and you can support them right back as we all work together to make this a place defined by good.

AFTERWORD

Compassion Is the Key

Everything you've just read comes from the voice of compassion. I don't mean my own voice—though I try to be as compassionate as possible, I don't mistake myself for the voice of it. I'm talking about Spirit of the Most High—Spirit of Compassion—my source for all of the information in this book. As I wrote in the introduction, Spirit is the living word *compassion*. Spirit is the expression of God's compassion for humanity. Spirit wants you to be happy and healthy so you can have a bright future. Spirit wants you to save yourself, to adapt, to change your life. It is directly out of this compassion that everything in the previous pages has made its way to you.

Hope is a popular topic these days. We all want hope. We all need hope. Hope is what fuels our dreams for ourselves and our families. Hope drives our will to live, our ambitions. Hope is the reason people get up in the morning; it's the glimmer in someone's eye. Hope is the spark of faith that your life can improve on every level. It's the determination in your heart that things can get better, they *will* get better. Without hope, we become empty shells of people.

Without compassion, though, there is no hope; compassion is hope's soul. Hope is the future, compassion is the present. Hope is the path forward, compassion is the torch that leads the way. Hope is the door, compassion is the key—and hope cannot be unlocked without compassion in hand.

When I was a child, overtaxed by Spirit inundating me with information about people's struggles, I wanted to choose not to care. It was heartbreaking to see into the suffering of everyone around me. Couldn't I just stop caring so much? I asked Spirit.

"You *must* care," Spirit told me. It wasn't an option to leave these people to their suffering. I had to take it to heart, to learn how to have compassion—to be with them in the present moment, so that they wouldn't feel alone, and so that they could feel hope again. We're all meant to have compassion for one another. It is one of the good works we do here, and it matters. It is part of our collective life path, part of surviving the Quickening and taking humanity to the next level.

Spirit defines compassion as the understanding of suffering. Compassion is looking past, around, or sometimes through our own experiences to connect with and express care for someone else.

In the best-case scenario, what's happened to us makes us better able to identify with someone else. A woman who's broken a leg in the past, for example, may be much more likely to offer help when she sees someone nearby on crutches, whereas if she'd never been in that position, she might not have even noticed a stranger's cast.

In the worst-case scenario, a life challenge hardens us. For example, someone who had a difficult home life growing up may later take it out on every intimate partner, using the false logic that making someone else hurt erases one's own damage. This is the source of bitterness and the rhetorical question, "You think *you've* got it bad?"

Then there's the middle ground, where our experiences can be like quicksand, preventing us from getting into someone else's head. Have you ever started to talk about a recent life event, and your companion says, "I know exactly what you mean"—then for the next 20 minutes, the conversation is about him? What started out as your companion's attempt to identify with you quickly sank into an evaluation of his own life.

If we're to make it through, we must remain open to others' perspectives. We have to truly share in their experiences.

Compassion is not empathy, though. Empathy has an expiration date, just like a carton of milk. If someone has been suffering for a long time, others' empathy starts to sour. I can't tell you how many people who have been ill for a long time tell me the same story: At first, their friends and family rallied around them, helping to shoulder their burdens. Months or years later, those onetime supporters are either nowhere to be found or suspicious and blameful about how long the suffering has lasted.

Compassion is also not sympathy. That's because sympathy has strings attached—it's like a loan. When you lend someone a sympathetic ear, it's with the implicit understanding that she or he will return the favor someday. "I owe you one," is something people find themselves saying so frequently to the friend who nurtures them through a breakup or visits them in the hospital, because we all understand that sympathy is transactional.

Compassion has no strings or sell-by date. It is timeless and can never spoil. When you've received compassion, there's no loan shark who will hunt you down and make you give it back with interest. Whereas empathy and sympathy can come with a violin playing, compassion has no melodrama. Compassion is on a plane beyond empathy and sympathy. It is strong, vital, and contagious in the best sense of the word. Compassion is life-changing. It opens up the heart and connects it to the soul.

Most of us have a compassionate source deep within us. It might have gotten buried along the way, yet it's there. And so often, we tap into this compassionate source on a conditional level. We decide that one situation warrants our compassion, while another doesn't. This arises out of an instinct to protect ourselves—which can be positive to a certain degree. When your trust has been broken, you're going to have some trepidation about trusting that a new situation is worth your compassion. Rightfully so.

When we become too frugal with our compassion, though, we get stuck in a pattern of withholding. We become afraid of feeling someone else's sadness, or understanding her or his perspective—we don't want to imagine that we could ever be in the same position. We treat our compassion like a precious commodity that has to be rationed, then we micromanage its distribution. We become trapped in our own heads, the barriers between us and others getting bigger and bigger, and we cut ourselves off from one of our most important human functions: to express compassion and help others heal.

More than ever before in history, we are getting the mainstream message to love ourselves. Only once you can appreciate the person you see in the mirror, the popular wisdom goes, can you express true caring for others. This is a step in the right direction. Self-hatred is a poison that's not going to help anybody.

We can't stop at loving ourselves, though. The next step is to rediscover compassion—first for ourselves, and then for others. When ignited and passed along, compassion has a force of its own. It exceeds every birthday and holiday present in hundreds of lifetimes put together. It breaks all material laws and supersedes everything seeable and tangible here on earth.

No matter what your beliefs and grounding principles are, compassion is critical. If you seek good karma, compassion is the foundation. If you want to attract abundance in your life, compassion is the only way for it to work. Compassion *is* abundance—abundance of spirit that reaches out from one person to another to express the sentiment we all want to hear: *You're not alone.*

And it's true: You are not alone. The life-changing foods in this book, the explanations of what's behind our modern-day epidemics, the life-changing angels—all of this is Spirit's message to you, so that you will know that you are being looked out for, you are being cared for, you are being witnessed.

Hold on to this knowledge. Let it change your life. Then pass it along. Together, we can adapt from Quickening to rebirth.

INDEX

Note: Page numbers in *italics* indicate recipes

A

B

C

E

F

G

I

J

K

L

M

N

O

P

Q

R

S

T

ACKNOWLEDGMENTS

Thank you to Patty Gift, Anne Barthel, Reid Tracy, Louise Hay, Margarete Nielsen, Diane Hill, Diane Ray and everyone at Hay House Radio, Aurora Rosas, Lindsay McGinty, and the rest of the Hay House team for your faith and commitment to getting Spirit's message out into the world.

Gwyneth Paltrow, Elise Loehnen, and your devoted GOOP crew, I am beyond grateful for your kindness and support.

Dr. Alejandro Junger, words cannot describe the appreciation I have for you.

Dr. Christiane Northrup, connecting with you brings true meaning to the saying, "I feel like I've known you forever."

Dr. Habib Sadeghi, your work is a beacon of light.

Dr. Deanna Minich, you are an inspiration to so many.

For your kindness, generosity, and friendship, my thanks go out to Grace Hightower, Robert De Niro, and family; Craig Kallman; Chelsea Field and Scott, Wil, and Owen Bakula; Nanci Chambers and David James, Stephanie, and Wyatt Elliott; Peggy Lipton, Kidada Jones, and Rashida Jones; Naomi Campbell; Jessica Seinfeld; Amanda de Cadenet; Sophia Bush; Maha Dakhil; Woody Fraser, Milena Monrroy, Midge Hussey, and everyone at Hallmark's *Home & Family*; Nena, Robert, and Uma Thurman; Morgan Fairchild; Demi Moore; Catherine, Sophia, and Laura Bach; Annabeth Gish; Robert Wisdom; Danielle LaPorte; Nick and Brenna Ortner; Jessica Ortner; Mike Dooley; Carol, Scott, and Christiana Ritchie; Dhru Purohit; Kris Carr; Kate Northrup; Kristina Carrillo-Bucaram; Ann Louise Gittleman; Jan and Panache Desai; Ami Beach and Mark Shadle; Robert and Michelle Colt; John Holland; Martin, Jean, Elizabeth, and Jacqueline Shafiroff; Jill Black Zalben; Alexandra Cohen; Christine Hill; Carol Donahue; Caroline Leavitt; Sally Arnold; Michael Sandler and Jessica Lee; Koya Webb; Jenny Hutt; Adam Cushman; Sonia Choquette; Colette Baron-Reid; Kelly Noonan; Denise Linn; and Carmel Joy Baird. I deeply value your encouragement.

To the doctors and other healers of the world who help so many: you have my profound admiration. Dr. Richard Sollazzo, Dr. Ron Steriti, Dr. Nicole Galante, Dr. Diana Lopusny, Dr. Dick and Noel Shepard, Dr. Aleksandra Phillips, Dr. Chris Maloney, Drs. Tosca and Gregory Haag, Dr. Dave Klein, Dr. Prudence Hall, Dr. Deborah Kern, Dr. Darren and Suzanne Boles, Dr.

Deirdre Williams and the late Dr. John McMahon, Dr. Jeff Feinman, and Dr. Robin Karlin—it's an honor to call you friends. Thank you for your dedication to the field of wellness.

Thanks to David Schmerler, Kimberly S. Grimsley, and Susan G. Etheridge for looking out for me.

Special thanks also to Muneeza Ahmed; Gretchen Manzer; Kimberly Spair; Stephanie Tisone; Megan Elizabeth McDonnell; Robby Barbaro; Ally Ertel; Victoria and Michael Arnstein; Nina Leatherer; Michelle Sutton; Haily Cataldo; Kerry; Alexandra Laws; Peggy Rometo; Ester Horn; Linda and Robert Coykendall; Tanya Akim; Heather Coleman; Glenn Klausner; Carolyn DeVito; Michael Monteleone; Bobbi and Leslie Hall; Katherine Belzowski; Matt and Vanessa Houston; David, Holly, and Ginnie Whitney; Lauren Henry; Olivia Amitrano and Nick Vazquez; Melody Lee Pence; Terra Appelman; Kate Hall; Eileen Crispell; Bianca Carrillo-Bucaram; Jennifer Rose Rossano; Kristin Cassidy; Catherine Lawton; Taylor Call; Alana DiNardo; and Eden Epstein Hill.

Thank you to the countless people, including those in the new Medical Medium communities, whom I've had the privilege of watching blossom and transform.

Ruby Scattergood, this book would not be possible without your writing and editing. Thank you for your literary counsel. Once again, you saved me.

Vibodha and Tila Clark, many thanks for all of your hard work and dedication and for being there through the years.

Philip and Casey McCluskey: *I saw four angels standing on the four corners of the earth . . . And I saw another angel ascending from the east.*

Ashleigh, Britton, and McClain Foster and Sterling Phillips, having you on my side makes everything so much brighter.

For your love and support, I thank my family: my luminous wife; Dad and Mom; my brothers, nieces, nephews, aunts, and uncles; my champions Indigo, Ruby, and Great Blue; Hope; Marjorie and Robert; Laura; Rhia Cataldo and Byron; Alayne Serle and Scott, Perri, Lissy, and Ari Cohn; David Somoroff; Kelly and Evy; Danielle, Johnny, and Declan; and all my loved ones who are on the other side.

Finally, thank you, Spirit, for being my constant companion and compassionate mentor.

ABOUT THE AUTHOR

Anthony William, *New York Times* best-selling author of *Medical Medium: Secrets Behind Chronic and Mystery Illness and How to Finally Heal*, was born with the unique ability to converse with a high-level spirit who provides him with extraordinarily accurate health information that's often far ahead of its time. Since age four, when he shocked his family by announcing that his symptom-free grandmother had lung cancer (which medical testing soon confirmed), Anthony has been using his gift to "read" people's conditions and tell them how to recover their health. His unprecedented accuracy and success rate as the Medical Medium have earned him the trust and love of hundreds of thousands worldwide, among them movie stars, rock stars, billionaires, professional athletes, best-selling authors, and countless other people from all walks of life who couldn't find a way to heal until he provided them with insights from Spirit. Anthony has also become an invaluable resource to doctors who need help solving their most difficult cases.

Learn more at www.medicalmedium.com.

Hay House Titles of Related Interest

YOU CAN HEAL YOUR LIFE, the movie,
starring Louise Hay & Friends
(available as a 1-DVD program, an expanded 2-DVD set, and an online streaming video)
Learn more at www.hayhouse.com/louise-movie

THE SHIFT, the movie,
starring Dr. Wayne W. Dyer
(available as a 1-DVD program, an expanded 2-DVD set, and an online streaming video)
Learn more at www.hayhouse.com/the-shift-movie

CRAZY SEXY KITCHEN: 150 Plant-Empowered Recipes to Ignite a Mouthwatering Revolution,
by Kris Carr with Chef Chad Sarno

GODDESSES NEVER AGE: The Secret Prescription for Radiance, Vitality, and Well-Being,
by Christiane Northrup, M.D.

REAL FOOD REVOLUTION: Healthy Eating, Green Groceries, and the Return of the American Family Farm, by Congressman Tim Ryan

All of the above are available at your local bookstore,
or may be ordered by contacting Hay House (see next page).

We hope you enjoyed this Hay House book. If you'd like to receive our online catalog featuring additional information on Hay House books and products, or if you'd like to find out more about the Hay Foundation, please contact:

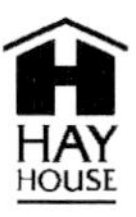

Hay House, Inc., P.O. Box 5100, Carlsbad, CA 92018-5100
(760) 431-7695 or (800) 654-5126
(760) 431-6948 (fax) or (800) 650-5115 (fax)
www.hayhouse.com® • www.hayfoundation.org

Published in Australia by:
Hay House Australia Pty. Ltd., 18/36 Ralph St., Alexandria NSW 2015
Phone: 612-9669-4299 • *Fax:* 612-9669-4144 • www.hayhouse.com.au

Published in the United Kingdom by:
Hay House UK, Ltd., Astley House, 33 Notting Hill Gate, London W11 3JQ
Phone: 44-20-3675-2450 • *Fax:* 44-20-3675-2451 • www.hayhouse.co.uk

Published in India by: Hay House Publishers India,
Muskaan Complex, Plot No. 3, B-2, Vasant Kunj, New Delhi 110 070
Phone: 91-11-4176-1620 • *Fax:* 91-11-4176-1630 • www.hayhouse.co.in

---

Access New Knowledge.
Anytime. Anywhere.

Learn and evolve at your own pace
with the world's leading experts.

www.hayhouseU.com

Free e-newsletters from Hay House, the Ultimate Resource for Inspiration

Be the first to know about Hay House's free downloads, special offers, giveaways, contests, and more!

Get exclusive excerpts from our latest releases and videos from ***Hay House Present Moments***.

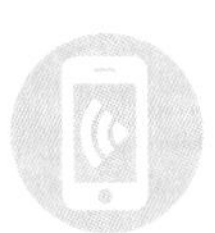

Our ***Digital Products Newsletter*** is the perfect way to stay up-to-date on our latest discounted eBooks, featured mobile apps, and Live Online and On Demand events.

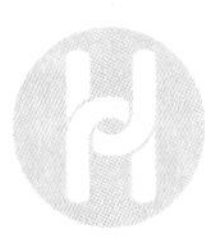

Learn with real benefits! ***HayHouseU.com*** is your source for the most innovative online courses from the world's leading personal growth experts. Be the first to know about new online courses and to receive exclusive discounts.

Enjoy uplifting personal stories, how-to articles, and healing advice, along with videos and empowering quotes, within ***Heal Your Life***.

Have an inspirational story to tell and a passion for writing? Sharpen your writing skills with insider tips from ***Your Writing Life***.

Sign Up Now!

Get inspired, educate yourself, get a complimentary gift, and share the wisdom!

Visit www.hayhouse.com/newsletters to sign up today!

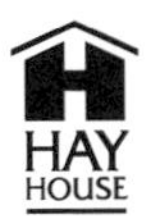

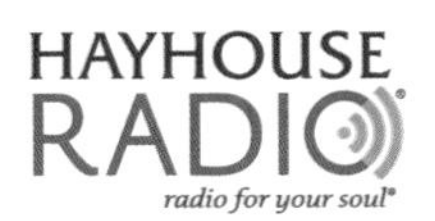

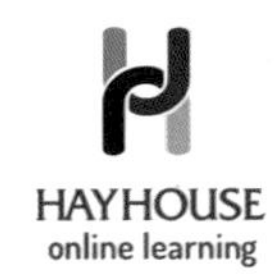